T0262179

Encyclopedia of Cancer Prevention and Management: Latest Researches in Cancer Treatment

Volume II

Encyclopedia of Cancer Prevention and Management: Latest Researches in Cancer Treatment Volume II

Edited by **Karen Miles and Richard Gray**

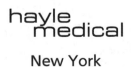

New York

Published by Hayle Medical,
30 West, 37th Street, Suite 612,
New York, NY 10018, USA
www.haylemedical.com

Encyclopedia of Cancer Prevention and Management:
Latest Researches in Cancer Treatment
Volume II
Edited by Karen Miles and Richard Gray

© 2015 Hayle Medical

International Standard Book Number: 978-1-63241-127-3 (Hardback)

This book contains information obtained from authentic and highly regarded sources. Copyright for all individual chapters remain with the respective authors as indicated. A wide variety of references are listed. Permission and sources are indicated; for detailed attributions, please refer to the permissions page. Reasonable efforts have been made to publish reliable data and information, but the authors, editors and publisher cannot assume any responsibility for the validity of all materials or the consequences of their use.

The publisher's policy is to use permanent paper from mills that operate a sustainable forestry policy. Furthermore, the publisher ensures that the text paper and cover boards used have met acceptable environmental accreditation standards.

Trademark Notice: Registered trademark of products or corporate names are used only for explanation and identification without intent to infringe.

Printed in the United States of America.

Contents

Preface

The main aim of this book is to educate learners and enhance their research focus by presenting diverse topics covering this vast field. This is an advanced book which compiles significant studies by distinguished experts in the area of analysis. This book addresses successive solutions to the challenges arising in the area of application, along with it; the book provides scope for future developments.

This book discusses various aspects of cancer treatment and its analysis, compiled by a team of experts from various parts of the world. Supportive care for patients, multidisciplinarity in cancer therapy: nutrition and beyond, perspectives in cancer biology and modeling are some of the topics covered. The ultimate objective of this book is to highlight the issues involved in fighting against cancer and provide insights about the mechanism involved in disease control and treatment. These efforts will together help in improving the methods adopted for welfare of patients who fight a daily battle against this fatal disease. The book would serve as an important reference for students and clinicians.

It was a great honour to edit this book, though there were challenges, as it involved a lot of communication and networking between me and the editorial team. However, the end result was this all-inclusive book covering diverse themes in the field.

Finally, it is important to acknowledge the efforts of the contributors for their excellent chapters, through which a wide variety of issues have been addressed. I would also like to thank my colleagues for their valuable feedback during the making of this book.

Editor

Multidisciplinarity in Cancer Therapy: Nutrition and Beyond

The Impact of Vitamin D in Cancer

Khanh vinh quoc Luong and Lan Thi Hoang Nguyen

Additional information is available at the end of the chapter

1. Introduction

The relationship between vitamin D and cancer has previously been reported in the literature. A systemic review and meta-analysis of prospective cohort studies revealed that a 20 nmol/L increase in the 25-hydroxyvitamin D_3 (25OHD) levels was associated with an 8% lower mortality in the elderly population (Schöttker et al., 2012). Oncology patients had significantly lower mean serum vitamin D levels than non-cancer primary care patients from the same geographic region (Churilla et al., 2011). In a community oncology experience, vitamin D deficiency is widespread in cancer patients and correlates with advanced stage disease (Churilla et al., 2012). A high prevalent of vitamin D deficiency has been associated with head and neck cancer (Orell-Kotikangas et al., 2011), breast cancer (Crew et al., 2009; Peppone et al., 2012), vulvar cancer (Salehin et al., 2012), prostate cancer (Varsavsky et al., 2011), pancreatic cancer (Wolpin et al., 2011), gastric cancer (Ren et al., 2012), colon and rectal cancer (Tangrea et al., 1997), ovarian cancer (Lefkowitz et al., 1994), oral cavity and esophagus cancers (Lipworth et al., 2009), myelo-proliferative neoplasms and myelo-dysplastic syndromes (Pardanani et al., 2011), multiple myeloma (Ng et at., 2009), non-Hodgkin's lymphoma (Drake et al., 2010), and chronic lymphocytic leukemia (Shamafelt et al., 2011). On the other hand, a serum 25OHD concentration of 25 nmol/L was associated with a 17% reduction in incidence of cancer, a 29% reduction in total cancer mortality, and a 45% reduction in digestive system cancer mortality (Giovannucci et al., 2006). Improving vitamin D status may also help lower the risk of colorectal cancer (Wu et al., 2011a). In a case-control study, a higher vitamin D intake is associated with a lower risk of esophageal squamous cell carcinoma (Launoy et al., 1998). A meta-analysis revealed that an increase of serum 25OHD by 50 nmol/L was associated with a risk reduction of 59% for rectal cancer and 22% for colon cancer (Yin et al., 2009). High 25OHD levels were associated with better prognosis in breast, colon, prostate cancer, and lung cancer relative to patients with lower 25OHD levels (Robsahm et al., 2004; Zhou et al., 2007). In a murine model, dietary vitamin D may play an important role as a preventive agent in androgen-insensitive human prostate tumor growth (Ray et al., 2012). The season in which patients were operated on seemed to have an effect on survival of patients undergoing resection of non-small cell lung cancer (Turna et al., 2012). The survival of patients who had surgery in winter was statistically significantly shorter than that of patients who underwent surgery in the summer. In Australia, prostate cancer mortality rates are inversely correlated with solar radiation exposure (Loke et al., 2011). Dietary vitamin D_3 and calcitriol have been shown to demonstrate equivalent anticancer activity in mouse xenograft models of breast and prostate cancers (Swani et al., 2012). The combination of calcitriol and dietary soy resulted in substantially greater inhibition of tumor growth than the inhibition achieved with either agent alone in a mouse xenograft model of prostate cancer (Wang et al., 2012a). Soy diets alone caused a modest elevation in serum calcitriol. Vitamin D_3 treatment significantly suppressed the viability of gastric cancer and cholangiocarcinoma cells and also had a synergistic effect with other anti-cancer drugs, such as paclitaxel, adriamycin, and vinblastine (Baek et al., 2011). The vitamin D analog, 19-Nor-2α-(3-hydroxypropyl)-1α,25-dihydroxyvitamin D_3, is a potent cell growth regulator with enhanced chemotherapeutic potency in liver cancer cells (Chiang et al., 2011). Alphacalcidol, a vitamin D analogue, has been demonstrated significant antitumor activity in patients with low-grade non-Hodgkin's lymphoma of the follicular, small-cleaved cell type (Raina et al., 1991). In patient with parathyroid cancer, vitamin D has been shown to prevent or delay the progression of recurrence (Palmieri-Sevier et al., 1993). In locally advanced or cutaneous metastatic breast cancer, topical calcipotriol treatment reduced the diameter of treated lesions that contained vitamin D receptor (*VDR*) (Bower et al., 1991). In a clinical trial, high-dose calcitriol decreased prostatic-specific antigen (PSA) levels by 50% and reduced thrombosis in prostate cancer patients (Beer et al., 2003 & 2006). In hepatocellular carcinoma, calcitriol and its analogs have been reported to reduce tumor volume, increase hepatocarcinoma cell apoptosis by 21.4%, and transient stabilize serum alpha-fetoprotein levels (Dalhoff et al., 2003; Luo et al., 2004; Morris et al., 2002). These findings suggested a relationship between vitamin D and cancer. In this chapter, we will discuss the role of vitamin D in cancer.

2. Genetic factors related to vitamin D and cancer

2.1. The Major Histocompatibility Complex (MHC) class II molecules

The major histocompatibility complex (MHC) class II molecules play an important role in the immune system and are essential in the defense against infection. The human MHC class II molecules are encoded by three different human leukocytic antigen (HLA) isotypes: HLA-DR, -DQ, and -DP. Studies have suggested that several genes within MHC region promote cancer susceptibility. A chimeric DR4 homozygous transgenic mouse line is reported to spontaneously develop diverse hematological malignancies at a high frequency (Raffegerst et al., 2009). Most of these neoplasms were highly similar to those found in human diseases. HLA-DR antigen expression was correlated with the histopathological type and to the degree of cell differentiation in cutaneous squamous cell carcinomas (Garcia-Plata et al., 1993). The DRB1*03 and DR-B1*13 alleles were significantly more frequent in patients with nasopharyngeal carcinoma compared with controls in southern Tunisia (Makni et al., 2010). The DR1 gene is strongly associated with thyroid carcinoma (Panza et al., 1982). The HLA-DR was also increased in poorly differentiated thyroid carcinoma, especially in the anaplastic type (Lindhorst et al., 2002). The DQA1*0102 and DPB1*0501 alleles were significantly more common in Chinese patients with hepatocellular carcinoma (HCC) (Donaldson et al., 2001). The frequency of DRB1*0404 allele was significantly higher in the gastric cancer group compared with the gastritis group in Koreans (Lee et al., 2009). However, the frequencies of the DRB1*0405 and DQB1*0401 alleles were increased in the Japanese patients with intestinal-type gastric cancer compared with controls (Ando et al., 2009). Somatic mutations affecting HLA class II genes may lead to loss of HLA class II expression due to the formation of microsatellites in unstable colorectal carcinomas (Michel et al., 2010). The DRB1*15 allele and the haplotype DRB1*15 DQB1*0602 were associated with human papillomavirus (HPV)-16 positive invasive cervical cancer in Mexican women (Hernández-Hernández et al., 2009). The DRB1*0410 allele was the susceptibility allele in Japanese patients with testicular germ cell carcinoma (Ozdemir et al., 1997). Furthermore, the frequencies of the DRB1*09 and DQB1*03 alleles were increased in patients with non-Hodgkin's lymphoma and diffuse large B cell lymphoma compared with normal controls (Choi et al., 2008). The frequencies of the DRB1*04 and DRB1*15 alleles were significantly higher in Turkish children with acute leukemia compared with controls (Ozdilli et al., 2010). The DRB1*16 allele was a marker for a signignificant risk of chronic myelogenous leukemia in Eastern Canada (Naugler and Liwski, 2009). The DRB1*04 and DRB5 alleles are associated with disease progression in Iranian patients with chronic lymphocytic leukemia (Hojattat-Farsangi et al., 2008). On the other hand, calcitriol is known to stimulate phagocytosis and suppress MHC class II antigen expression in human mononuclear phagocytes (Tokuda et al., 1992 & 1996), thereby preventing antigen-specific T cell proliferation. In addition, calcitriol exerts effects that opposes the effect of IL-4 on MHC class II antigen expression in human monocytes (Xu et al., 1993) and specifically modulates human monocyte phenotype and function by altering HLA-DR antigen expression and antigen presentation, while leaving lytic function intact (Rigby et al., 1990). Calcitriol also decreases interferon-γ-induced HLA-DR antigen expression in normal and transformed human keratinocytes (Tamaki et al., 1990-1991 & Tone et al., 1991) and reduces the levels of HLA-DR mRNA in cultured epithelial tumor cell lines (Tone et al., 1993). In addition, 1α-calcidol significantly modulates the expression of HLA-DR in human peripheral blood monocytes (Scherberich et al., 2005). These findings suggest that calcitriol may have an effect on cancer by suppressing the expression of MHC class II antigens.

2.2. Vitamin D Receptor (VDR)

The expression of VDR in a variety of cell lines, coupled with increased evidence of VDR involvement in cell differentiation, inhibition of cellular proliferation and angiogenesis in many tumor types, suggest that vitamin D plays a role in cancer (Luong and Nguyen, 2010 & Luong and Nguyễn, 2012). VDR ablation is associated with ductal ectasia of the primary mammary ducts, loss of secondary and tertiary branches and atrophy of the mammary fad pad (Welsh et al., 2011). Breast cancer patients with high VDR expression showed significant better in progression-free survival and overall survival than patients with moderate/negative VDR expression scores (Ditch et al., 2012). Certain allelic variations in the VDR may also be genetic risk factors for developing tumors. There are five important common polymorphisms within the *VDR* gene region that are likely to exert functional effects on *VDR* expression. The anti-carcinogenic potential of vitamin D might be mediated by VDR expression. The association between plasma 25OHD levels and colorectal adenoma was modified by the *TaqI* polymorphism of the VDR gene (Yamaji et al., 2011). There is a significant association between single nucleotide polymorphisms (SNPs) in the VDR gene and vitamin D intake in African Americans with colorectal cancer (Kupfer et al., 2011). The *BsmI* polymorphism of the VDR gene also modified the association between dietary vitamin D intake and breast cancer (Rollison et al., 2012). The *AA* genotype of VDR is reported to be associated with colorectal cancer, with a stronger association in female patients (Mahmoudi et al., 2012). The *FokI* and *BsmI* genotypes of VDR gene are implicated in the pathogenesis of renal cell carcinoma (RCC) in a North Indian population (Arjumand et al., 2012). Altered VDR expression was associated with RCC carcinogenesis via the expression of epithelial Ca^{2+} channel transient receptor potential vanilloid subfamily 5 and 6 (TRPV5/6) (Wu et al., 2011b). There is a significant association between shorter progression-free survival time in patients with head and neck squamous cell carcinoma and the *FokI TT* genotype, as well as the *Cdx2-FoxI-ApaI* haplotype (Hama et al., 2011). In Spanish children, osteosarcoma patients showed a significantly higher frequency of the *Ff* genotype of the *FokI VDR* gene than the control group (Ruza et al., 2003). In a German population, the *AaTtBb* genotype of the VDR gene is associated with basal cell carcinoma risk, whereas the *aaTTbb* genotype is found at a high frequency in both basal cell carcinomas and cutaneous squamous cell carcinomas compared with controls (Köststner et al., 2012). In a systematic review, *TaqI*, *BsmI* and *FokI* polymorphisms of the VDR gene were found to be associated with malignant melanoma (Denzer et al., 2011). Furthermore, the presence of specific VDR *BsmI* and *TaqI* alleles was associated with a higher C-reactive protein (CRP) level in cancer patients with cachectic syndrome (Punzi et al., 2012). In another prospective study, plasma 25OHD levels and common variation among several vitamin D-related genes (*CYP27A1, CYP2R1, CYP27B1, CYP24A1, GC, RXRA,* and *VDR*) were associated with lethal prostate cancer risk (Shui et al., 2012). Slattery et al. (2009) examined genetic variants that are linked to the pathway that contribute to colon cancer. They revealed that *FoxI VDR* polymorphism was associated with CpG Island methylator phenotype (CIMP) positive/Ki-ras mutated tumors, whereas the Poly *A* and *Cdx2 VDR* polymorphisms were associated only with Ki-ras mutated tumors.

2.3. MicroRNA (miRNA)

MiRNAs are endogenous noncoding RNAs that regulate gene expression through the translational repression or degradation of target mRNA (Bartel, 2004). Aberrant miRNA expression has been well characterized in cancer (Lu et al., 2005). Circulating miRNAs are suggested to be diagnostic and prognostic markers in breast cancer (Cortez et al., 2012). Circulating miR-NA-125b expression is associated with chemotherapeutic resistance of breast cancer (Wang et al., 2012b). Several miRNAs are found to share 125b complementarity with a sequence in the 3'-unstranslated region of human VDR mRNA. The overexpression miRNA-125b significantly decreased the endogenous VDR protein level in human breast adenocarcinoma cells lines (MCF-7) to 40% of the control (Mohri et al., 2009). This miRNA is down-regulated in cancer tissue and causes high CYP24 protein expression, which catalyzes the inactivation of calcitriol (Komagata et al., 2009). Stress induced by serum starvation caused significant alteration in the expression of multiple miRNAs including miRNA-182, but calcitriol effectively reversed this alteration in breast epithelial cells (Peng et al., 2010). Vitamin D_3 up-regulated protein 1 (VDUP1) is regulated by miRNA-17-5p at the post-transcriptional levels in senescent fibroblasts (Zhuo et al., 2010). VDUP1 expression is increased in cancer cells (Takahashi et al., 2002; Dutta et al., 2005). In melanoma cell lines, the endogenous VDR mRNA level is inversely associated with expression of miRNA-125b (Essa et al., 2010), and calcitriol also reduced the miRNA-27b expression in these cell lines. In human colon cells, calcitriol induced miRNA-22 and may contribute to its antitumor action against this neoplasm (Alvarez-Diaz et al., 2012). Fifteen miRNAs are also differentially regulated by calcitriol in prostate cancer cells (LNCaP) (Wang et al 2011a). Furthermore, calcitriol regulated miRNA-32 and miRNA-181 expressions in human myeloid leukemia cells (Gocek et al., 2011; Zimmerman et al., 2011; Wang et al., 2009a).

2.4. Renin-Angiotensin System (RAS)

The primary function of the renin-angiotensin system (RAS) is to maintain fluid homeostasis and regulate blood pressure. The angiotensin converting enzyme (ACE) is a key enzyme in the RAS and converts angiotensin (AT) I to the potent vasoconstrictor AT II (Johnston, 1994). The local RAS may influence tissue angiogenesis, cellular proliferation, apoptosis, and inflammation (Deshayes and Nahmias, 2005). Epidemiological and experimental studies suggested that the RAS may contribute to the paracrine regulation of tumor growth. The renin levels are elevated in patients with liver cirrhosis and HCC and positively correlated with α-fetoprotein (Lotfy et al., 2010). The over-expression of ACE is reported in extrahepatic cholangiocarcinoma (Beyazit et al., 2011), leukemic myeloid blast cells (Aksu et al., 2006), and macrophages in the lymph nodes of Hodgkin's disease patients (Koca et al., 2007). The AT II receptors were also expressed in all human gastric cancer lines (Huang et al., 2008), pre-malignant and malignant prostate cells (Louis et al., 2007), human lung cancer xenografts (Feng et al., 2011a), and ovarian cancer (Ino et al., 2006). The RAS mutation in codon 61 was the most common genetic alteration in poorly differentiated thyroid carcinomas (Volante et al., 2009). The ACE *I/D* polymorphism is a possible target for developing genetic markers for breast cancer in Brazilian women (Alves Corrêa et al., 2009). The ACE *I/D* polymorphisms play an important role in breast cancer risk and disease-free survival in Caucasian postmenopausal women (González-Zuloeta Ladd et al., 2012). Carriers of the high-activity *DD* genotype had an increased risk of breast cancer compared with low activity *II/ID* genotype carriers (van der Knaap et al., 2008). The *DD* genotype was associated with patients with an aggressive stage of prostate cancer (Wang et al., 2011b). ACE2 expression was decreased in non-small-cell lung cancer and pancreatic ductal adenocarcinoma in which AT II levels were higher than those in controls (Feng et al., 2010; Zhou et al., 2009). ACE2 has been suggested as a potential molecular target for pancreatic cancer therapy (Zhou et al., 2011). The AT II concentration in gastric cancer region was significantly higher than those of normal region (Kinoshita et al., 2009). Furthermore, AT II receptor blockers (ARB) suppress the cell proliferation effects of AT II in breast cancer cells (Du et al., 2012). The addition of ACE inhibitor or ARB to platinum-based first line chemotherapy contributed to prolong survival in patients with advanced lung cancer (Wilop et al., 2009) and affected the prognosis of advanced pancreatic cancer patients receiving gemcitabine (Nakai et al., 2010). The RAS inhibitors also improved the outcome of sunitinib treatment in metastatic renal cell carcinoma (Keizman et al., 2011). On the other hand, the administration of ACE inhibitors in patients with the ACE *DD* genotype has been shown to decrease the level of calcitriol required (Pérez-Castrillón et al., 2006). In a hypertensive Turkish population, the presence of the ACE *D* allele, which correlates negatively with serum 25OHD levels, is linked to a higher left ventricular mass index value and elevated ambulatory blood pressure measurements (Kulah et al., 2007). In addition, genetic disruption of the *VDR* gene resulted in overstimulation of the RAS with increased renin and angiotensin II production, which lead to high blood pressure and cardiac hypertrophy. However, treatment with captopril reduced cardiac hypertrophy in VDR-knockout mice (Xiang et al., 2005), suggesting that calcitriol may function as an endocrine suppressor of renin biosynthesis. Moreover, calcitriol suppresses renin gene transcription by blocking the activity of the cyclic AMP response element in the renin core promoter (Yuan et al., 2007) and decreases ACE activity in bovine endothelial cells (Higiwara et al., 1988).

2.5. Toll-Like Receptor (TLR)

Toll-like receptors (TLRs) are a group of glycoproteins that functions as surface trans-membrane receptors and are involved in the innate immune responses to exogenous pathogenic microorganisms. Substantial evidence exists for an important role of TLRs in the pathogenesis and outcomes of cancer. TLR2 expression was significantly higher in sporadic colorectal cancerous tissue than in non-cancerous tissue (Nihon-Yanagi et al., 2012). The TLR5 play an important role in tumor progression of gastric cancer (Song et al., 2011). The TLR7 and TLR9 showed high expression in laryngeal carcinoma cells (Shikora et al., 2010). The over-expression of TLR9 was reported oral squamous cell carcinoma (Min et al., 2011), esophageal squamous cell carcinoma (Takala et al., 2011), and breast cancer cells (Qiu et al., 2011; Sandholm et al., 2012). The expression levels of TLR1, TLR2, TLR4, TLR5, TLR6, TLR8, and TLR10 are significantly higher in the human renal carcinoma cell line (780-6) than those in normal renal cell (HK-2) line (Yu et al., 2011). Chronic lymphocytic leukemia cells express all TLRs expressed by normal activated B cells, with a high expression of TLR9 and CD180 and an intermediate expression of TLR1, TLR6, and TLR10 (Arvaniti et al., 2011). The TLR4 polymorphisms are reported in patients with the risk of prostate cancer (Kim et al., 2012), head and neck squamous cell carcinomas (Bergmann et al., 2011), HCC (Minmin et al., 2011), and colon cancer (Eyking et al., 2011). Furthermore, multiple SNPs in TLR2 and TLR4 were associated with colon cancer survival (Slattery et al., 2012). On the other hand, vitamin D deficiency increases the expression of hepatic mRNA levels of TLR2, TLR4, and TLR9 in obese rats (Roth et al., 2011). However, calcitriol suppresses the expression of TLR2 and TLR4 protein and mRNA in human monocytes and triggers hypo-responsiveness to pathogen-associated molecular patterns (Sadeghi et al., 2006). Calcitriol has also been shown to down-regulate intracellular TLR2, TLR4 and TLR9 expression in human monocytes (Dickie et al., 2010). TLR activation results in the expression of the VDR and 1α-vitamin D hydroxylase in human monocytes (Liu et al., 2006). Additionally, calcitriol can cause the vitamin D-induced expression of cathelicidin in bronchial epithelial cells (Yim et al., 2007) and may enhance the production of cathelicidin LL-37 (Rivas-Santiago et al., 2008). The addition of a VDR antagonist has also been shown to inhibit the induction of cathelicidin mRNA by more than 80%, thereby reducing the protein expression of this antimicrobial agent by approximately 70% (Yim et al., 2007). Cathelicidin was abundant in tumor-infiltrating NK1.1⁺ cells in mice. Cathelicidin knockout mice (*Camp⁻/⁻*) permitted faster tumor growth than wild type controls; NK cells derived from *Camp⁻/⁻* mice showed impaired cytotoxic activity toward tumor targets compared with wild-type mice (Büchau et al., 2010). The human cathelicidin LL-37, which inhibits gastric cancer cell proliferation, is down-regulated in gastric adenocarcinomas (Wu et al., 2010). Gastrointestinal cancer cells lacked LL-37 expression; Cathelicidin expression is modulated by histone-deacetylase (HDAC) inhibitors in various gastrointestinal cells, including gastric and hepatocellular cells (Schauer et al., 2004). HDAC inhibitors enhance the acetylation of core proteins, which is linked to the formation of transcriptionally active chromatin in various cells. The expression of the LL-37/hCAP-18 gene was also reduced in some leukemia cells (Yang et al., 2003). In patients with acute myeloid leukemia, there was a marked reduction of LL-37/hCAP-18 expression in the peripheral blood compared with the level in healthy donors (An et al., 2005). In myeloid cells, cathelicidin gene is a direct target of the VDR and is strongly up-regulated by calcitriol (Gombart et al., 2005). The combination of TLR ligands (CpG oligodeoxynucleotides, CpG-ODN) LL-37 generated significantly better therapeutic tumor effects and enhanced survival in murine ovarian tumor-bearing mice compared with CpG-ODN or LL-37 alone (Chuang et al., 2009).

3. Role of vitamin D and its analog in cancer

3.1. The bacillus Calmette-Guerin (BCG) vaccination

The BCG vaccine was developed to provide protection against tuberculosis and has also been demonstrated to offer protection against cancer. The combination of BCG and ionizing radiation resulted in the induction of autophagy in colon cancer cells (Yuk et al., 2010). Intravesical BCG therapy has been demonstrated to reduce the recurrence rate and the risk of progression to muscle-invasive disease in patients with superficial bladder tumors (Herr et al., 1988). The BCG vaccination significantly prolongs the survival of patients with a malignant melanoma after initial surgical removed (Kölmel et al., 2005) and improved survival rates in patients with resected lung cancer (Repin, 1992). BCG inoculation delayed the tumor growth and prolonged the survival time in nude mice with leukemia (Wang et al., 2011c). BCG vaccination reduced the risk of lymphomas in a Danish population (Villumsen et al., 2009) and demonstrated to reduce the mortality, morbidity, and frequency of myeloic and chronic leukemia in children (Ambrosch et al., 1981). On the other hand, BCG-vaccinated infants are almost 6 times more likely to have sufficient vitamin D concentrations than unvaccinated infants 3 months after BCG vaccination, and this association remains strong even after adjusting for season, ethnic group and sex (Lalor et al., 2011). Among the vaccinated group, there was also a strong inverse correlation between the IFN-γ response to *M. tuberculosis* PPD and vitamin D concentration; infants with higher vitamin D concentrations had lower IFN-γ responses. Similarly, tuberculosis in cattle usually presents with a rapid transient increase in serum calcitriol within the first two weeks following infection (Rhodes et al., 2003). 1,25OHD-positive mononuclear cells were later identified in all of the tuberculous granulomas. During tuberculosis infection, alveolar macrophage-produced calcitriol plays a beneficial role by limiting inflammation-mediated tissue injury, potentiating NO production by stimulated monocytes/macrophages, inhibiting INF-γ production by stimulated CD4$^+$ cells, and suppressing the growth of *M. tuberculosis* (Ametaj et al., 1996; Rockett et al., 1998).

3.2. Matrix Metalloproteinase (MMPs)

MMPs are proteolytic enzymes responsible for extracellular matrix remodeling and the regulation of leukocyte migration through the extracellular matrix, which is an important step in inflammatory and infectious pathophysiology. MMPs are produced by many cell types including lymphocytes, granulocytes, astrocytes and activated macrophages. The MMP-1 expression is linked to sarcoma cell invasion (Garamszegi et al., 2011). MMP-2 expression is increased in gastric cancer cells (Partyka et al., 2012) and colorectal cancer (Dong et al., 2011). MMP-9 is expressed in many cancer cells, such as those associated with non-small-cell lung cancer (Peng et al., 2012), ovarian cancer invasion and metastasis (Zhang et al., 2011a), glioblastoma multiforme (Yan et al., 2011), and adamantinous craniopharyndioma (Xia et al., 2011). The MMP-2 and MMP-9 secreted by leukemic cells increase the permeability of blood brain barrier of the CNS by disrupting tight junction proteins (Feng et al., 2011b). In gastric cancer, MMP-2 and MMP-9 play an important role in tumor invasion and metastasis (Parsons et al., 1998). The risks for the development of hypophyseal adenoma and cervical neoplasia are greater in patients with MMP-1 polymorphisms (Altaş et al., 2010; Tee et al., 2012) than those with the wild-type allele. The MMP-2 polymorphism contributed to prostate cancer susceptibility in North India (Srivastava et al., 2012) and to the clinical outcome of Chinese patients with non-small cell lung cancer treated with first-line, platinum-based chemotherapy (Zhao et al., 2011). The MMP-7 polymorphisms are associated with esophageal squamous cell carcinoma and colorectal cancers (Manzoor et al., 2011; Dziki et al., 2011). The SPNs in the MMP-2 and MMP-9 region are associated with susceptibility to head and neck squamous cell carcinoma in an Indian population (Chaudhary et al., 2011). The SNPs of genes encoding MMPs (-1, -2, -3, -7, -8, -9, -12, -13, and -21) are related to breast cancer risk, progression, and survival (Wieczorek et al., 2012). Based on meta-analysis studies, the MMP-2 allele (-1306T) is a protective factor for digestive cancer risk (Zhang and Ren, 2011), the MMP-9 polymorphism is associated with a lower risk of colorectal cancer (Zhang et al., 2012a), and polymorphisms in the promoter regions of MMP-1, -3, -7, and -9 are associated with metastasis in some cancers (Liu et al., 2012). On the other hand, VDR-knock-out mice were shown to have an influx of inflammatory cells, phospho-acetylation of NF-κB, and up-regulated expression of MMP-2, MMP-9, and MMP-12 in the lung (Sundar et al., 2011). The *VDR TaqI* polymorphism is associated with decreased production of TIMP-1, a natural inhibitor of MMP-9 (Timms et al., 2002). In addition, calcitriol modulates tissue MMP expression under experimental conditions (Dean et al., 1996), down-regulates MMP-9 levels in keratinocytes, and may attenuate the deleterious effects of excessive TNF-α-induced proteolytic activity associated with cutaneous inflammation (Bahar-Shang et al., 2010). Calcitriol decreased the invasive properties of breast carcinoma cells and decreased MMP-9 levels in association with the increased levels of the tissue inhibitor of MMP-1 activity (Koli and Keshi-Oja, 2000). Calcitriol also inhibits endometrial cancer cell growth and is associated with decreased MMP-2 and MMP-9 expression

(Nguyen et al., 2011). Moreover, calciferol, calcitriol, and vitamin D analogs decreased MMP-2 and MMP-9 activities and inhibited prostate cancer cell invasion (Tokar and Webber, 2005; Schartz et al., 1997; Iglesias-Gato et al., 2011; Stio et al., 2011). A vitamin D analog has also been reported to reduce the expression of MMP-2, MMP-9, vascular endothelial growth factor (VEGF) and PTH-related peptide in Lewis lung carcinoma cells (Nakagawa et al., 2005). Taken together, these studies suggest that calcitriol may play an important role in the pathological processes in cancer by down-regulating the level of MMPs and regulating the level of TIMPs.

3.3. Wnt/β-catenin

The Wnt/β-catenin signaling pathway plays a pivotal role in the regulation of cell growth, cell development and the differentiation of normal stem cells. Wnt/β-catenin signaling is implicated in many human cancers, including gastrointestinal cancer, gastric cancer, colon cancer, melanoma, HCC, endometrial carcinoma, ovarian carcinoma, cervical cancer, papillary thyroid carcinoma, renal cell carcinoma, prostate cancer, parathyroid carcinoma, and hematological malignancies (White et al., 2012; Nuñez et al., 2011; Polakis, 2000; Li et al., 2012; Yoshioka et al., 2012; Guturi et al., 2012; Bulut et al., 2011; Gilber-Sirieix et al., 2011; Ueno et al., 2011; Svedlund et al., 2010; Ge and Wang, 2010). Calcitriol inhibits β-catenin transcriptional activity by promoting VDR binding to β-catenin and the induction of E-cadherin expression (Palmer et al., 2001). Paricalcitol, a vitamin D analog, suppressed β-catenin-mediated gene transcription and ameliorated proteinuria and kidney injury in adriamycin nephropathy (He et al., 2011). Most VDR variants fail to activate the vitamin D-responsive promoter and also fail to bind β-catenin or regulate its activity (Byers and Shah, 2007). VDR depletion enhances Wnt/β-catenin signaling and the tumor burden in colon cancer (Larriba et al., 2011). The action of cacitriol on colon carcinoma cells depends on the dual action of VDR as a transcription factor and a nongenomic activator of RhoA-ROCK and p38MAPK-MSK1, which are required for the inhibition of the Wnt/β-catenin signaling pathway and cell proliferation (Ordóñez-Morán et al., 2008). The DICKKOFF-4 gene induces a malignant phenotype, promotes tumor cell invasion, and angiogenesis in colon cancer cells and is repressed by calcitriol (Pendás-Franco et al., 2008a); whereas DICKKOFF-1 gene acts as a tumor suppressor in human colon cells and is up-regulated by calcitriol (Aguilera et al., 2007; Pendás-Franco et al., 2008b). The transcription factor TCF-4 acts as transcriptional repressor in breast and colorectal cancer cell growth. The TCF-4 and β-catenin binding partner are indirect targets of the VDR pathway. In the VDR knockout mouse, TCF-4 is decreased in the mammary gland when compared with a wild-type mouse. In addition, calcitriol increases TCF-4 RNA and protein levels in several human colorectal cancer cell lines (Beildeck et al., 2009). Furthermore, the Snail1 gene is associated with gastric cancer, melanoma, breast cancer, HCC, and colon carcinoma. Calcitriol inhibits the Wnt/β-catenin signaling pathway and is abrogated by Snail1 in human colon cancer cells (Larriba et al., 2007).

3.4. The Mitogen-Activated Protein Kinase (MAPK) pathways

The MAPK pathways provide a key link between the membrane bound receptors that receive these cues and changes in the pattern of gene expression, including the extracellular signal-regulated kinase (ERK) cascade, the stress activated protein kinases/c-jun N-terminal kinase

(SAPK/JNK) cascade, and the p38MAPK/RK/HOG cascade (Hipskind and Bilbe, 1998). In human colon cancer cells, calcitriol increases cytosolic Ca^{2+} concentration and transiently activates RhoA-ROCK, and then activates the p38MAPK-MSK signaling pathway (Ordóñez-Morán et al., 2008). In breast cancer cells, the MARK (JNK and p38) signaling pathway involved in calcitriol-induced breast cell death (Brosseau et al., 2010) and potentiated the cytotoxic action of calcitriol and TNF-α (Weitsman, et al., 2004). In murine squamous cell carcinoma cells, vitamin D induced apoptosis and selective induction of caspase-dependent MEK cleavage (McGuire et al., 2001). In an ovarian cancer animal model, vitamin D induced cell death and is mediated by the p38MAPK signaling pathway (Lange et al., 2010). In human promyeloblastic leukemia cells (HL60), vitamin D derivatives had anti-proliferative activity and activated MAPK signaling pathways (Ji et al., 2002). In human acute myeloid leukemia cells, calcitriol-induced differentiation is enhanced by the activation of MAPK signaling pathways (Zhang et al., 2011b).

3.5. The Prostaglandins (PGs)

Prostaglandins (PGs) play a role in inflammatory processes, and cyclooxygenase (COX) participates in the conversion of arachidonic acid in PGs. A variety studies have shown that prostaglandin signaling stimulates cancer cell growth and cancer progression. The regulation of PG metabolism and biological actions contribute to its anti-proliferation effects in prostate cells and calcitriol has been reported to regulate the expression of several key genes involved in the PG pathway, resulting in decreased PG synthesis (Moreno et al., 2005). The expression of the COX-2 gene is significantly increased in human gastric adenocarcinoma tissues compared with adjuvant normal gastric mucosal specimens (Ristimäki et al., 1997). There is inversely association between elevated COX-2 levels and decreased VDR expression in patients with breast and ovarian cancers compared with healthy women (Cordes et al., 2012). Calcitriol differentiated the human leukemic cell line (HL-60) and metabolized exogenous arachidonic acid to both COX products (predominantly thromboxane B_2 and PG E_2) and lipoxygenase products, including leukotriene B_4 (Stenson et al., 1988). In a mouse xenograft model of prostate cancer, the combination of cacitriol and dietary soy enhanced cacitriol activity in regulating target gene expression and increased the suppression of PG synthesis and signaling, such as COX-2, 15-hydroxyprostaglandin dehydrogenase (15-PGDH), and PG receptors. (Wang et al., 2012a). Calcitriol and its analogs have also been shown to selectively inhibit the activity of COX-2 (Aparna et al., 2008), and an inverse correlation exists between the expression of PG-metabolizing enzymes and reduced VDR expression in malignant breast cell lines (Thill et al., 2012). Taken together, these findings suggest that vitamin D may play a role in modulating the inflammatory process in cancer.

3.6. Oxidative stress

Reactive oxygen species (ROS) play a major role in various cell-signaling pathways. ROS activates various transcription factors and increases in the expression of proteins that control cellular transformation, tumor cell survival, tumor cell proliferation and invasion, angiogenesis, and metastasis. ROS has an important role in the initiation and progression of many cancers (Gupta et al., 2012; Marra et al., 2011; Zhang et al., 2011c; Wang et al., 2011c; Rogalska et al., 2011; Gupta-

Elera et al., 2012). Single nucleotide polymorphisms of antioxidant defense genes may significantly modify the functional activity of the encoded proteins. Women with genetic variability in the iron-related oxidative stress pathways may be at increased risk of post-menopausal breast cancer (Hong et al., 2007). The *ala* variant of superoxide dismutase (SOD) is associated with a moderately increased risk of prostate cancer (Woodson et al., 2003). Based on meta-analysis studies, manganese SOD (MnSOD) polymorphisms may contribute to cancer development (Val-9Ala) (Wang et al., 2009b), prostate cancer susceptibility (Val-16Ala) (Mao et al., 2010), but not to breast cancer susceptibility (Val-16Ala) (Ma et al., 2010a). Calcitriol can also protect nonmalignant prostate cells from oxidative stress-induced cell death through the prevention of reactive oxygen species (ROS)-induced cellular injuries (Bao et al., 2008). Vitamin D metabolites and vitamin D analogs have been reported to induce lipoxygenase mRNA expression, lipoxygenase activity and ROS in a human bone cell line (Somjen et al., 2011). Vitamin D can also reduce the extent of lipid peroxidation and induce SOD activity in the hepatic anti-oxidant system of rats (Sardar et al., 1996). Moreover, the activation of macrophage 1α-hydroxylase results in an increase in 1,25OHD, which inhibits iNOS expression and reduces nitric oxide (NO) production by LPS-stimulated macrophages (Chang et al., 2004). This calcitriol production by macrophages may provide protection against the oxidative injuries caused by the NO burst. Calcitriol is known to inhibit LPS-induced immune activation in human endothelial cells (Equil et al., 2005), and calcitriol has also been shown to enhance intracellular glutathione pools and significantly reduce the nitrite production induced by the LPS (Garcion et al., 1999). Furthermore, overproduction of ROS induces DNA damage and leads to carcinogenesis. In the mouse colon, there was an inverse relationship between VDR levels and colonic hyperproliferation; the expression of 8-hydroxy-2'-deoxyguanosine (8-OHdG), a maker of oxidative DNA damage, significantly increased with complete loss of VDR (Kállay et al., 2002). Vitamin D decrease 8-OHdG by 22% in the normal human colorectal mucosa (Fedirko et al., 2012). Calcitriol contributes to a reduction of the DNA intensify replication stress in lymphocytes (Halicka et al., 2012). In addition, vitamin D_3 up-regulated protein 1(VDUP1) is a regular for redox signaling and stress-mediated diseases (Chung et al., 2006). Taken together, these findings suggest that vitamin D modulates oxidative stress in cancer.

4. The use of vitamin D in cancer treatment

A number of clinical trials have used vitamin D_3 and calcitriol alone or in combination with anti-tumor agents. Most preclinical suggest that that the optimal anti-tumor effect of calcitriol and other analogs is seen with the administration of high dose calcitriol on intermittent schedule. A small number of single agent trials utilizing vitamin D_3 and calcitriol hace been conducted with limited success.

4.1. Vitamin D_3 trials

Fifteen patients were given 2,000 IU (50 microg) of cholecalciferol daily and monitored prospectively every 2-3 mo. There was a statistically significant decrease in the rate of PSA rise after administration of cholecalciferol compared with that before cholecalciferol. The median PSA doubling time increased from 14.3 months prior to commencing cholecalciferol to 25 months after commencing cholecalciferol. Fourteen of 15 patients had a prolongation of PSA doubling time after commencing cholecalciferol (Woo et al., 2005). Breast cancer patients with bone metastases received 10,000 IU of vitamin D_3 daily for 4 months. There was a significant reduction in the number of sites of pain (Amir et al., 2010). Arlet al. (2012) reported on an unexpected observation of a spectacular 13-month remission of chronic lymphocytic leukemia after the administration of cholecalciferol in an elderly patient. Dietary vitamin D_3 and calcitriol have been shown to demonstrate equivalent anticancer activity in mouse xenograft models of breast and prostate cancers (Swani et al., 2012).

4.2. Calcitriol trials — Single agent

In a clinical trial, high-dose calcitriol decreased prostatic-specific antigen (PSA) levels by 50% and reduced thrombosis in prostate cancer patients (Beer et al., 2003 & 2006). In hepatocellular carcinoma, calcitriol and its analogs have been reported to reduce tumor volume, increase hepatocarcinoma cell apoptosis by 21.4%, and transient stabilize serum alpha-fetoprotein levels (Dalhoff et al., 2003; Luo et al., 2004; Morris et al., 2002). The vitamin D analog, 19-Nor-2α-(3-hydroxypropyl)-1α,25-dihydroxyvitamin D_3, is a potent cell growth regulator with enhanced chemotherapeutic potency in liver cancer cells (Chiang et al., 2011). Alphacalcidol, a vitamin D analogue, has been demonstrated significant antitumor activity in patients with low-grade non-Hodgkin's lymphoma of the follicular, small-cleaved cell type (Raina et al., 1991). In patient with parathyroid cancer, vitamin D has been shown to prevent or delay the progression of recurrence (Palmieri-Sevier et al., 1993). Treatment with paricalcitol inhibited gastric cancer cell growth and peritoneal metastatic gastric cancer volume was significantly lower in paricalcitol treated mice (Park et al., 2012). Calcitriol treatment of breast cancer cell lines led to significantly fewer inflammatory breast cancer experimental metastases as compared to control (Hillyer et al., 2012).

4.3. Calcitriol trials — In combination

Calcitriol additively or synergistically potentiates the antitumor of other types of chemotherapeutic agents. Calcitriol enhances cellular sensitivity of human colon cancer cells to 5-fluorouracil (Liu et al., 2010). Combination of calcitriol and cytarabine prolonged remission in elderly patients with acute myeloid leukemia (AML) and myelodysplastic syndrome (MDS) (Slapak et al., 1992; Ferrero, et al., 2004). A renal cell carcinoma patient with multiple bone metastases that were almost completely resolved after treatment with vitamin D and interferon-α (Fujioka et al., 1988). In a prospective study, a combination of active vitamin D and α-interferon has shown to be effective in patients with metastatic renal cell carcinoma (Obara et al., 2008). Calcitriol promotes the anti-proliferative effects of gemcitabine and cisplatin in human bladder cancer models (Ma et al., 2010b), and also potentiates antitumor activity of paclitaxel and docetaxel (Hershberger et al., 2001; Ting et al. 2007). A phase II study showed that high-dose calcitriol with docetaxel may increase time to progression in patients with incurable pancreatic cancer when compared with docetaxel monotherapy (Blanke, 2009). Vitamin D_3 treatment significantly suppressed the viability of gastric cancer and cholangiocarcinoma cells and also had a synergistic effect with other anti-cancer drugs, such as paclitaxel, adriamycin, and vinblastine (Baek et al., 2011). In locally advanced or cutaneous metastatic breast cancer, topical calcipotriol treatment reduced the diameter of treated lesions that contained vitamin D receptor (*VDR*) (Bower et al., 1991). Calcitriol potentiates both carboplatin and cisplatin-mediated growth inhibition in breast and prostate cancer cell lines (Cho et al., 1991; Moffatt et al., 1999). Tamoxifen and calcitriol or its analog used together to enhance growth inhibition in breast cancer cells than either agent alone (Vink-van Wijngaarden et al., 1994). Cacitriol sensitizes breast cancer cells to doxorubicin through the inhibition of the expression and activity of cytoplasmic antioxidant enzyme (Ravid et al., 1999). Calcitriol may increase cisplatin sensitivity in chemotherapy-resistant testicular germ cell cancer-derived cell lines (Jørgensen et al., 2012). Combination of retinoic acid and vitamin D analog exert synergistic growth inhibition and apoptosis induction on hepatocellular cancers cells (Zhang et al., 2012b). The combination of calcitriol and dietary soy resulted in substantially greater inhibition of tumor growth than the inhibition achieved with either agent alone in a mouse xenograft model of prostate cancer (Wang et al., 2012a).

5. Conclusion

Vitamin D has a role in the prevention and treatment of cancer. Genetic studies have provided the opportunity to determine what proteins link vitamin D to the pathology of cancer. Vitamin D also exerts its effect on cancer via non-genomic mechanisms. As a result, it is imperative that vitamin D levels in patients with cancer be followed. Many studies use the relationship between serum PTH and 25OHD to define the normal range of serum 25OHD. According to the report on Dietary Reference Intakes for vitamin D and calcium by the Institute of Medicine (IOM), persons are at risk of deficiency at serum 25OHD levels less than 30 nmol/L. Saliba et al. (2011) suggested that a 25OHD threshold of 50 nmol/L is sufficient for PTH suppression and prevention of secondary hyperparathyroidism in persons with normal renal function. It is necessary to check serum $25OHD_3$ and parathyroid hormone (PTH) status in cancer patients. Serum levels of PTH have been reported to correlate with PSA levels and colorectal cancer (Skinner & Schwartz, 2009; Charalampopoulos et al., 2010). Some authors proposed that, in patients with normal calcium levels, the serum $25OHD_3$ levels should be stored to > 55ng/ml in cancer patients (colon, breast, and ovary) (Garland et al., 2007). Calcitriol, $1,25OHD_3$, is best used for cancer treatment, because of its active form of vitamin D_3 metabolite, suppression of PTH levels (acted as cellular growth factor), and their receptors presented in most of human cells. However, monitor of serum $25OHD_3$ after taking calcitriol is not necessary because calcitriol inhibits the production of serum $25OHD_3$ by the liver (Bell et al., 1984; Luong & Nguyen, 1996). The main limitation to the clinical widespread evolution of $1,25OHD_3$ is its hypercalcemic side-effects.

Author details

Khanh vinh quoc Luong and Lan Thi Hoang Nguyen

Vietnamese American Medical Research Foundation, Westminster, California, USA

References

[1] Aguilera, O, Peña, C, García, J. M, Larriba, M. J, Ordóñez-morán, P, Navarro, D, & Barbáchano, A. López de Silanes I, Ballestar E, Fraga MF, Esteller M, Gamallo C, Bonilla F, González-Sancho JM, Muñoz A. The Wnt antagonist DICKKOPF-1 gene is induced by 1alpha,25-dihydroxyvitamin D_3 associated to the differentiation of human colon cancer cells. Carcinogenesis. (2007). Sep;, 28(9), 1877-84.

[2] Aksu, S, Beyazit, Y, Haznedaroglu, I. C, Canpinar, H, Kekilli, M, Uner, A, Sayinalp, N, Büyükasik, Y, Goker, H, & Ozcebe, O. I. Over-expression of angiotensin-converting enzyme (CD 143) on leukemic blasts as a clue for the activated local bone marrow RAS in AML. Leuk Lymphoma. (2006). May;, 47(5), 891-6.

[3] Ambrosch, F, Wiedermann, G, Krepler, P, Kundi, M, & Ambrosch, P. Effect of BCG vaccination of the newborn infant on the incidence and course of juvenile leukemias]. Fortschr Med. (1981). Sep 17;Article in German], 99(35), 1389-93.

[4] Ametaj, B, Beitz, D, Reihardt, T, & Nonnecke, B. (1996). dihydroxyvitamin D_3 inhibits secretion of interferon-gamma by mitogen- and antigen-stimulated bovine mononuclear leukocytes. Vet Immunol Imnunopathol. 52, 77-90., 1, 25.

[5] Amir, E, Simmons, C. E, Freedman, O. C, Dranitsaris, G, Cole, D. E, Vieth, R, Ooi, W. S, & Clemons, M. A phase 2 trial exploring the effects of high-dose (10,000 IU/day) vitamin D_3 in breast cancer patients with bone metastases. Cancer. (2010). Jan 15;, 116(2), 284-91.

[6] An, L. L, Ma, X. T, Yang, Y. H, Lin, Y. M, Song, Y. H, & Wu, K. F. Marked reduction of LL-37/hCAP-18, an antimicrobial peptide, in patients with acute myeloid leukemia. Int J Hematol. (2005). Jan;, 81(1), 45-7.

[7] Ando, T, Ishikawa, T, Kato, H, Yoshida, N, Naito, Y, Kokura, S, Yagi, N, Takagi, T, Handa, O, Kitawaki, J, Nakamura, N, Hasegawa, G, Fukui, M, Imamoto, E, Nakamura, C, Oyamada, H, Isozaki, Y, Matsumoto, N, Nagao, Y, Okita, M, Nakajima, Y, Kurokawa, M, Nukina, M, Ohta, M, Mizuno, S, Ogata, M, Obayashi, H, Park, H, Kitagawa, Y, Nakano, K, & Yoshikawa, T. Synergistic effect of HLA class II loci and cytokine gene polymorphisms on the risk of gastric cancer in Japanese patients with Helicobacter pylori infection. Int J Cancer. (2009). Dec 1;, 125(11), 2595-602.

[8] Altas, M, Bayrak, O. F, Ayan, E, Bolukbasi, F, Silav, G, Coskun, K. K, Culha, M, Sahin, F, Sevli, S, & Elmaci, I. The effect of polymorphisms in the promoter region of the MMP-1 gene on the occurrence and invasiveness of hypophyseal adenoma. Acta Neurochir (Wien). (2010). Sep;, 152(9), 1611-7.

[9] Alvarez-díaz, S, Valle, N, Ferrer-mayorga, G, Lombardía, L, Herrera, M, Domínguez, O, Segura, M. F, Bonilla, F, Hernando, E, & Muñoz, A. MicroRNA-22 is induced by vitamin D and contributes to its antiproliferative, antimigratory and gene regulatory effects in colon cancer cells. Hum Mol Genet. (2012). May 15;, 21(10), 2157-65.

[10] Alves Corrêa SA, Ribeiro de Noronha SM, Nogueira-de-Souza NC, Valleta de Carvalho C, Massad Costa AM, Juvenal Linhares J, Vieira Gomes MT, Guerreiro da Silva ID. Association between the angiotensin-converting enzyme (insertion/deletion) and angiotensin II type 1 receptor (A1166C) polymorphisms and breast cancer among Brazilian women. J Renin Angiotensin Aldosterone Syst. (2009). Mar;, 10(1), 51-8.

[11] Arjumand, W, Ahmad, S. T, Seth, A, Saini, A. K, & Sultana, S. Vitamin D receptor FokI and BsmI gene polymorphism and its association with grade and stage of renal cell carcinoma in North Indian population. Tumour Biol. (2012). Feb;, 33(1), 23-31.

[12] Arlet, J. B, Callens, C, Hermine, O, Darnige, L, Macintyre, E, Pouchot, J, & Capron, L. Chronic lymphocytic leukaemia responsive to vitamin D administration. Br J Haematol. (2012). Jan;, 156(1), 148-9.

[13] Arvaniti, E, Ntoufa, S, Papakonstantinou, N, Touloumenidou, T, Laoutaris, N, Anagnostopoulos, A, Lamnissou, K, Caligaris-cappio, F, Stamatopoulos, K, Ghia, P, Muzio, M, & Belessi, C. Toll-like receptor signaling pathway in chronic lymphocytic leukemia: distinct gene expression profiles of potential pathogenic significance in specific subsets of patients. Haematologica. (2011). Nov;, 96(11), 1644-52.

[14] Baek, S, Lee, Y. S, Shim, H. E, Yoon, S, Baek, S. Y, Kim, B. S, Oh, S. O, & Vitamin, D. regulates cell viability in gastric cancer and cholangiocarcinoma. Anat Cell Biol. (2011). Sep;, 44(3), 204-9.

[15] Bahar-shany, K, Ravid, A, & Koren, R. Upregulation of MMP-production by TNFalpha in keratinocytes and its attenuation by vitamin D. J Cell Physiol. (2010). , 222, 729-37.

[16] Bao, B. Y, Ting, H. J, Hsu, J. W, & Lee, Y. F. Protective role of 1α-dihydroxyvitamin D_3 against oxidative stress in nonmalignant human prostate epithelial cells. Int J Cancer. (2008). , 122, 2699-706.

[17] Bartel, D. P. (2004). MicroRNAs: genomics, biogenesis, mechanism, and function. Cell. , 116, 281-297.

[18] BeerTM; Lemmon, D; Lowe, BA; et al. ((2003). High-dose weekly oral calcitriol in patients with a rising PSA after prostatectomy or radiation for prostate carcinoma. Cancer. , 97, 1217-1224.

[19] BeerTM; Venner, PM; Ryan, CW; et al. ((2006). High dose calcitriol may reduce thrombosis in cancer patients. Br J Hematol. , 135, 392-394.

[20] Beildeck, M. E, Islam, M, Shah, S, Welsh, J, & Byers, S. W. Control of TCF-4 expression by VDR and vitamin D in the mouse mammary gland and colorectal cancer cell lines. PLoS One. (2009). Nov 17;4(11):e7872.

[21] Bell, N. H, Shaw, S, & Turner, R. T. Evidence that 1,25-dihydroxyvitamin D_3 inhibits the hepatic production of 25-hydroxyvitamin D in man. J Clin Invest. (1984). , 74, 1540-1544.

[22] Bergmann, C, Bachmann, H. S, Bankfalvi, A, Lotfi, R, Pütter, C, Wild, C. A, Schuler, P. J, Greve, J, Hoffmann, T. K, Lang, S, Scherag, A, & Lehnerdt, G. F. Toll-like receptor 4 single-nucleotide polymorphisms Asp299Gly and Thr399Ile in head and neck squamous cell carcinomas. J Transl Med. (2011). Aug 21;9:139.

[23] Beyazit, Y, Purnak, T, Suvak, B, Kurt, M, Sayilir, A, Turhan, T, Tas, A, Torun, S, Celik, T, Ibis, M, & Haznedaroglu, I. C. Increased ACE in extrahepatic cholangiocarcinoma as a clue for activated RAS in biliary neoplasms. Clin Res Hepatol Gastroenterol. (2011). Oct;, 35(10), 644-9.

[24] BlankeCD; Beer, TM; Todd; et al. ((2009). Phase II study of calcitriol-enhanced docetaxel in patients with previously untreated metastatic or locally advanced pancreatic cancer. Investigational New Drugs. , 27(4), 374-378.

[25] BowerM; Colston, KW; Stein, RC; et al. ((1991). Topical calcipotriol treatment in advanced breast cancer. Lancet. , 337(8743), 701-702.

[26] Brosseau, C. M, Pirianov, G, & Colston, K. W. Involvement of stress activated protein kinases (JNK and in 1,25 dihydroxyvitamin D3-induced breast cell death. Steroids. (2010). Dec 12;75(13-14):1082-8., 38.

[27] Büchau, A. S, Morizane, S, Trowbridge, J, Schauber, J, Kotol, P, Bui, J. D, & Gallo, R. L. The host defense peptide cathelicidin is required for NK cell-mediated suppression of tumor growth. J Immunol. (2010). Jan 1;, 184(1), 369-78.

[28] Bulut, G, Fallen, S, Beauchamp, E. M, Drebing, L. E, Sun, J, Berry, D. L, Kallakury, B, Crum, C. P, Toretsky, J. A, Schlegel, R, & Üren, A. Beta-catenin accelerates human papilloma virus type-16 mediated cervical carcinogenesis in transgenic mice. PLoS One. (2011). e27243.

[29] Byers, S, Shah, S, & Vitamin, D. and the regulation of Wnt/beta-catenin signaling and innate immunity in colorectal cancer. Nutr Rev. (2007). Aug;65(8 Pt 2):S, 118-20.

[30] Chang, J, Kuo, M, Kuo, H, Hwang, S, Tsai, J, et al. alpha,25-hydroxyvitamin D_3 regulates inducible nitric oxide synthase messenger RNA expression and nitric oxide release in macrophage-like RAW 264.7 cells. J Lab Clin Med. (2004). , 143, 14-22.

[31] Charalampopoulos A; Charalabopoulos, A; Batistatou, A; et al. ((2010). Parathormone and $1,25(OH)_2D_3$ but not $25(OH)D_3$ serum levels, in an inverse correlation, reveal an association with advanced stages of colorectal cancer. Clin Exp Med. , 10, 69-72.

[32] Chaudhary, A. K, Pandya, S, Mehrotra, R, Singh, M, & Singh, M. Role of functional polymorphism of matrix metalloproteinase-2 (-1306 C/T and-168 G/T) and MMP-9 (-1562 C/T) promoter in oral submucous fibrosis and head and neck squamous cell carcinoma in an Indian population. Biomarkers. (2011). Nov;, 16(7), 577-86.

[33] Chiang, K. C, Yeh, C. N, Chen, H. Y, Lee, J. M, Juang, H. H, Chen, M. F, Takano, M, Kittaka, A, & Chen, T. C. Nor-2α-(3-hydroxypropyl)-1α,25-dihydroxyvitamin D_3

(MART-10) is a potent cell growth regulator with enhanced chemotherapeutic potency in liver cancer cells. Steroids. (2011). Dec 11;, 76(13), 1513-9.

[34] Cho, Y. L, Christensen, C, Saunders, D. E, Lawrence, W. D, Deppe, G, Malviya, V. K, & Malone, J. M. Combined effects of 1,25-dihydroxyvitamin D_3 and platinum drugs on the growth of MCF-7 cells. Cancer Res. (1991). Jun 1;, 51(11), 2848-53.

[35] Choi, H. B, Roh, S. Y, Choi, E. J, Yoon, H. Y, Kim, S. Y, Hong, Y. S, Kim, D. W, & Kim, T. G. Association of HLA alleles with non-Hodgkin's lymphoma in Korean population. Int J Hematol. (2008). Mar;, 87(2), 203-9.

[36] Chuang, C. M, Monie, A, Wu, A, Mao, C. P, & Hung, C. F. Treatment with LL-37 peptide enhances antitumor effects induced by CpG oligodeoxynucleotides against ovarian cancer. Hum Gene Ther. (2009). Apr;, 20(4), 303-13.

[37] Chung, J. W, Jeon, J. H, Yoon, S. R, & Choi, I. Vitamin D upregulated protein 1 (VDUP1) is a regulator for redox signaling and stress-mediated diseases. J Dermatol. (2006). Oct;, 33(10), 662-9.

[38] Churilla, T. M, Lesko, S. L, Brereton, H. D, Klem, M, Donnelly, P. E, & Peters, C. A. Serum vitamin D levels among patients in a clinical oncology practice compared to primary care patients in the same community: a case-control study. BMJ Open. (2011). Dec 19;1(2):e000397.

[39] Churilla, T. M, Brereton, H. D, Klem, M, & Peters, C. A. Vitamin D Deficiency Is Widespread in Cancer Patients and Correlates With Advanced Stage Disease: A Community Oncology Experience. Nutr Cancer. (2012). Mar 27. [Epub ahead of print]

[40] Cordes, T, Hoellen, F, Dittmer, C, Salehin, D, Kümmel, S, Friedrich, M, Köster, F, Becker, S, Diedrich, K, & Thill, M. Correlation of prostaglandin metabolizing enzymes and serum PGE_2 levels with vitamin D receptor and serum $25(OH)_2D_3$ levels in breast and ovarian cancer. Anticancer Res. (2012). Jan;, 32(1), 351-7.

[41] Cortez, M. A, Welsh, J. W, & Calin, G. A. Circulating MicroRNAs as Noninvasive Biomarkers in Breast Cancer. Recent Results Cancer Res. (2012). , 195, 151-61.

[42] Crew, K. D, Shane, E, Cremers, S, Mcmahon, D. J, Irani, D, & Hershman, D. L. High prevalence of vitamin D deficiency despite supplementation in premenopausal women with breast cancer undergoing adjuvant chemotherapy. J Clin Oncol. (2009). May 1;, 27(13), 2151-6.

[43] Dalhoff K; Dancey, J; Astrup, L; et al. ((2003). A phase II study of the vitamin D analogue Seocalcitol in patients with inoperable hepatocellular carcinoma. Br J Cancer. , 89, 252-257.

[44] Dean, D. D, Schwartz, Z, Schmitz, J, Muniz, O. E, Lu, Y, et al. Vitamin D regulation of metalloproteinase activity in matrix vesicles. Connect Tissue Res. (1996). , 35, 331-6.

[45] Denzer, N, Vogt, T, & Reichrath, J. Vitamin D receptor (VDR) polymorphisms and skin cancer: A systematic review. Dermatoendocrinol. (2011). Jul;, 3(3), 205-10.

[46] Deshayes, F, & Nahmias, C. Angiotensin receptors: a new role in cancer? Trends Endocrinol Metab. (2005). Sep;, 16(7), 293-9.

[47] Dickie, L, Church, L, Coulthard, L, Mathews, R, Emery, P, & Mcdermott, M. Vitamin D downregulates intracellular toll-like receptor 9 expression and toll-like receptor 9-induced IL-6 production in human monocytes. Rheumatol. (2010). , 48, 1466-71.

[48] Ditsch, N, Toth, B, Mayr, D, Lenhard, M, Gallwas, J, Weissenbacher, T, Dannecker, C, Friese, K, & Jeschke, U. The association between vitamin D receptor expression and prolonged overall survival in breast cancer. J Histochem Cytochem. (2012). Feb;, 60(2), 121-9.

[49] Donaldson, P. T, Ho, S, Williams, R, & Johnson, P. J. HLA class II alleles in Chinese patients with hepatocellular carcinoma. Liver. (2001). Apr;, 21(2), 143-8.

[50] Dong, W, Li, H, Zhang, Y, Yang, H, Guo, M, Li, L, & Liu, T. Matrix metalloproteinase 2 promotes cell growth and invasion in colorectal cancer. Acta Biochim Biophys Sin (Shanghai). (2011). Nov;, 43(11), 840-8.

[51] Drake, M. T, Maurer, M. J, Link, B. K, Habermann, T. M, Ansell, S. M, Micallef, I. N, Kelly, J. L, Macon, W. R, Nowakowski, G. S, Inwards, D. J, Johnston, P. B, Singh, R. J, Allmer, C, Slager, S. L, Weiner, G. J, Witzig, T. E, & Cerhan, J. R. Vitamin D insufficiency and prognosis in non-Hodgkin's lymphoma. J Clin Oncol. (2010). Sep 20;, 28(27), 4191-8.

[52] Du, N, Feng, J, Hu, L. J, Sun, X, Sun, H. B, Zhao, Y, Yang, Y. P, & Ren, H. Angiotensin II receptor type 1 blockers suppress the cell proliferation effects of angiotensin II in breast cancer cells by inhibiting AT1R signaling. Oncol Rep. (2012). Jun;, 27(6), 1893-903.

[53] Dziki, L, Przybylowska, K, Majsterek, I, Trzcinski, R, & Sygut, M. A. A. G Polymorphism of the MMP-7 Gene Promoter Region in Colorectal Cancer. Pol Przegl Chir. (2011). Nov 1;, 83(11), 622-6.

[54] Equils, O, Naiki, Y, Shapiro, A. M, Michelsen, K, Lu, D, et al. hydroxyvitamin D_3 inhibits liposaccharide-induced immune activation in human endothelial cells. Clin Exp Immunol. (2005). , 143, 58-64.

[55] Essa, S, Denzer, N, Mahlknecht, U, Klein, R, Collnot, E. M, Tilgen, W, & Reichrath, J. VDR microRNA expression and epigenetic silencing of vitamin D signaling in melanoma cells. J Steroid Biochem Mol Biol. (2010). Jul;121(1-2):110-3.

[56] Essa, S, Reichrath, S, Mahlknecht, U, Montenarh, M, Vogt, T, & Reichrath, J. Signature of VDR miRNAs and epigenetic modulation of vitamin D signaling in melanoma cell lines. Anticancer Res. (2012). Jan;, 32(1), 383-9.

[57] Eyking, A, Ey, B, Rünzi, M, Roig, A. I, Reis, H, Schmid, K. W, Gerken, G, Podolsky, D. K, & Cario, E. Toll-like receptor 4 variant D299G induces features of neoplastic progression in Caco-2 intestinal cells and is associated with advanced human colon cancer. Gastroenterology. (2011). Dec;, 141(6), 2154-65.

[58] Fedirko, V, Bostick, R. M, Flanders, W. D, Long, Q, Shaukat, A, Rutherford, R. E, Daniel, C. R, Cohen, V, & Dash, C. Effects of vitamin D and calcium supplementation on markers of apoptosis in normal colon mucosa: a randomized, double-blind, placebo-controlled clinical trial. Cancer Prev Res (Phila). (2009). Mar;, 2(3), 213-23.

[59] Feng, Y, Wan, H, Liu, J, Zhang, R, Ma, Q, Han, B, Xiang, Y, Che, J, Cao, H, Fei, X, & Qiu, W. The angiotensin-converting enzyme 2 in tumor growth and tumor-associated angiogenesis in non-small cell lung cancer. Oncol Rep. (2010). Apr;, 23(4), 941-8.

[60] Feng, Y, Ni, L, Wan, H, Fan, L, Fei, X, Ma, Q, Gao, B, Xiang, Y, Che, J, & Li, Q. Overexpression of ACE2 produces antitumor effects via inhibition of angiogenesis and tumor cell invasion in vivo and in vitro. Oncol Rep. (2011). a Nov;, 26(5), 1157-64.

[61] Feng, S, Cen, J, Huang, Y, Shen, H, Yao, L, Wang, Y, & Chen, Z. Matrix metalloproteinase-2 and-9 secreted by leukemic cells increase the permeability of blood-brain barrier by disrupting tight junction proteins. PLoS One. (2011b). e20599.

[62] Ferrero, D, Campa, E, Dellacasa, C, et al. (2004). Differentiating agents + low-dose chemotherapy in the management of old/poor prognosis patients with acute myeloid leukemia or myelodysplastic syndrome. Haematologica. , 89, 619-620.

[63] Fujioka, T, Hasegawa, M, Ishikura, K, Matsushita, Y, Sato, M, & Tanji, S. Inhibition of tumor growth and angiogenesis by vitamin D3 agents in murine renal cell carcinoma. J Urol. (1998). , 160, 247-51.

[64] Garamszegi, N, Garamszegi, S. P, & Scully, S. P. Matrix metalloproteinase-1 contribution to sarcoma cell invasion. J Cell Mol Med. (2011). Jul 31. doi:j.x. [Epub ahead of print], 1582-4934.

[65] García-plata, D, Mozos, E, Carrasco, L, & Solana, R. HLA molecule expression in cutaneous squamous cell carcinomas: an immunopathological study and clinical-immunohistopathological correlations. Histol Histopathol. (1993). Apr;, 8(2), 219-26.

[66] Garcion, E, Sindji, L, Leblondel, G, Brachet, P, & Darcy, F. hydroxyvitamin D_3 regulates the synthesis of γ-glutamyl transpeptidase and glutathione levels in rat primary astrocytes. J Neurochem. (1999). , 73, 859-66.

[67] GarlandCF; Grant, WB; Mohr, SB; et al. ((2007). What is the dose-response relationship between vitamin D and cancer risk? Nutr Rev. Pt.2, , 65(8), S91-S95.

[68] Ge, X, & Wang, X. Role of Wnt canonical pathway in hematological malignancies. J Hematol Oncol. (2010). Sep 15;3:33

[69] Gilbert-sirieix, M, Makoukji, J, Kimura, S, Talbot, M, Caillou, B, Massaad, C, & Massaad-massade, L. Wnt/β-catenin signaling pathway is a direct enhancer of thyroid

transcription factor-1 in humanpapillary thyroid carcinoma cells. PLoS One. (2011). e22280.

[70] Giovannucci E; Liu, Y; Rimm, EB; et al. ((2008). Prospective study of predictors of vitamin D status and cancer incidence and mortality in men. J Natl Cancer Inst. , 98, 451-459.

[71] Gocek, E, Wang, X, Liu, X, Liu, C. G, & Studzinski, G. P. MicroRNA-32 upregulation by 1,25-dihydroxyvitamin D_3 in human myeloid leukemia cells leads to Bim targeting and inhibition of AraC-induced apoptosis. Cancer Res. (2011). Oct 1;, 71(19), 6230-9.

[72] Gombart, A. F, Borregaard, N, & Koeffler, H. P. Human cathelicidin antimicrobial peptide (CAMP) gene is a direct target of the vitamin D receptor and is strongly upregulated in myeloid cells by 1,25-dihydroxyvitamin D_3. FASEB J. (2005). Jul;, 19(9), 1067-77.

[73] González-Zuloeta Ladd AM, Arias Vásquez A, Sayed-Tabatabaei FA, Coebergh JW, Hofman A, Njajou O, Stricker B, van Duijn C. Angiotensin-converting enzyme gene insertion/deletion polymorphism and breast cancer risk. Cancer Epidemiol Biomarkers Prev. (2005). Sep;, 14(9), 2143-6.

[74] Gupta, S. C, Hevia, D, Patchva, S, Park, B, Koh, W, & Aggarwal, B. B. Upsides and Downsides of Reactive Oxygen Species for Cancer: The Roles of Reactive Oxygen Species in Tumorigenesis, Prevention, and Therapy. Antioxid Redox Signal. (2012). Jan 16. [Epub ahead of print]

[75] Gupta-elera, G, Garrett, A. R, Robison, R. A, & Neill, O. KL. The role of oxidative stress in prostate cancer. Eur J Cancer Prev. (2012). , 21, 155-62.

[76] Guturi, K. K, Mandal, T, Chatterjee, A, Sarkar, M, Bhattacharya, S, Chatterjee, U, & Ghosh, M. K. Mechanism of β-catenin mediated transcriptional regulation of EGFR expression in GSK3β inactivated prostate cancer cells. J Biol Chem. (2012). Apr 5. [Epub ahead of print]

[77] Hama, T, Norizoe, C, Suga, H, Mimura, T, Kato, T, Moriyama, H, & Urashima, M. Prognostic significance of vitamin D receptor polymorphisms in head and neck squamous cell carcinoma. PLoS One. (2011). e29634.

[78] Halicka, H. D, Zhao, H, Li, J, Traganos, F, Studzinski, G. P, & Darzynkiewicz, Z. Attenuation of constitutive DNA damage signaling by dihydroxyvitamin D_3. Aging (Albany NY). (2012). Apr 11. [Epub ahead of print], 1, 25.

[79] He, W, Kang, Y. S, Dai, C, & Liu, Y. Blockade of Wnt/β-catenin signaling by paricalcitol ameliorates proteinuria and kidney injury. J Am Soc Nephrol. (2011). Jan;, 22(1), 90-103.

[80] Hernández-hernández, D. M, Cerda-flores, R. M, Juárez-cedillo, T, Granados-arriola, J, Vargas-alarcón, G, Apresa-garcía, T, Alvarado-cabrero, I, García-carrancá, A, Salce-

do-vargas, M, & Mohar-betancourt, A. Human leukocyte antigens I and II haplo-types associated with human papillomavirus 16-positive invasive cervical cancer in Mexican women. Int J Gynecol Cancer. (2009). Aug;, 19(6), 1099-106.

[81] Herr, H. W, Laudone, V. P, Badalament, R. A, Oettgen, H. F, Sogani, P. C, Freedman, B. D, & Melamed, M. R. Whitmore WF Jr. Bacillus Calmette-Guérin therapy alters the progression of superficial bladder cancer. J Clin Oncol. (1988). Sep;, 6(9), 1450-5.

[82] Hershberger PA; Yu, WD; Modzelewski, RA; et al. ((2001). Calcitriol (1,25-dihydroxy-cholecalciferol) enhances paclitaxel antitumor activity in vitro and in vivo and accelerates paclitaxel-induced apoptosis. Clin Cancer Res. , 7, 1043-1051.

[83] Higiwara, H, Furuhashi, H, Nakaya, K, & Nakamura, Y. Effects of vitamin D_3 and related compounds on angiotensin converting activity of endothelial cells and on release of plasminogen activator from them. Chem Pharm Bull. (1988). , 36, 4858-64.

[84] Hillyer, R. L, Sirinvasin, P, Joglekar, M, Sikes, R. A, Van Golen, K. L, & Nohe, A. Differential effects of vitamin D treatment on inflammatory and non-inflammatory breast cancer cell lines. Clin Exp Metastasis. (2012). Dec;, 29(8), 971-9.

[85] Hipskind, R. A, & Bilbe, G. MAP kinase signaling cascades and gene expression in osteoblasts. Front Biosci. (1998). Aug 1;3:d, 804-16.

[86] Hojjat-farsangi, M, Jeddi-tehrani, M, Amirzargar, A. A, Razavi, S. M, Sharifian, R. A, Rabbani, H, & Shokri, F. Human leukocyte antigen class II allele association to disease progression in Iranian patients with chronic lymphocytic leukemia. Hum Immunol. (2008). Oct;, 69(10), 666-74.

[87] Hong, C. C, Ambrosone, C. B, Ahn, J, Choi, J. Y, Mccullough, M. L, Stevens, V. L, et al. Genetic variability in iron-related oxidative stress pathways (Nrf2, NQ01, NOS3, and HO-1), iron intake, and risk of postmenopausal breast cancer. Cancer Epidemiol Biomarkers Prev. (2007). , 16, 1784-94.

[88] Huang, W, Yu, L. F, Zhong, J, Qiao, M. M, Jiang, F. X, Du, F, Tian, X. L, & Wu, Y. L. Angiotensin II type 1 receptor expression in human gastric cancer and induces MMP2 and MMP9 expression in MKN-28 cells. Dig Dis Sci. (2008). Jan;, 53(1), 163-8.

[89] Ino, K, Shibata, K, Kajiyama, H, Yamamoto, E, Nagasaka, T, Nawa, A, Nomura, S, & Kikkawa, F. Angiotensin II type 1 receptor expression in ovarian cancer and its correlation with tumour angiogenesis and patient survival. Br J Cancer. (2006). Feb 27;, 94(4), 552-60.

[90] Iglesias-gato, D, Zheng, S, Flanagan, J. N, Jiang, L, Kittaka, A, Sakaki, T, Yamamoto, K, Itoh, T, Lebrasseur, N. K, Norstedt, G, & Chen, T. C. Substitution at carbon 2 of nor-1α,25-dihydroxyvitamin D_3 with 3-hydroxypropyl group generates an analogue with enhanced chemotherapeutic potency in PC-3 prostate cancer cells. J Steroid Biochem Mol Biol. (2011). Nov;127(3-5):269-75., 19.

[91] Ji, Y, Kutner, A, Verstuyf, A, Verlinden, L, & Studzinski, G. P. Derivatives of vitamins D_2 and D_3 activate three MAPK pathways and upregulate pRb expression in differentiating HL60 cells. Cell Cycle. (2002). Nov-Dec;, 1(6), 410-5.

[92] Johnston, C. I. Tissue angiotensin converting enzyme in cardiac and vascular hypertrophy, repair, and remodeling. Hypertension. (1994). , 23, 258-68.

[93] Jørgensen, A. Blomberg Jensen M, Nielsen JE, Juul A, Rajpert-De Meyts E. Influence of vitamin D on cisplatin sensitivity in testicular germ cell cancer-derived cell lines and in a NTera2 xenograft model. J Steroid Biochem Mol Biol. (2012). Oct 23. pii: S0960-0760(12)00208-7. doi:j.jsbmb.2012.10.008. [Epub ahead of print]

[94] Kállay, E, Bareis, P, Bajna, E, Kriwanek, S, Bonner, E, Toyokuni, S, & Cross, H. S. Vitamin D receptor activity and prevention of colonic hyperproliferation and oxidative stress. Food Chem Toxicol. (2002). Aug;, 40(8), 1191-6.

[95] Keizman, D, Huang, P, Eisenberger, M. A, Pili, R, Kim, J. J, Antonarakis, E. S, Hammers, H, & Carducci, M. A. Angiotensin system inhibitors and outcome of sunitinib treatment in patients with metastatic renal cell carcinoma: a retrospective examination. Eur J Cancer. (2011). Sep;, 47(13), 1955-61.

[96] Kim, H. J, Bae, J. S, Chang, I. H, Kim, K. D, Lee, J, Shin, H. D, Lee, J. Y, Kim, W. J, Kim, W, & Myung, S. C. Sequence variants of toll-like receptor 4 (TLR4) and the risk of prostate cancer in Korean men. World J Urol. (2012). Apr;, 30(2), 225-32.

[97] Kinoshita, J, Fushida, S, Harada, S, Yagi, Y, Fujita, H, Kinami, S, Ninomiya, I, Fujimura, T, Kayahara, M, Yashiro, M, Hirakawa, K, & Ohta, T. Local angiotensin II-generation in human gastric cancer: correlation with tumor progression through the activation of ERK1/2, NF-kappaB and survivin. Int J Oncol. (2009). Jun;, 34(6), 1573-82.

[98] Koca, E, Haznedaroglu, I. C, Uner, A, Sayinalp, N, Saglam, A. E, Goker, H, & Ozcebe, O. I. Angiotensin-converting enzyme expression of the lymphoma-associated macrophages in the lymph nodes of Hodgkin's disease. J Natl Med Assoc. (2007). Nov; 99(11):1243-4, 1246-7.

[99] Kölmel, K. F, Grange, J. M, Krone, B, Mastrangelo, G, Rossi, C. R, Henz, B. M, Seebacher, C, Botev, I. N, Niin, M, Lambert, D, Shafir, R, Kokoschka, E. M, Kleeberg, U. R, Gefeller, O, & Pfahlberg, A. Prior immunisation of patients with malignant melanoma with vaccinia or BCG is associated with better survival. An European Organization for Research and Treatment of Cancer cohort study on 542 patients. Eur J Cancer. (2005). Jan;, 41(1), 118-25.

[100] Komagata, S, Nakajima, M, Takagi, S, Mohri, T, Taniya, T, & Yokoi, T. Human CYP24 catalyzing the inactivation of calcitriol is post-transcriptionally regulated by miR-125b. Mol Pharmacol. (2009). Oct;, 76(4), 702-9.

[101] Koli, K, & Keski-oja, J. Alpha, 25-dihydroxyvitamin D and its analogues down-regu-
       late cell invasion-associated proteases in cultured malignant cells. Cell Growth Dif-
       fer. (2000). Apr;, 11(4), 221-9.

[102] Köstner, K, Denzer, N, Koreng, M, Reichrath, S, Gräber, S, Klein, R, Tilgen, W, Vogt,
       T, & Reichrath, J. Association of genetic variants of the vitamin D receptor (VDR)
       with cutaneous squamous cell carcinomas (SCC) and basal cell carcinomas (BCC): a
       pilot study in a German population. Anticancer Res. (2012). Jan;, 32(1), 327-33.

[103] Kulah, E, Dursun, A, Aktunc, E, Acikgoz, S, Aydin, M, et al. Effects of angiotensin-
       converting enzyme gene polymorphism and serum vitamin D levels on ambulatory
       blood pressure measurement and left ventricular mass in Turkish hypertensive pop-
       ulation. Blood Press Monit. (2007). , 12, 207-13.

[104] Kupfer, S. S, Anderson, J. R, Ludvik, A. E, Hooker, S, Skol, A, Kittles, R. A, Keku, T.
       O, Sandler, R. S, Ruiz-ponte, C, Castellvi-bel, S, Castells, A, Carracedo, A, & Ellis, N.
       A. Genetic associations in the vitamin D receptor and colorectal cancer in African
       Americans and Caucasians. PLoS One. (2011). e26123.

[105] Ma, X, Chen, C, Xiong, H, Fan, J, Li, Y, Lin, H, et al. No association between SOD2
       Val16Ala polymorphism and breast cancer susceptibility: a meta-analysis based on
       9,710 cases and 11,041 controls. Breast Cancer Res Treat. (2010a). , 122, 509-14.

[106] Ma Y; Yu, WD; Trump, DL; et al. ((2010b). Enhances antitumor activity of gemcita-
       bine and cisplatin in human bladder cancer models. *Cancer.* , 116, 3294-3303.

[107] Mahmoudi, T, Arkani, M, Karimi, K, Safaei, A, Rostami, F, Arbabi, E, Pourhoseing-
       holi, M. A, Mohebbi, S. R, Nikzamir, A, Romani, S, Almasi, S, Abbaszadeh, M, Va-
       faei, M, & Zali, M. R. The-4817 G>A (rs2238136) variant of the vitamin D receptor
       gene: a probable risk factor for colorectal cancer. Mol Biol Rep. (2012). May;, 39(5),
       5277-82.

[108] Makni, H, & Daoud, J. Ben Salah H, Mahfoudh N, Haddar O, Karray H, Boudawara
       T, Ghorbel A, Khabir A, Frikha M. HLA association with nasopharyngeal carcinoma
       in southern Tunisia. Mol Biol Rep. (2010). Jun;, 37(5), 2533-9.

[109] Malik, M. A, Sharma, K. L, Zargar, S. A, & Mittal, B. Association of matrix metallo-
       proteinase-7 (-181A>G) polymorphism with risk of esophageal squamous cell carci-
       noma in Kashmir Valley. Saudi J Gastroenterol. (2011). Sep-Oct;, 17(5), 301-6.

[110] Mao, C, Qiu, L. X, Zhan, P, Xue, K, Ding, H, Du, F. B, et al. MnSOD Val16Ala poly-
       morphism and prostate cancer susceptibility: a meta-analysis involving 8,962 sub-
       jects. J Cancer Res Clin Oncol. (2010). , 136, 975-9.

[111] Marra, M, Sordelli, I. M, Lombardi, A, Lamberti, M, Tarantino, L, Giudice, A, et al.
       Molecular targets and oxidative stress biomarkers in hepatocellular carcinoma: an
       overview. J Transl Med. (2011).

[112] Mcguire, T. F, Trump, D. L, & Johnson, C. S. Vitamin D induced apoptosis of murine squamous cell carcinoma cells. Selective induction of caspase-dependent MEK cleavage and up-regulation of MEKK-1. J Biol Chem. (2001). Jul 13;, 276(28), 26365-73.

[113] Michel, S, Linnebacher, M, Alcaniz, J, Voss, M, Wagner, R, Dippold, W, & Becker, C. von Knebel Doeberitz M, Ferrone S, Kloor M. Lack of HLA class II antigen expression in microsatellite unstable colorectal carcinomas is caused by mutations in HLA class II regulatory genes. Int J Cancer. (2010). Aug 15;, 127(4), 889-98.

[114] Min, R, Zun, Z, Siyi, L, Wenjun, Y, Lizheng, W, & Chenping, Z. Increased expression of Toll-like receptor-9 has close relation with tumour cell proliferation in oral squamous cell carcinoma. Arch Oral Biol. (2011). Sep;, 56(9), 877-84.

[115] Minmin, S, Xiaoqian, X, Hao, C, Baiyong, S, Xiaxing, D, Junjie, X, Xi, Z, Jianquan, Z, & Songyao, J. Single nucleotide polymorphisms of Toll-like receptor 4 decrease the risk of development of hepatocellular carcinoma. PLoS One. (2011). Apr 29;6(4):e19466.

[116] Moffatt, K. A, Johannes, W. U, & Miller, G. J. α Dihydroxyvitamin D_3 and platinum drugs act synergistically to inhibit the growth of prostate cancer cell lines. Clin Cancer Res. (1999). Mar;, 5(3), 695-703.

[117] Mohri, T, Nakajima, M, Takagi, S, Komagata, S, & Yokoi, T. MicroRNA regulates human vitamin D receptor. Int J Cancer. (2009). Sep 15;, 125(6), 1328-33.

[118] Moreno, J, Krishnan, A. V, Swami, S, Nonn, L, Peehl, D. M, & Feldman, D. Regulation of prostaglandin metabolism by calcitriol attenuates growth stimulation in prostate cancer cells. Cancer Res. (2005). Sep 1;, 65(17), 7917-25.

[119] Morris DL; Jourdan, JL; Finlay, I; et al. ((2002). Hepatic intra-arterial injection of 1,25-dihydroxyvitamin D_3 in lipiodol: pilot study in patients with hepatocellular carcinoma. Int J Oncol. , 21, 901-906.

[120] Nuñez, F, Bravo, S, Cruzat, F, Montecino, M, & De Ferrari, G. V. Wnt/β-catenin signaling enhances cyclooxygenase-2 (COX2) transcriptional activity in gastric cancer cells. PLoS One. (2011). Apr 6;6(4):e18562.

[121] Nakagawa, K, Sasaki, Y, Kato, S, Kubodera, N, & Okano, T. Oxa-1α,25-dihydroxyvitamin D_3 inhibits metastasis and angiogenesis in lung cancer. Carcinogenesis. (2005). , 26, 1044-54.

[122] Nakai, Y, Isayama, H, Ijichi, H, Sasaki, T, Sasahira, N, Hirano, K, Kogure, H, Kawakubo, K, Yagioka, H, Yashima, Y, Mizuno, S, Yamamoto, K, Arizumi, T, Togawa, O, Matsubara, S, Tsujino, T, Tateishi, K, Tada, M, Omata, M, & Koike, K. Inhibition of renin-angiotensin system affects prognosis of advanced pancreatic cancer receiving gemcitabine. Br J Cancer. (2010). Nov 23;, 103(11), 1644-8.

[123] Naugler, C, & Liwski, R. HLA risk markers for chronic myelogenous leukemia in Eastern Canada. Leuk Lymphoma. (2009). Feb;, 50(2), 254-9.

[124] Ng, A. C, Kumar, S. K, Rajkumar, S. V, & Drake, M. T. Impact of vitamin D deficien-
       cy on the clinical presentation and prognosis of patients with newly diagnosed multi-
       ple myeloma. Am J Hematol. (2009). Jul;, 84(7), 397-400.

[125] Nguyen, H, Ivanova, V. S, Kavandi, L, Rodriguez, G. C, Maxwell, G. L, & Syed, V.
       Progesterone and 1,25-dihydroxyvitamin D3 inhibit endometrial cancer cell growth
       by upregulating semaphorin 3B and semaphorin 3F. Mol Cancer Res. (2011). Nov;,
       9(11), 1479-92.

[126] Nihon-yanagi, Y, Terai, K, Murano, T, Matsumoto, T, & Okazumi, S. Tissue expres-
       sion of Toll-like receptors 2 and 4 in sporadic human colorectal cancer. Cancer Im-
       munol Immunother. (2012). Jan;, 61(1), 71-7.

[127] Lange, T. S, Stuckey, A. R, Robison, K, Kim, K. K, Singh, R. K, Raker, C. A, Brard, L,
       Lange, T. S, Stuckey, A. R, Robison, K, Kim, K. K, Singh, R. K, Raker, C. A, & Brard,
       L. Effect of a vitamin D$_3$ derivative (B3CD) with postulated anti-cancer activity in an
       ovarian cancer animal model. Invest New Drugs. (2010). Oct;, 28(5), 543-53.

[128] Lalor, M, Floyd, S, Gorak-stolinska, P, Weir, R, Blitz, R, Branson, K, et al. (2011). BCG
       vaccination: a role for vitamin D? PLos ONE. 6, 216709.

[129] Larriba, M. J, Valle, N, Pálmer, H. G, Ordóñez-morán, P, Alvarez-díaz, S, Becker, K.
       F, Gamallo, C, De Herreros, A. G, González-sancho, J. M, & Muñoz, A. The inhibition
       of Wnt/beta-catenin signalling by 1alpha,25-dihydroxyvitamin D$_3$ is abrogated by
       Snail1 in human colon cancer cells. Endocr Relat Cancer. (2007). Mar;, 14(1), 141-51.

[130] Larriba, M. J, Ordóñez-morán, P, Chicote, I, Martín-fernández, G, Puig, I, Muñoz, A,
       & Pálmer, H. G. Vitamin D receptor deficiency enhances Wnt/β-catenin signaling
       and tumor burden in colon cancer. PLoS One. (2011). e23524.

[131] Launoy, G, Milan, C, Day, N. E, Pienkowski, M. P, Gignoux, M, & Faivre, J. Diet and
       squamous-cell cancer of the oesophagus: a French multicentre case-control study. Int
       J Cancer. (1998). Mar 30;, 76(1), 7-12.

[132] Lee, H. W, Hahm, K. B, Lee, J. S, Ju, Y. S, Lee, K. M, & Lee, K. W. Association of the
       human leukocyte antigen class II alleles with chronic atrophic gastritis and gastric
       carcinoma in Koreans. J Dig Dis. (2009). Nov;, 10(4), 265-71.

[133] Lefkowitz, E. S, & Garland, C. F. Sunlight, vitamin D, and ovarian cancer mortality
       rates in US women. Int J Epidemiol. (1994). Dec;, 23(6), 1133-6.

[134] Li, Z. Q, Ding, W, Sun, S. J, Li, J, Pan, J, Zhao, C, Wu, W. R, & Si, W. K. Cyr61/CCN1
       Is Regulated by Wnt/β-Catenin Signaling and Plays an Important Role in the Pro-
       gression of Hepatocellular Carcinoma. PLoS One. (2012). e35754.

[135] Lindhorst, E, Schumm-draeger, P. M, Bojunga, J, Usadel, K. H, & Herrmann, G. Dif-
       ferences in tumor cell proliferation, HLA DR expression and lymphocytic infiltration
       in various types of thyroid carcinoma. Exp Clin Endocrinol Diabetes. (2002). Jan;,
       110(1), 27-31.

[136] Lipworth, L, Rossi, M, Mclaughlin, J. K, Negri, E, Talamini, R, Levi, F, & Franceschi, S. La Vecchia C. Dietary vitamin D and cancers of the oral cavity and esophagus. Ann Oncol. (2009). Sep;, 20(9), 1576-81.

[137] Liu, P. T, Stenger, S, Li, H, Wenzel, L, Tan, B. H, Krutzik, S. R, et al. Toll-like receptor triggering of a vitamin D-mediated human antimicrobial response. Science. (2006). , 311, 1770-3.

[138] LiuG; Hu, X; Chakrabarty, S; et al. ((2010). Vitamin D mediates its action in human colon carcinoma cells in a calcium-sensing receptor-dependent manner: downregulates malignant cell behavior and the expression of thymidylate synthase and surviving and promotes cellular sensitivity to 5-FU. Int J Cancer. , 126, 631-639.

[139] Liu, D, Duan, W, Guo, H, Xu, X, & Bai, Y. Meta-analysis of associations between polymorphisms in the promoter regions of matrix metalloproteinases and the risk of colorectal cancer. Int J Colorectal Dis. (2011). Sep;, 26(9), 1099-105.

[140] Liu, D, Guo, H, Li, Y, Xu, X, Yang, K, & Bai, Y. Association between polymorphisms in the promoter regions of matrix metalloproteinases (MMPs) and risk of cancer metastasis: a meta-analysis. PLoS One. (2012). e31251.

[141] Loke, T. W, Sevfi, D, & Khadra, M. Prostate cancer incidence in Australia correlates inversely with solar radiation. BJU Int. (2011). Nov;108 Suppl , 2, 66-70.

[142] Lotfy, M. El-Kenawy Ael-M, Abdel-Aziz MM, El-Kady I, Talaat A. Elevated renin levels in patients with liver cirrhosis and hepatocellular carcinoma. Asian Pac J Cancer Prev. (2010). , 11(5), 1263-6.

[143] Louis, S. N, Wang, L, Chow, L, Rezmann, L. A, & Imamura, K. MacGregor DP, Casely D, Catt KJ, Frauman AG, Louis WJ. Appearance of angiotensin II expression in non-basal epithelial cells is an early feature of malignant change in human prostate. Cancer Detect Prev. (2007). , 31(5), 391-5.

[144] Lu, J, Getz, G, Miska, E. A, Alvarez-saavedra, E, Lamb, J, Peck, D, Sweet-cordero, A, Ebert, B. L, Mak, R. H, Ferrando, A. A, Downing, J. R, Jacks, T, Horvitz, H. R, & Golub, T. R. MicroRNA expression profiles classify human cancers. Nature. (2005). Jun 9;, 435(7043), 834-8.

[145] LuoWJ; Chen, JY; Xu, W; et al. ((2004). Effects of vitamin D analogue EB1089 on proliferation and apoptosis of hepatic carcinoma cells. Zhonghua Yu Fang Yi Xue Za Zhi. article in Chinese], 38, 415-418.

[146] Luong, K. V, & Nguyen, L. T. Coexisting hyperparathyroidism and primary hyperparathyroidism with vitamin D-deficient osteomalacia in a Vietnamese immigrant. Endocrine Practice. (1996). , 2, 250-254.

[147] Luong, K, & Nguyen, L. T. The beneficial role of vitamin D and its analogs in cancer treatment and prevention. Crit Rev Oncol Hematol. (2010). Mar;, 73(3), 192-201.

[148] Lương KVQNguyễn LTH. ((2012). Vitamin D and cancer. In "Advanced in Cancer Management". InTech Publishing Co. January 2012. , 1-16.

[149] ObaraW; Mizutani, Y; Oyama, C; et al. ((2008). Prospective study of combined treatment with interferon-alpha and active vitamin D_3 for Japanese patients with metastatic renal cell carcinoma. *Int J Urol.* , 15, 794-799.

[150] Ordóñez-Morán, P, Larriba, MJ, Pálmer, HG, Valero, RA, Barbáchano, A, Duñach, M, de Herreros, AG, Villalobos, C, Berciano, MT, Lafarga, M, & Muñoz, A. 1 mediate vitamin D effects on gene expression, phenotype, and Wnt pathway in colon cancer cells. J Cell Biol. 2008 Nov 17;183(4):697-710.

[151] Orell-kotikangas, H, Schwab, U, Osterlund, P, Saarilahti, K, Mäkitie, O, & Mäkitie, A. A. High prevalence of vitamin D insufficiency in patients with head and neck cancer at diagnosis. Head Neck. (2012). Jan 27. doi:hed.21954. [Epub ahead of print]

[152] Ozdemir, E, Kakehi, Y, Mishina, M, Ogawa, O, Okada, Y, Ozdemir, D, & Yoshida, O. High-resolution HLA-DRB1 and DQB1 genotyping in Japanese patients with testicular germ cell carcinoma. Br J Cancer. (1997). , 76(10), 1348-52.

[153] Ozdilli, K, Oguz, F. S, Anak, S, Kekik, C, Carin, M, & Gedikoglu, G. The frequency of HLA class I and II alleles in Turkish childhood acute leukaemia patients. J Int Med Res. (2010). Sep-Oct;, 38(5), 1835-44.

[154] Panza, N. Del Vecchio L, Maio M, De Felice M, Lombardi G, Minozzi M, Zappacosta S. ong association between an HLA-DR antigen and thyroid carcinoma. Tissue Antigens. (1982). Aug;, 20(2), 155-8.

[155] Pálmer, H. G, González-sancho, J. M, Espada, J, Berciano, M. T, Puig, I, Baulida, J, Quintanilla, M, Cano, A, De Herreros, A. G, Lafarga, M, Muñoz, A, & Vitamin, D. promotes the differentiation of colon carcinoma cells by the induction of E-cadherin and the inhibition of beta-catenin signaling. J Cell Biol. (2001). Jul 23;, 154(2), 369-87.

[156] Palmieri-SevierA; Palmieri, GM; Baumgartner, CJ; Britt, LG. ((1993). Case report: long-term remission of parathyroid cancer: possible relation to vitamin D and calcitriol therapy. *Am J Med Sci.* , 306(5), 309-312.

[157] Pardanani, A, Drake, M. T, Finke, C, Lasho, T. L, Rozell, S. A, Jimma, T, & Tefferi, A. Vitamin D insufficiency in myeloproliferative neoplasms and myelodysplastic syndromes: clinical correlates and prognostic studies. Am J Hematol. (2011). Dec;, 86(12), 1013-6.

[158] Park, M. R, Lee, J. H, Park, M. S, Hwang, J. E, Shim, H. J, Cho, S. H, Chung, I. J, & Bae, W. K. Suppressive effect of 19-nor-1α-25-dihydroxyvitamin D_2 on gastric cancer cells and peritoneal metastasis model. J Korean Med Sci. (2012). Sep;, 27(9), 1037-43.

[159] Parsons, S. L, Watson, S. A, Collins, H. M, Griffin, N. R, Clarke, P. A, & Steele, R. J. Gelatinase (MMP-2 and-9) expression in gastrointestinal malignancy. Br J Cancer. (1998). Dec;, 78(11), 1495-502.

[160] Partyka, R, Gonciarz, M, Jalowiecki, P, Kokocinska, D, & Byrczek, T. VEGF and met-alloproteinase 2 (MMP 2) expression in gastric cancer tissue. Med Sci Monit. (2012). Apr 1;18(4):BR, 130-134.

[161] Pendás-franco, N, García, J. M, Peña, C, Valle, N, Pálmer, H. G, Heinäniemi, M, Carlberg, C, Jiménez, B, Bonilla, F, Muñoz, A, & González-sancho, J. M. DICKKOPF-4 is induced by TCF/beta-catenin and upregulated in human colon cancer, promotes tumour cell invasion and angiogenesis and is repressed by 1alpha,25-dihydroxyvitamin D_3. Oncogene. (2008). a Jul 24;, 27(32), 4467-77.

[162] Pendás-franco, N, Aguilera, O, Pereira, F, González-sancho, J. M, Muñoz, A, & Vitamin, D. and Wnt/beta-catenin pathway in colon cancer: role and regulation of DICKKOPF genes. Anticancer Res. (2008). Sep-Oct;28(5A):, 2613-23.

[163] Peng, X, Vaishnav, A, Murillo, G, Alimirah, F, Torres, K. E, & Mehta, R. G. Protection against cellular stress by 25-hydroxyvitamin D_3 in breast epithelial cells. J Cell Biochem. (2010). Aug 15;, 110(6), 1324-33.

[164] Peng, W. J, Zhang, J. Q, Wang, B. X, Pan, H. F, Lu, M. M, Wang, J, Peng, W. J, Zhang, J. Q, Wang, B. X, Pan, H. F, Lu, M. M, & Wang, J. Prognostic value of matrix metalloproteinase 9 expression in patients with non-small cell lung cancer. Clin Chim Acta. (2012). Jul 11;413(13-14):1121-6.

[165] Peppone, L. J, Rickles, A. S, Janelsins, M. C, Insalaco, M. R, Skinner, K. A, Peppone, L. J, Rickles, A. S, Janelsins, M. C, Insalaco, M. R, & Skinner, K. A. The Association Between Breast Cancer Prognostic Indicators and Serum OH Vitamin D Levels. Ann Surg Oncol. (2012). Mar 24. [Epub ahead of print], 25.

[166] Pérez-castrillón, J. L, Justo, I, Sanz, A, De Luis, D, & Dueñas, A. Effect of angiotensin converting enzyme inhibitors on $1,25(OH)_2$ D levels of hypertensive patients. Relationship with ACE polymorphisms. Horm Metab Res. (2006). , 38, 812-6.

[167] Polakis, P. (2000). Wnt signaling and cancer. Genes Dev , 14, 1837-1851.

[168] Punzi, T, Fabris, A, Morucci, G, Biagioni, P, Gulisano, M, & Ruggiero, M. Pacini S. C-reactive protein levels and vitamin d receptor polymorphisms as markers in predicting cachectic syndrome in cancer patients. Mol Diagn Ther. (2012). Apr 1;, 16(2), 115-24.

[169] Qiu, J, Shao, S, Yang, G, Shen, Z, & Zhang, Y. Association of Toll like receptor 9 expression with lymph node metastasis in human breast cancer. Neoplasma. (2011). , 58(3), 251-5.

[170] Raffegerst, S. H, Hoelzlwimmer, G, Kunder, S, Mysliwietz, J, Quintanilla-martinez, L, & Schendel, D. J. Diverse hematological malignancies including hodgkin-like lymphomas develop in chimeric MHC class II transgenic mice. PLoS One. (2009). Dec 31;4(12):e8539.

[171] RainaV; Cunninham, D; Gilchrist, N; Soukop, M. ((1991). Alphacalcidol is a nontoxic, effective treatment of follicular small-cleaved cell lymphoma. *Br J Cancer.* , 63, 463-465.

[172] Ray, R, Banks, M, Abuzahra, H, Eddy, V. J, Persons, K. S, Lucia, M. S, Lambert, J. R, & Holick, M. F. Effect of dietary vitamin D and calcium on the growth of androgen-insensitive human prostate tumor in a murine model. Anticancer Res. (2012). Mar;, 32(3), 727-31.

[173] Ravid, A, Rocker, D, Machlenkin, A, Rotem, C, Hochman, A, Kessler-icekson, G, Liberman, U. A, & Koren, R. Dihydroxyvitamin D_3 enhances the susceptibility of breast cancer cells to doxorubicin-induced oxidative damage. Cancer Res. (1999). Feb 15;, 59(4), 862-7.

[174] Ren, C, Qiu, M. Z, Wang, D. S, Luo, H. Y, Zhang, D. S, Wang, Z. Q, Wang, F. H, Li, Y. H, Zhou, Z. W, & Xu, R. H. Prognostic effects of hydroxyvitamin D levels in gastric cancer. J Transl Med. (2012). Jan 27;10:16., 25.

[175] Repin IuMBCG vaccine immunotherapy after radical operations for lung cancer]. Vestn Khir Im I I Grek. (1992). Jul-Aug;149(7-8):11-6. [Article in Russian]

[176] Rhodes, S. G, Terry, L. A, Hope, J, Hewinson, R. G, & Vordermeier, H. M. dihydroxy-vitamin D_3 and development of tuberculosis in cattle. Clin Diagn Lab Immunol. (2003). Nov;, 10(6), 1129-35.

[177] Ristimäki, A, Honkanen, N, Jänkälä, H, Sipponen, P, & Härkönen, M. Expression of cyclooxygenase-2 in human gastric carcinoma. Cancer Res. (1997). Apr 1;, 57(7), 1276-80.

[178] Rivas-santiago, B, Hernandez-pando, R, Carranza, C, Juarez, E, Contreras, J. L, et al. Expression of cathelicidin LL-37 during Mycobacterium tuberculosis infection in human alveolar macrophages, monocytes, neutrophils, and epithelial cells. Infect Immunity. (2008). , 76, 935-41.

[179] Robsahm, T. E, Tretli, S, Dahlback, A, Moan, J, & Vitamin, D. from sunlight may improve the prognosis of breast-, colon- and prostate cancer (Norway). Cancer Causes Control. (2004). Mar;, 15(2), 149-58.

[180] Rockett, K, Brookes, R, Udalova, I, Vidal, V, Hill, A, & Kwiatkowski, D. (1998). hydroxyvitamin D_3 induces nitric oxide synthase and suppresses growth of *Mycobacterium tuberculosis* in a human macrophage-like cell line. Infect Immun. 66, 5314-5321., 1, 25.

[181] Rogalska, A, Gajek, A, Szwed, M, Józwiak, Z, & Marczak, A. The role of reactive oxygen species in WP 631-induced death of human ovarian cancer cells: a comparison with the effect of doxorubicin. Toxicol In Vitro. (2011). , 25, 1712-20.

[182] Rollison, D. E, Cole, A. L, Tung, K. H, Slattery, M. L, Baumgartner, K. B, Byers, T, Wolff, R. K, & Giuliano, A. R. Vitamin D intake, vitamin D receptor polymorphisms,

and breast cancer risk among women living in the southwestern U.S. Breast Cancer Res Treat. (2012). Apr;, 132(2), 683-91.

[183] Roth, C. L, Elfers, C. T, Figlewicz, D. P, Melhorn, S. J, Morton, G. J, et al. Vitamin D deficiency in obese rats exacerbates NAFLD and increases hepatic resistin and toll-like receptor activation. Hepatol. (2011). Oct 12. [Epub ahead of print].

[184] Ruza, E, Sotillo, E, Sierrasesúmaga, L, Azcona, C, & Patiño-garcía, A. Analysis of polymorphisms of the vitamin D receptor, estrogen receptor, and collagen Ialpha1 genes and their relationship with height in children with bone cancer. J Pediatr Hematol Oncol. (2003). Oct;, 25(10), 780-6.

[185] Sadeghi, K, Wessner, B, Laggner, U, Ploder, M, Tamandl, D, et al. Vitamin D_3 down-regulates monocyte TLR expression and triggers hyporesponsiveness to pathogen-associated molecular patterns. Eur J Immunol. (2006). , 36, 361-70.

[186] Sandholm, J, Kauppila, J. H, Pressey, C, Tuomela, J, Jukkola-vuorinen, A, Vaarala, M, Johnson, M. R, Harris, K. W, & Selander, K. S. Estrogen receptor-α and sex steroid hormones regulate Toll-like receptor-9 expression and invasive function in human breast cancer cells. Breast Cancer Res Treat. (2012). Apr;, 132(2), 411-9.

[187] Salehin, D, Haugk, C, Thill, M, Cordes, T, William, M, Hemmerlein, B, & Friedrich, M. Serum 25-hydroxyvitamin D levels in patients with vulvar cancer. Anticancer Res. (2012). Jan;, 32(1), 265-70.

[188] Saliba, W, Barnett, O, Rennert, H. S, Lavi, I, & Rennert, G. The relationship between serum 25(OH)D and parathyroid hormone levels. Am J Med. (2011). , 124, 1165-70.

[189] Sardar, S, Chakraborty, A, & Chatterjee, M. Comparative effectiveness of vitamin D_3 and dietary vitamin E on peroxidation of lipids and enzymes of the hepatic antioxidant system in Sprague-Dawley rats. Int J Vitam Nutr Res. (1996). , 66, 39-45.

[190] Schauber, J, Iffland, K, Frisch, S, Kudlich, T, Schmausser, B, Eck, M, Menzel, T, Gostner, A, Lührs, H, & Scheppach, W. Histone-deacetylase inhibitors induce the cathelicidin LL-37 in gastrointestinal cells. Mol Immunol. (2004). Jul;, 41(9), 847-54.

[191] Scherberich, J, Kellermeyer, M, Ried, C, & Hartinger, A. alpha-calcidol modulates major human monocyte antigens and toll-like receptors TRL2 and TRL4 in vitro. Eur J Med Res. (2005). , 10, 179-82.

[192] Schöttker, B, Ball, D, Gellert, C, & Brenner, H. Serum hydroxyvitamin D levels and overall mortality. A systematic review and meta-analysis of prospective cohort studies. Ageing Res Rev. (2012). Feb 17. [Epub ahead of print], 25.

[193] Schwartz, G. G, Wang, M. H, Zang, M, Singh, R. K, & Siegal, G. P. alpha,25-Dihydroxyvitamin D (calcitriol) inhibits the invasiveness of human prostate cancer cells. Cancer Epidemiol Biomarkers Prev. (1997). Sep;, 6(9), 727-32.

[194] Shanafelt, T. D, Drake, M. T, Maurer, M. J, Allmer, C, Rabe, K. G, Slager, S. L, Weiner, G. J, Call, T. G, Link, B. K, Zent, C. S, Kay, N. E, Hanson, C. A, Witzig, T. E, & Cer-

han, J. R. Vitamin D insufficiency and prognosis in chronic lymphocytic leukemia. Blood. (2011). Feb 3;, 117(5), 1492-8.

[195] Shui, I. M, Mucci, L. A, Kraft, P, Tamimi, R. M, Lindstrom, S, Penney, K. L, Nimptsch, K, Hollis, B. W, Dupre, N, Platz, E. A, Stampfer, M. J, & Giovannucci, E. Vitamin D-Related Genetic Variation, Plasma Vitamin D, and Risk of Lethal Prostate Cancer: A Prospective Nested Case-Control Study. J Natl Cancer Inst. (2012). May 2;, 104(9), 690-699.

[196] Sikora, J, Frydrychowicz, M, Kaczmarek, M, Brzezicha, B, Mozer-lisewska, I, Szcze-panski, M, & Zeromski, J. TLR receptors in laryngeal carcinoma- immunophenotypic, molecular and functional studies. Folia Histochem Cytobiol. (2010). Dec;, 48(4), 624-31.

[197] Skinner, H. G, & Schwartz, G. G. (2009). The relation of serum parathyroid hormone and serum calcium to serum levels of Prostatic-specific antigen: a population-based study. *Cancer Epidemiol Biomarkers Prev.* , 18(11), 2869-2873.

[198] Slapek, C. A, Desforges, J. F, Fogaren, T, et al. (1992). Treatment of acute myeloid leu-kemia in the elderly with low-dose cytarabine, hydroxyurea, and calcitriol. Am J Hematol. , 41, 178-183.

[199] Slattery, M. L, Wolff, R. K, Curtin, K, Fitzpatrick, F, Herrick, J, Potter, J. D, Caan, B. J, & Samowitz, W. S. Colon tumor mutations and epigenetic changes associated with genetic polymorphism: insight into disease pathways. Mutat Res. (2009). Jan 15;660(1-2):12-21.

[200] Slattery, M. L, Herrick, J. S, Bondurant, K. L, & Wolff, R. K. Toll-like receptor genes and their association with colon and rectal cancer development and prognosis. Int J Cancer. (2012). Jun 15;, 130(12), 2974-80.

[201] Somjen, D, Katzburg, S, Grafi-cohen, M, Knoll, E, Sharon, O, & Posner, G. H. Vitamin D metabolites and analogs induce lipoxygenase mRNA expression and as well as re-active oxygen species (ROS) production in human bone cell line. J Steroid Biochem Mol Biol. (2011). , 123, 85-9.

[202] Song, E. J, Kang, M. J, Kim, Y. S, Kim, S. M, Lee, S. E, Kim, C. H, Kim, D. J, & Park, J. H. Flagellin promotes the proliferation of gastric cancer cells via the Toll-like recep-tor 5. Int J Mol Med. (2011). Jul;, 28(1), 115-9.

[203] Srivastava, P, Lone, T. A, Kapoor, R, & Mittal, R. D. Association of Promoter Poly-morphisms in MMP 2 and TIMP2 with Prostate Cancer Susceptibility in North India. Arch Med Res. (2012). Feb 25. [Epub ahead of print]

[204] Stenson, W. F, Teitelbaum, S. L, & Bar-shavit, Z. Arachidonic acid metabolism by a vitamin D_3-differentiated human leukemic cell line. J Bone Miner Res. (1988). Oct;, 3(5), 561-71.

[205] Stio, M, Martinesi, M, Simoni, A, Zuegel, U, Steinmeyer, A, Santi, R, Treves, C, & Nesi, G. The novel vitamin D analog ZK191784 inhibits prostate cancer cell invasion. Anticancer Res. (2011). Dec;, 31(12), 4091-8.

[206] Sundar, I, Hwang, J, Wu, S, Sun, J, & Rahman, I. Deletion of vitamin D receptor leads to premature emphysema/COPD by increased matrix metalloproteinase and lymphoid aggregates formation. Biochem Biophys Res Commun. (2011). , 406, 127-33.

[207] Swami, S, Krishnan, A. V, Wang, J. Y, Jensen, K, Horst, R, Albertelli, M. A, & Feldman, D. Dietary Vitamin D_3 and Dihydroxyvitamin D_3 (Calcitriol) Exhibit Equivalent Anticancer Activity in Mouse Xenograft Models of Breast and Prostate Cancer. Endocrinology. (2012). Mar 27. [Epub ahead of print], 1, 25.

[208] Svedlund, J, Aurén, M, Sundström, M, Dralle, H, Akerström, G, Björklund, P, & Westin, G. Aberrant WNT/β-catenin signaling in parathyroid carcinoma. Mol Cancer. (2010). Nov 15;9:294.

[209] Takala, H, Kauppila, J. H, Soini, Y, Selander, K. S, Vuopala, K. S, Lehenkari, P. P, Saarnio, J, & Karttunen, T. J. Toll-like receptor 9 is a novel biomarker for esophageal squamous cell dysplasia and squamous cell carcinoma progression. J Innate Immun. (2011). , 3(6), 631-8.

[210] Tamaki, K, Saitoh, A, & Kubota, Y. hydroxyvitamin D_3 decreases the interferon-gamma (IFN-gamma) induced HLA-DR expression but not intercellular adhesion molecule 1 (ICAM-1) on human keratinocytes. Reg Immunol. (1990). , 3, 223-7.

[211] Tangrea, J, Helzlsouer, K, Pietinen, P, Taylor, P, Hollis, B, Virtamo, J, & Albanes, D. Serum levels of vitamin D metabolites and the subsequent risk of colon and rectal cancer in Finnish men. Cancer Causes Control. (1997). Jul;, 8(4), 615-25.

[212] Tee, Y. T, Liu, Y. F, Chang, J. T, Yang, S. F, Chen, S. C, Han, C. P, Wang, P. H, & Liao, C. L. Single-Nucleotide Polymorphisms and Haplotypes of Membrane Type 1 Matrix Metalloproteinase in Susceptibility and Clinical Significance of Squamous Cell Neoplasia of Uterine Cervix in Taiwan Women. Reprod Sci. (2012). Apr 23. [Epub ahead of print]

[213] Thill, M, Hoellen, F, Becker, S, Dittmer, C, Fischer, D, et al. Expression of prostaglandin- and vitamin D-metabolising enzymes in benign and malignant breast cells. Anticancer Res. (2012). , 32, 367-72.

[214] Timms, P. M, Mannan, N, Hitman, G. A, Noonan, K, Mills, P. G, et al. Circulating MMP9, vitamin D and variation in the TIMP-1 response with VDR genotype: mechanisms for inflammatory damage in chronic disorders? Q J Med. (2002). , 95, 787-96.

[215] Ting HJ; Hsu, J; Bao,BY; Lee, YF. ((2007). Docetaxel-induced growth inhibition an apoptosis in androgen indepenpent prostate cancer cells are enhanced by 1alpha,25-dihydroxyvitamin D_3. Cancer Lett. , 247, 122-129.

[216] Tokar, E. J, & Webber, M. M. Cholecalciferol (vitamin D_3) inhibits growth and invasion by up-regulating nuclear receptors and 25-hydroxylase (CYP27A1) in human prostate cancer cells. Clin Exp Metastasis. (2005)., 22(3), 275-84.

[217] Tokuda, N, Mizuki, N, Kasahara, M, & Levy, R. B. hydroxyvitamin D_3 down-regulation of HLA-DR on human peripheral blood monocytes. Immunol. (1992)., 75, 349-54.

[218] Tokuda, N, & Levy, R. hydroxyvitamin D_3 stimulates phagocytosis but suppresses HLA-DR and CD13 antigen expression in human mononuclear phagocytes. Proc Soc Exp Biol Med. (1996)., 211, 244-50.

[219] Tone, T, Eto, H, Katsuoka, K, Nishioka, K, & Nishiyama, S. Suppression of gamma-interferon induced HLA-DR antigen expression on normal and transformed keratinocytes by 1,25 $(OH)_2$ vitamin D_3. Nippon Hifuka Gakkai Zasshi. (1991). Article in Japanese]., 101, 519-25.

[220] Tone, T, Eto, H, Katou, T, Otani, F, & Nishiyama, S. Alpha,25-dihydroxyvitamin D modulation of HLA-DR mRNA induced by gamma-interferon in cultured epithelial tumor cell lines. J Dermatol. (1993)., 20, 581-4.

[221] Turna, A, Pekçolaklar, A, Metin, M, Yaylim, I, & Gurses, A. The effect of season of operation on the survival of patients with resected non-small cell lung cancer. Interact Cardiovasc Thorac Surg. (2012). Feb;, 14(2), 151-5.

[222] Ueno, K, Hirata, H, Majid, S, Chen, Y, Zaman, M. S, Tabatabai, Z. L, Hinoda, Y, & Dahiya, R. Wnt antagonist DICKKOPF-3 (Dkk-3) induces apoptosis in human renal cell carcinoma. Mol Carcinog. (2011). Jun;, 50(6), 449-57.

[223] Wang, X, Gocek, E, Liu, C. G, & Studzinski, G. P. MicroRNAs181 regulate the expression of 27Kip1in human myeloid leukemia cells induced to differentiate by 1,25-dihydroxyvitamin D_3. Cell Cycle. (2009). a Mar 1;8(5):736-41.

[224] Wang, S, Wang, F, Shi, X, Dai, J, Peng, Y, Guo, X, et al. Association between manganese superoxide dismutase (MnSOD) Val-9Ala polymorphism and cancer risk- A meta-analysis. Eur J Cancer. (2009b)., 45, 2874-81.

[225] Wang, H. C, & Choudhary, S. Reactive oxygen species-mediated therapeutic control of bladder cancer. Nat Rev Urol. (2011)., 8, 608-16.

[226] Wang, W. L, Chatterjee, N, Chittur, S. V, Welsh, J, & Tenniswood, M. P. Effects of 1α, 25 dihydroxyvitamin D_3 and testosterone on miRNA and mRNA expression in LNCaP cells. Mol Cancer. (2011). a May 18;10:58.

[227] Wang, S, Wang, X, Wu, J, Lin, Y, Chen, H, Zheng, X, Zhou, C, & Xie, L. Association of vitamin D receptor gene polymorphism and calcium urolithiasis in the Chinese Han population. Urol Res. (2011). b Nov 25. [Epub ahead of print]

[228] Wang, Y. Y, Wang, L. Z, & Sun, L. R. Antitumor effect of BCG on growth of trans-planted human myeloid leukemia HL-60 cells in nude mice]. Zhongguo Shi Yan Xue Ye Xue Za Zhi. (2011). c Jun;, 19(3), 725-9.

[229] Wang, J. Y, Swami, S, Krishnan, A. V, & Feldman, D. Combination of calcitriol and dietary soy exhibits enhanced anticancer activity and increased hypercalcemic toxici-ty in a mouse xenograft model of prostate cancer. Prostate. (2012). a Mar 27. doi:pros. 22516. [Epub ahead of print]

[230] Wang, H, Tan, G, Dong, L, Cheng, L, Li, K, Wang, Z, & Luo, H. Circulating MiR-125b as a Marker Predicting Chemoresistance in Breast Cancer. PLoS One. (2012b). e34210.

[231] Weitsman, G. E, Ravid, A, Liberman, U. A, & Koren, R. The role of MAP kinase in the synergistic cytotoxic action of calcitriol and TNF-alpha in human breast cancer cells. J Steroid Biochem Mol Biol. (2004). May;89-90(1-5):361-4., 38.

[232] Welsh, J, Zinser, L. N, Mianecki-morton, L, Martin, J, Waltz, S. E, James, H, & Zinser, G. M. Age-related changes in the epithelial and stromal compartments of the mam-mary gland in normocalcemic mice lacking the vitamin D_3 receptor. PLoS One. (2011). Jan 26;6(1):e16479

[233] White, B. D, Chien, A. J, & Dawson, D. W. Dysregulation of Wnt/β-catenin signaling in gastrointestinal cancers. Gastroenterology. (2012). Feb;, 142(2), 219-32.

[234] Wieczorek, E, Reszka, E, Gromadzinska, J, & Wasowicz, W. Genetic polymorphism of matrix metalloproteinases in breast cancer. Neoplasma. (2012). , 59(3), 237-47.

[235] Wilop, S, Von Hobe, S, Crysandt, M, Esser, A, Osieka, R, & Jost, E. Impact of angio-tensin I converting enzyme inhibitors and angiotensin II type 1 receptor blockers on survival in patients with advanced non-small-cell lung cancer undergoing first-line platinum-based chemotherapy. J Cancer Res Clin Oncol. (2009). Oct;, 135(10), 1429-35.

[236] Wolpin, B. M, Ng, K, Bao, Y, Kraft, P, Stampfer, M. J, Michaud, D. S, Ma, J, Buring, J. E, Sesso, H. D, Lee, I. M, Rifai, N, Cochrane, B. B, Wactawski-wende, J, Chlebowski, R. T, Willett, W. C, Manson, J. E, Giovannucci, E. L, & Fuchs, C. S. Plasma 25-hydrox-yvitamin D and risk of pancreatic cancer. Cancer Epidemiol Biomarkers Prev. (2012). Jan;, 21(1), 82-91.

[237] Woo, T. C, Choo, R, Jamieson, M, Chander, S, & Vieth, R. Pilot study: potential role of vitamin D (Cholecalciferol) in patients with PSA relapse after definitive therapy. Nutr Cancer. (2005). , 51(1), 32-6.

[238] Woodson, K, Tangrea, J. A, Lehman, T. A, Modali, R, Taylor, K. M, Snyder, K, et al. Manganese superoxide dismutase (MnSOD) polymorphism, alpha-tocopherol sup-plementation and prostate cancer risk in the alpha-tocopherol, beta-carotene cancer prevention study (Finland). Cancer Causes Control. (2003). , 14, 513-8.

[239] Wu, W. K, Sung, J. J, To, K. F, Yu, L, Li, H. T, Li, Z. J, Chu, K. M, Yu, J, & Cho, C. H. The host defense peptide LL-37 activates the tumor-suppressing bone morphogenetic

protein signaling via inhibition of proteasome in gastric cancer cells. J Cell Physiol. (2010). Apr;, 223(1), 178-86.

[240] Wu, K, Feskanich, D, Fuchs, C. S, Chan, A. T, Willett, W. C, Hollis, B. W, Pollak, M. N, & Giovannucci, E. Interactions between plasma levels of hydroxyvitamin D, insu-lin-like growth factor (IGF)-1 and C-peptide with risk of colorectal cancer. PLoS One. (2011a). e28520., 25.

[241] Wu, Y, Miyamoto, T, Li, K, Nakagomi, H, Sawada, N, Kira, S, Kobayashi, H, Zakohji, H, Tsuchida, T, Fukazawa, M, Araki, I, & Takeda, M. Decreased expression of the ep-ithelial Ca2+ channel TRPV5 and TRPV6 in human renal cell carcinoma associated with vitamin D receptor. J Urol. (2011b). Dec;, 186(6), 2419-25.

[242] Yamaji, T, Iwasaki, M, Sasazuki, S, Sakamoto, H, Yoshida, T, & Tsugane, S. Associa-tion between plasma 25-hydroxyvitamin D and colorectal adenoma according to di-etary calcium intake and vitamin D receptor polymorphism. Am J Epidemiol. (2012). Feb 1;, 175(3), 236-44.

[243] Yan, W, Zhang, W, Sun, L, Liu, Y, You, G, Wang, Y, Kang, C, You, Y, & Jiang, T. Identification of MMP-9 specific microRNA expression profile as potential targets of anti-invasion therapy in glioblastoma multiforme. Brain Res. (2011). Sep 9;, 1411, 108-15.

[244] Yang, Y. H, Zheng, G. G, Li, G, Zhang, B, Song, Y. H, & Wu, K. F. Expression of LL-37/hCAP-18 gene in human leukemia cells. Leuk Res. (2003). Oct;, 27(10), 947-50.

[245] Yim, S, Dhawan, P, Ragunath, C, Christakos, S, & Diamond, G. Induction of cathelici-din in normal and CF bronchial epithelial cells by 1,25-dihydroxyvitamin D_3. J Cys Fibros. (2007). , 6, 403-410.

[246] Yin, L, Grandi, N, Raum, E, Haug, U, Arndt, V, & Brenner, H. Meta-analysis: longitu-dinal studies of serum vitamin D and colorectal cancer risk. Aliment Pharmacol Ther. (2009). Jul 1;, 30(2), 113-25.

[247] Yoshioka, S, King, M. L, Ran, S, & Okuda, H. MacLean JA 2nd, McAsey ME, Sugino N, Brard L, Watabe K, Hayashi K. WNT7A regulates tumor growth and progression in ovarian cancer through the WNT/β-catenin pathway. Mol Cancer Res. (2012). Mar;, 10(3), 469-82.

[248] Yu, H, Xu, S. S, Cheng, Q. Q, He, L. M, & Li, Z. Expression and clinical significance of Toll-like receptors in human renal carcinoma cell 786-0 and normal renal cell HK-2]. Zhonghua Yi Xue Za Zhi. (2011). Jan 11;Article in Chinese], 91(2), 129-31.

[249] Yuan, W, Pan, W, Kong, J, Zheng, W, Szeto, F, et al. dihydroxyvitamin D_3 suppresses renin gene transcription by blocking the activity of the cyclic AMP response element in the renin gene promoter. J Biol Chem. (2007). , 282, 29821-30.

[250] Yuk, J. M, Shin, D. M, Song, K. S, Lim, K, Kim, K. H, Lee, S. H, Kim, J. M, Lee, J. S, Paik, T. H, Kim, J. S, & Jo, E. K. Bacillus calmette-guerin cell wall cytoskeleton enhan-

ces colon cancer radiosensitivity through autophagy. Autophagy. (2010). Jan;, 6(1), 46-60.

[251]   Xia, Z, Liu, W, Li, S, Jia, G, Zhang, Y, Li, C, Ma, Z, Tian, J, & Gong, J. Expression of matrix metalloproteinase-9, type IV collagen and vascular endothelial growth factor in adamantinous craniopharyngioma. Neurochem Res. (2011). Dec;, 36(12), 2346-51.

[252]   Xiang, W, Kong, J, Chen, S, Cao, L, Qiao, G, et al. Cardiac hypertrophy in vitamin D receptor knockout mice: role of the systemic and cardiac renin-angiotensin systems. Am J Phys Endocrinol Met. (2005). E, 125-32.

[253]   Xu, H, Soruri, A, Gieseler, R. K, & Peters, J. H. dihydroxyvitamin D$_3$ exerts opposing effects to IL-4 on MHC class-II antigen expression, accessory activity, and phagocytosis of human monocytes. Scand J Immunol. (1993). , 38, 535-60.

[254]   Zhao, X, Wang, X, Wu, W, Gao, Z, Wu, J, Garfield, D. H, Wang, H, Wang, J, Qian, J, Li, H, Jin, L, Li, Q, Han, B, Lu, D, & Bai, C. Matrix metalloproteinase-2 polymorphisms and clinical outcome of Chinese patients with nonsmall cell lung cancer treated with first-line, platinum-based chemotherapy. Cancer. (2011). Nov 9. doi:cncr. 26669. [Epub ahead of print]

[255]   Zhang, L. Y, & Ren, K. W. Meta-analysis of MMP2-1306T allele as a protective factor in digestive cancer. Arch Med Res. (2011). Apr;, 42(3), 239-43.

[256]   Zhang, W, Yang, H. C, Wang, Q, Yang, Z. J, Chen, H, Wang, S. M, Pan, Z. M, Tang, B. J, Li, Q. Q, & Li, L. Clinical value of combined detection of serum matrix metalloproteinase-9, heparanase, and cathepsin for determining ovarian cancer invasion and metastasis. Anticancer Res. (2011). a Oct;, 31(10), 3423-8.

[257]   Zhang, J, Harrison, J. S, & Studzinski, G. P. Isoforms of gamma and delta contribute to differentiation of human AML cells induced by 1,25-dihydroxyvitamin D₃. Exp Cell Res. (2011). b Jan 1;317(1):117-30., 38MAPK.

[258]   Zhang, Q, Ma, Y, Cheng, Y. F, Li, W. J, Zhang, Z, & Chen, S. Y. Involvement of reactive oxygen species in 2-methoxyestradiol-induced apoptosis in human neuroblastoma cells. Cancer Lett. (2011c). , 313, 201-10.

[259]   Zhang, L. F, Mi, Y. Y, Cao, Q, Wang, W, Qin, C, Wei, J. F, Zhou, Y. J, Li, Y. F, Tang, M, Liu, W. M, Zhang, W, & Zou, J. G. Update analysis of studies on the MMP-9-1562 C>T polymorphism and cancer risk. Mol Biol Rep. (2012). a Apr;, 39(4), 3435-41.

[260]   Zhang, J, Zhang, H, Zhang, X, & Yu, Z. Synergistic effect of retinoic acid and vitamin D analog EBinduced apoptosis of hepatocellular cancer cells. Cytotechnology. (2012). b Oct 16. [Epub ahead of print], 1089.

[261]   Zhou, W, Heist, R. S, Liu, G, Asomaning, K, Neuberg, D. S, Hollis, B. W, Wain, J. C, Lynch, T. J, Giovannucci, E, Su, L, & Christiani, D. C. Circulating 25-hydroxyvitamin D levels predict survival in early-stage non-small-cell lung cancer patients. J Clin Oncol. (2007). Feb 10;, 25(5), 479-85.

[262] Zhou, L, Zhang, R, Yao, W, Wang, J, Qian, A, Qiao, M, Zhang, Y, & Yuan, Y. Decreased expression of angiotensin-converting enzyme 2 in pancreatic ductal adenocarcinoma is associated with tumor progression. Tohoku J Exp Med. (2009). Feb;,
217(2), 123-31.

[263] Zhou, L, Zhang, R, Zhang, L, Yao, W, Li, J, & Yuan, Y. Angiotensin-converting enzyme 2 acts as a potential molecular target for pancreatic cancer therapy. Cancer Lett.
(2011). Aug 1;, 307(1), 18-25.

[264] Zhuo de X, Niu XH, Chen YC, Xin DQ, Guo YL, Mao ZB. Vitamin D_3 up-regulated
protein 1(VDUP1) is regulated by FOXO3A and miR-17-5p at the transcriptional and
post-transcriptional levels, respectively, in senescent fibroblasts. J Biol Chem. (2010).
Oct 8;, 285(41), 31491-501.

[265] Zimmerman, E. I, Dollins, C. M, Crawford, M, Grant, S, Nana-sinkam, S. P, Richards,
K. L, Hammond, S. M, & Graves, L. M. Lyn kinase-dependent regulation of miR181
and myeloid cell leukemia-1 expression: implications for drug resistance in myelogenous leukemia. Mol Pharmacol. (2010). Nov;, 78(5), 811-7.

[266] Van Der Knaap, R, Siemes, C, Coebergh, J. W, Van Duijn, C. M, Hofman, A, & Stricker, B. H. Renin-angiotensin system inhibitors, angiotensin I-converting enzyme gene
insertion/deletion polymorphism, and cancer: the Rotterdam Study. Cancer. (2008).
Feb 15;, 112(4), 748-57.

[267] Varsavsky, M, Reyes-garcía, R, Cortés-berdonces, M, García-martin, A, Rozas-more-
no, P, & Muñoz-torres, M. Serum 25 OH vitamin D concentrations and calcium intake are low in patients with prostate cancer. Endocrinol Nutr. (2011). Nov;, 58(9),
487-91.

[268] Vink-van Wijngaarden T, Pols HA, Buurman CJ, van den Bemd GJ, Dorssers LC, Bir-
kenhäger JC, van Leeuwen JP. Inhibition of breast cancer cell growth by combined
treatment with vitamin D_3 analogues and tamoxifen. Cancer Res. (1994). Nov 1;,
54(21), 5711-7.

[269] Villumsen, M, Sørup, S, Jess, T, Ravn, H, Relander, T, Baker, J. L, Benn, C. S, Søre-
nsen, T. I, Aaby, P, & Roth, A. Risk of lymphoma and leukaemia after bacille Calmette-Guérin and smallpox vaccination: a Danish case-cohort study. Vaccine. (2009).
Nov 16;, 27(49), 6950-8.

[270] Volante, M, Rapa, I, Gandhi, M, Bussolati, G, Giachino, D, Papotti, M, & Nikiforov,
Y. E. RAS mutations are the predominant molecular alteration in poorly differentiat-
ed thyroid carcinomas and bear prognostic impact. J Clin Endocrinol Metab. (2009).
Dec;, 94(12), 4735-41.

Chapter 2

Nutrigenomics and Cancer Prevention

Júlio César Nepomuceno

Additional information is available at the end of the chapter

1. Introduction

Cancer is fundamentally a genetic disease. At the beginning of the process is an alteration in the DNA of a single cell. This change in DNA can be caused by several factors, chemical, physical or biological phenomena. The stage of promotion is the second stage of carcinogenesis. The genetically altered cells, ie, "initiated," suffer the effects of carcinogens classified as oncopromotores. The initiated cell is transformed into a malignant cell, a slow and gradual process. For this transformation to occur, you need a long and continuous contact with the carcinogen promoter. The stage of progression is the third and final stage and is characterized by uncontrolled proliferation of cells and irreversibly changed. At this stage cancer is already installed, progressing to the emergence of the first clinical manifestations of the disease [1]. In this sense, the diet plays a key role in various stages of cancer development. The process of carcinogenesis may be affected by nutritional factors through mechanisms that promote or inhibit its development. Some foods can contain not only carcinogens, but also other substances that act to reduce the damage to the cell's genetic material caused by environmental mutagens. The observation of cancer in an individual does not identify the causative agent(s). However, epidemiological data on populations do indicate that a large fraction of human cancers are associated with lifestyle/ diet. Such studies may also help identify the etiologic agents but unless there are good dose-response data for humans and/or animal models, the probability of identifying the agent is not high. Cancers may result from endogenous reactions, such as oxidations or from exogenous agents, such as tobacco smoke (lung cancer), sunlight exposure (skin cancer), aflatoxin (liver cancer), and relatively high doses of ionizing radiations (many types of cancers) [2].

The importance of nutrition in health is not a new idea. More than two thousand years ago, Hippocrates, the father of Western medicine, wrote: "Let food be thy medicine and medicine be thy food." What has changed since the time of Hippocrates is our understanding of the details of how nutrition affects our health. Researchers are getting more knowledge as to what foods or bioactive food compounds and how they can interact with our bodies promoting health. The Human Genome Project was one of the key factors that enable the study of gene-food interactions and promotion of health. Discoveries in genetics make it possible to understand the effects of nutrients in processes at the molecular level in the body and also the variable effects of dietary components on each individual. Research has shown that the nutrients affect gene expression and formation of several proteins that are important in the formation and maintenance of tissues. So, faced with this interaction genomics and nutrition, emerges Nutrigenomics aiming to understand the functions of all genes and their interactions with food, in order to promote health and reduce the risk of developing diseases [3].

Nutrigenomics studies the modulating effect of the chemical compounds in foods and on the stability of DNA synthesis and gene expression. The nutrients are able to affect the genome and its expression through the synthesis of nucleotides, prevention and repair of DNA damage, or through epigenetic mechanisms including methylation of histones, proteins responsible for chromatin structure that play an important role in regulating gene expression. Those methodological approaches are based on nutrition, molecular biology, and genomics. Integration of these disciplines is leading to identification and understanding of individual and population differences and similarities in gene expression, or phenotype, in response to diet. We can consider nutrigenomics as a multidisciplinary science that applies the genomic techniques besides the biochemical and epidemiological aspects, with the aim to understand the etiologic aspects of chronic diseases such as cardiovascular diseases, diabetes, obesity and cancer [4].

An understanding of scientific information about the composition and functions of genomes, has created unprecedented opportunities for increasing our understanding of how nutrients modulate gene and protein expression and ultimately influence cellular and organismal metabolism. On that basis, the purpose of this chapter is to make a broad review study to evaluate the modulation between compounds found in nutrients and their interactions with on the genomic stability and control of gene expression.

2. Nutrition and epigenetics

All the cells in the body have identical genomes. However, each cell has one of many "epigenomes", unique sets of epigenetic instructions for establishing and maintaining lineage-specific expression profiles. The genome is programmed to express appropriate sets of genes, in particular tissues, at specific time points during the individual's life. Epigenetic events create a memory of cell identity, maintaining genomic functions such as the maintenance of cell identity after differentiation, the propagation of essential features of chromosomal architecture and dosage compensation [5]. Epigenetic mechanisms are capable of modulating gene expression through changes in the chromosomes structure. Chromosomes are formed from the condensation of the chromatin, which is formed by a complex of DNA, and unique proteins called histone. Examples of epigenetic mechanisms may be mentioned as DNA methylation and histone acetylation [3].

DNA methylation occurs at the cytosine bases of eukaryotic DNA, which are converted to 5-methylcytosine. The altered cytosine residues are usually immediately adjacent to a guanine nucleotide, resulting in two methylated cytosine residues sitting diagonally to each other on opposing DNA strands [6]. DNA methylation, which modifies a cytosine base at the CpG dinucleotide residues with methyl groups, is catalyzed by DNA methyltransferases (Dnmt) and regulates gene expression patterns by altering chromatin structures. Currently, 5 different Dnmt are known: Dnmt1, Dnmt2, Dnmt 3a, Dnmt3b and DnmtL [7]. The Polycomb group protein EZH2 directly controls DNA methylation (Figure 1). EZH2 serves as a recruitment platform for DNA methyltransferases, thus highlighting a previously unrecognized direct connection between two key epigenetic repression systems [8].

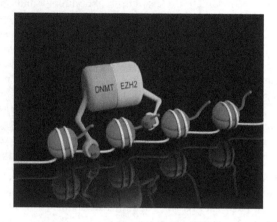

Figure 1. Polycomb Group (PcG) protein EZH2 serves as a recruitment platform for DNA methyltransferases (http://www.ulb.ac.be/medecine/fukslab/research.htm).

DNA methylation is essential for cell differentiation and embryonic development. Moreover, in some cases, methylation has observed to play a role in mediating gene expression. In mammals, methylation is found sparsely but globally, distributed in definite CpG sequences throughout the entire genome, with the exception of CpG islands, or certain stretches (approximately 1 kilobase in length) where high CpG contents are found. The methylation of these sequences can lead to inappropriate gene silencing, such as the silencing of tumor suppressor genes in cancer cells [6]. A large amount of research on DNA methylation and disease has focused on cancer and tumor suppressor genes. Tumor suppressor genes are often silenced in cancer cells due to hypermethylation. In contrast, the genomes of cancer cells have been shown to be hypomethylated overall when compared to normal cells, with the exception of hyper-methylation events at genes involved in cell cycle regulation, tumor cell invasion, DNA repair, and other events in which silencing propagates metastasis. In fact, in certain cancers, such as that of the colon, hypermethylation is detectable early and might serve as a biomarker for the disease [6] (See Figure 2).

In the nutritional field, epigenetics is exceptionally important, because nutrients and bioactive food components can modify epigenetic phenomena and alter the expression of genes at the transcriptional level. Nutrients can reverse or change epigenetic phenomena such as DNA

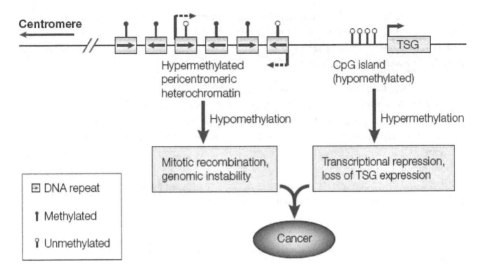

Figure 2. DNA methylation and cancer. This diagram shows a representative region of genomic DNA in a normal cell. The region contains repeat-rich, hypermethylated pericentromeric heterochromatin and an actively transcribed tumor suppressor gene (TSG) associated with a hypomethylated CpG island (indicated in red). In tumor cells, repeat-rich heterochromatin becomes hypomethylated, and this contributes to genomic instability (a hallmark of tumor cells) through increased mitotic recombination events. *De novo* methylation of CpG islands also occurs in cancer cells, and it can result in the transcriptional silencing of growth-regulatory genes. These changes in methylation are early events in tumorigenesis. (See reference [9].)

methylation and histone modifications, thereby modifying the expression of critical genes associated with physiologic and pathologic processes, including embryonic development, aging, and carcinogenesis [7].

The most interesting study linking diet and epigenetics was made by Kucharski et al. [10], about nutritional control of reproductive status in honeybees via DNA methylation. Fertile queens and sterile workers are alternative forms of the adult female honeybee that develop from genetically identical larvae following differential feeding with royal jelly. Royal jelly is a complex, protein-rich substance secreted from glands on the heads of worker bees. A larva destined to become a queen is fed large quantities of royal jelly inside a specially constructed compartment called a queen cup. The authors observed that larvae fed with royal jelly developed functional ovaries and a larger abdomen for egg laying, while worker bees remain sterile. She'll also develop the necessary behaviors to act as queen, such as killing rival queens, making communication sounds known as "piping," and going on "mating flights." The queen is fed royal honey exclusively for the rest of her life. They showed that royal jelly silences a key gene (Dnmt3), which codes for an enzyme involved in genome-wide gene silencing. When Dnmt3 is active in bee larvae, the queen genes are epigenetically silenced and the larvae develop into the default "worker" variety. But when royal jelly turns Dnmt3 off, certain genes jump into action that turn the lucky larvae into queens. The authors suggested that DNA methylation in *Apis* is used for storing epigenetic information, that the use of that information can be differentially altered by nutritional input, and that the flexibility of epigenetic modifications underpins, profound shifts in developmental fates, with massive implications for reproductive and behavioral status.

During our lifetime, nutrients can modify physiologic and pathologic processes through epigenetic mechanisms that are critical for gene expression (summarized in Table 1). Modulation of these processes through diet or specific nutrients may prevent diseases and maintain health. However, it is very hard to delineate the precise effect of nutrients or bioactive food components on each epigenetic modulation and their associations with physiologic and pathologic processes in our body, because the nutrients also interact with genes, other nutrients, and other lifestyle factors. Furthermore, each epigenetic phenomenon also interacts with the others, adding to the complexity of the system [7].

	Nutrient or diet	Epigenetic mechanism
Embryonic development	Folate	DNA methylation, imprinting
	Choline	DNA methylation
	Protein restriction	DNA methylation, histone modifications
	Alcohol	DNA methylation
Stem cell	Butyrate	Histone acetylation, DNA methylation
	Retinoic acid	PRC
Aging	Folate	DNA methylation
	Calorie restriction	Histone acetylation
Immune function	Folate	DNA methylation
Cancer	Methyl-deficient diet	Histone modification, microRNA
	Genistein	DNA methylation, microRNA
	(-)-Epigallocatechin-3-gallate	DNA methylation, PRC
	Curcumin	microRNA
Obesity, insulin resistance	High-fat diet	DNA methylation, microRNA
	Methyl-deficient diet	DNA methylation
	Curcumin	Histone acetylation
Inflammation	Resveratrol	Histone acetylation
	AdoMet	Histone methylation
	Methyl-deficient diet	microRNA
Neurocognition	Choline	DNA methylation, histone methylation

Data in reference [7].

Table 1. Epigenetic roles of nutrition in physiologic and pathologic processes

2.1. Diet and genomic stability

Eukaryotic DNA replication starts at multiple sites throughout the genome and is necessarily coordinated with transcription, sister chromatid cohesion, nucleosome assembly and cell cycle progression. In addition to the complexity of the replication reaction it, during replication cells need to deal with DNA damage and stalled forks, originated inevitably by the action of exogenous and endogenous agents. The success of this process is crucial to preserve genome stability, and the inability to deal with DNA lesions during replication or to protect or restart stalled forks leads to DNA breaks, chromosomal rearrangements, and mutations that can cause the loss of cell viability, but in addition errors in DNA replication result in a large number of human syndromes, including premature aging, various cancer predispositions and genetic abnormalities. To solve or reduce these problems, cells use repair and detoxification pathways as well as surveillance mechanisms, called checkpoints, which serve to detect the problem and coordinate repair with chromosome segregation and progression through the cell cycle (see Figure 3. www.genomic-instability.org/).

Maintaining genomic stability in the face of replication and recombination requires a huge variety of different damage response proteins. A cell's ability to decide when and where to deploy this DNA repair kit is critical to prevent tumor development [11].

There is evidence that inappropriate nutrient supply can cause sizeable levels of genome mutation and alter expression of genes required for genome maintenance. Deficiencies in several micronutrients have been shown to cause DNA damage and are thought to be associated with a number of serious human diseases: folic acid, niacin, vitamin B6 and B12 deficiency may increase the risk of colon cancer, heart disease and neurological dysfunction due to chromosome breaks and disabled DNA repair [12]. On the other hand, as seen in reference [13], the authors believe that caloric restriction (CR) is an 'intervention' that alters the activation of specific 'stress response genes', key enzymes in DNA repair pathways, which then results in upregulation of 'DNA repair' capacity. Enhanced DNA repair reduces the levels of DNA damage, consequently reducing mutation frequency, which would result in maintenance of genomic stability.

Recommended dietary allowances (RDAs) of micronutrients have been traditionally defined as those levels necessary to prevent symptoms of deficiency diseases. There is increasing evidence that higher levels of many such micronutrients may be necessary for various DNA maintenance reactions, and that the current RDAs for some micronutrients may be inadequate to protect against genomic instability. Dietary imbalance may increase gene mutation and chromosome aberrations in human populations, similar to exposure to radiation, mutagens and carcinogens. Diet may well be a key factor in determining genomic stability since it impacts on all relevant pathways, i.e. exposure to dietary carcinogens, activation/detoxification of carcinogens, DNA repair, DNA synthesis and apoptosis, as mentioned previously. Many micronutrient minerals and vitamins act as substrates and/or co-factors in key DNA maintenance reactions, and the exact concentration of these in the cell may be critical. Sub-optimal levels of key micronutrients required for DNA maintenance will reduce genomic stability, producing similar effects to inherited genetic disorders or exposure to carcinogens [14].

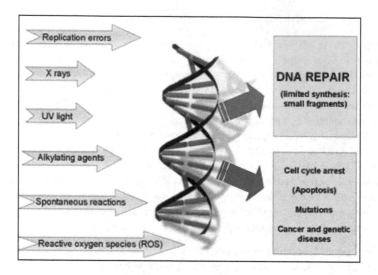

Figure 3. A general view of DNA insults and consequences on cell cycle and DNA repair (www.genomic-instability.org/).

3. Diet and cancer prevention

Current cancer models comprise those that are inherited through the germline and represent only ~5% of total cases of human cancers. These tumors originate because of mutational events. The remaining ~95% originate as sporadic events and evolve as a result of exposure to the environment, which includes exposure to both environmental contaminants and dietary agents. The multistage model of carcinogenesis identifies various phases, initiation, promotion, and progression, appears to be influenced by tissue microenvironment and organization. Significant opportunities in nutrition and cancer prevention exist in the early stages of initiation and promotion prior to clonal expansion of heterogeneous populations. Nutrigenomics represents a strategy that can be applied to the study and prevention of many diseases including cancer. DNA methylation and histone modifications are epigenetic events that mediate heritable changes in gene expression and chromatin organization in the absence of changes in the DNA sequence. The age-increased susceptibility to cancer may derive from accumulation of epigenetic changes and represents a potential target for therapies with bioactive compounds. Factors that mediate the response to dietary factors include nuclear receptors and transcription factors, which function as sensors to dietary components and determine changes in the profile of transcripts [15]. Milner and Romagnolo [15] affirm that the opportunity of targeting nutrients–gene interactions to influence the cancer process is modulated by genetic variations in human populations, epigenetic modifications that selectively and permanently alter gene expression, by complex interactions/associations among dietary components, and heterogeneity of cells within a certain tumor. Therefore, integration of information about gene polymorphisms, identification of gene targets that regulate cell and tissue specific pathways, and development of diagnostic strategies to control for clinical heterogeneity are important to understand how nutrigenomics may be used in cancer prevention.

Berrino, Krogh and Riboli [16] were made a review which showed an epidemiology studies on diet and cancer (see Table 2 that summarizes the results of the randomized studies published). The authors summarized (Table 3) the results of the World Cancer Research Fund (WCRF) evaluation on major foods and nutrients and major cancer sites. The 'probable' and 'possible' judgements provide a frame of hypotheses to be addressed in further studies. The overall pattern indicates that vegetarian food, except sugar and alcoholic beverages, is usually associated with cancer prevention, whereas animal food is frequently associated with cancer risk. The first WCRF dietary recommendation to reduce cancer, indeed, is: "Choose predominantly plant-based diets rich in a variety of vegetables and fruits, pulses (legumes) and minimally processed starchy staple foods". This seems to open a new perspective in nutrition and cancer research: from chemoprevention studies based on a single or a few micronutrients to an experimental strategy requiring a comprehensive modification of dietary habits.

Study and year of publication	Agent	Primary end point	Relative risk	Relative risk for secondary end points
ECPOS, 2000	Ispaghula fiber	Colon adenoma	1.67**	
APPP, 1995	Beta-carotene	Colon adenoma	1.50**	
CARET, 1996	Beta-carotene	Lung cancer	1.28**	
APPP, 1995	Cereal fibre	Colon adenoma	1.20	
TPPT, 1994	Cereal fibre*	Colon adenoma	1.20	
ATBC, 1994	Beta-carotene	Lung cancer	1.18**	0.98 for colon adenoma 1.05 for colorectal cancer 1.26 for stomach cancer 1.23 for prostate cancer
NPCS, 1996	Selenium	Skin, squamous cell	1.14	0.50** for all cancers
NPCS, 1996	Selenium	Skin, basal cell	1.10	
PPS, 1994	Vit C + Vit E	Colon adenoma	1.08	
SWCPS, 1997	Retinol	Skin, basal cell	1.06	
Linxian, China, 1993	Vit C + Mb	All cancers	1.06	1.10 for stomach cancer
SCPS, 1990	Beta-carotene	Skin	1.05	
PPS, 1994	Beta-carotene	Colon adenoma	1.01	

Study and year of publication	Agent	Primary end point	Relative risk	Relative risk for secondary end points
Linxian, China, 1993	Retinol + Zn	All cancers	1.00	0.96 for stomach cancer
EUROSCAN, 2000	Retinilpalmitate	Lung cancer	1.00	
Alberts et al., 2000	Cereal fiber	Colon adenoma	0.99	
ATBC, 1994	Alpha tocopherol	Lung cancer	0.99	0.64** for prostate cancer
				1.66** for colon adenoma
				0.83 for colorectal cancer
				1.26 for stomach cancer
				1.18** for stomach cancer
Linxian, China, 1993	14 vitamins + 12 minerals***	Esophagus/cardias	0.98	
PHS, 1996	Beta-carotene	All cancers	0.98	0.95 for lung cancer
Linxian, China, 1993	Riboflavin+niacin	All cancers	0.95	1.04 for stomach cancer
Linxian, China, 1993	Se + Vit E + beta-carotene	All cancers	0.93	0.79** for stomach cancer
				0.91** for total mortality
Baron et al., 1999	Calcium	Colon adenoma	0.83	
SWCPS, 1997	Retinol	Skin, squamous cell	0.74**	
ECPOS, 2000	Calcium	Colon adenoma	0.66	

*and low fat diet; **P < 0.05; ***including selenium, vitamin E and beta-carotene.
APPP, Australian Polyp Prevention Project; ATBC, Alpha Tocopherol Beta Carotene study; CARET, Carotene and Retinol Efficacy Trial; ECPOS, European Cancer Prevention Organisation Study Group; EUROSCAN, European Organization for Research and Treatment of Head and Neck Cancer and Lung Cancer Cooperative Group; NPCS, Nutritional Prevention of Skin Cancer; PHS, Physicians Health Study; PPS, Polyp Prevention Study Group; PPT, Polyp Prevention Trial; SCPS, Skin Cancer Prevention Study Group; SWCPS, Sothwest Skin Cancer Prevention Study; TPPT, Toronto Polyp Prevention Trial. Adapted from reference [16].

Table 2. Randomized controlled trials of dietary supplements to prevent cancer or colorectal adenomas, ordered by relative risk

American Cancer Society Guidelines on Nutrition and Physical Activity for Cancer Prevention [17] says that many epidemiologic studies have reported a modest but significant association

	Vegetables	Fruits	Grains, fibers	Tea	Sugar	Alcohol	Salt & salting	Meat	Eggs	Milk & dairy
Mouth, pharynx	---	---				+++				
Nasopharynx							+++			
Esophagus	---	---	+			+++				
Stomach	---	---	-	-			++			
Pancreas	--	--	-						+	
Gallbladder										
Liver	-					+++				
Colon, rectum	---		-					++	+	
Larynx	--	--				+++				
Lung	---	---				+				
Breast	--	--	-			++		+		
Cervix	-	-								
Endometrium	-	-								
Ovary	-	-								
Prostate	-							+		+
Bladder	--	--								
Kidney	-							+		+
Thyroid	-									

Increased risk: +++, convincing; ++, probable; +, possible; decreased risk: ---, convincing; --, probable; -, possible. Data adapted from reference [16].

Table 3. Matrix summary of the WCRF/AICR judgments on the role of various foods in the risk of cancer

between high intakes of processed meats (such as bacon, sausage, luncheon meats) and red meats (defined as beef, pork, or lamb) and increases in cancer incidence and mortality as well as death from other causes. The American Cancer Society says that current evidence supports approximately a 15% to 20% increased risk of cancers of the colon and/or rectum per 100 grams (g) of red meat or 50 g of processed meat consumed per day, while the evidence for some other cancers (those of the esophagus, stomach, lung, pancreas, breast, prostate, stomach, endometrium, renal, and ovarian) is considered limited and suggestive. According to American Cancer Society meat contains several constituents that could increase the risk of cancer. Mutagens and carcinogens (heterocyclic amines and polycyclic aromatic hydrocarbons) are produced by cooking meat at high temperatures and/or by charcoal grilling. Nitrates/nitrites and salt used to process meat contribute to the formation of nitrosamines, which are known mutagens and carcinogens in animals. Iron from the heme group of myoglobin in red meat may act as a catalyst to nitrosamine formation, and generate free radicals that may damage DNA. It is also possible that the fat content in meat contributes to risk through increasing the concentration of secondary bile acids and other compounds in the stool that could be carcinogens or promoters of carcinogenesis [17].

According to Davis [18] epidemiologic evidence suggests that regular consumption of fruits, vegetables, and whole grains may reduce cancer risk in some individuals. This association has been attributed to these foods being rich sources of numerous bioactive compounds. Plant foods contain a variety of components, including, but not limited to, essential nutrients, polyunsaturated fatty acids, and phytochemicals such as glucosinolates and flavonoids, many of which can inhibit cell proliferation and induce apoptosis, and which may act additively or synergistically when combined in the human diet.

3.1. Polyphenols

Polyphenols are common constituents of foods of plant origin and major antioxidants of our diet. The main dietary sources of polyphenols are fruits and beverages. Fruits like apple, grape, pear, cherry, and various berries contain up to 200–300 mg polyphenols per 100 g fresh weight. Typically, a glass of red wine or a cup of tea or coffee contains about 100 mg polyphenols. Cereals, chocolate, and dry legumes also contribute to the polyphenol intake [19]. Red wine polyphenols, which consisted of various powerful antioxidants such as flavonoids and stilbenes, have been implicated in cancer prevention and that promote human health without recognizable side effects. Experimental studies have shown that polyphenols from red wine, like resveratrol, quercetin, (+)-catechin and gallic acid, were potential cancer chemopreventive agents. However, red wine contains a wide range of different polyphenols and protective effects have not been assigned to a specific fraction or compound, so it is not yet clear which compounds present in red wine are endowed with protective activity [20]. Among the most highly cited class of polyphenols are the flavonoids, which comprise a large and diverse family of compounds synthesized by plants. Flavonoid subclasses include anthocyanidins in berries and grapes, flavanols in tea, flavanones in citrus fruits, flavonols in onions, flavones in herbs and peppers, and isoflavones in soy [21].

Zhou et al. [22] evaluated combined effects of soy phytochemical concentrate (SPC) and tea (green tea and black tea) components on the growth and metastasis of androgen-sensitive LNCaP human prostate cancer. The authors find that both black tea and green tea inhibited tumorigenicity rates of LNCaP tumors. For them the combination of soy phytochemicals and tea synergistically inhibited tumorigenicity, final tumor weight and metastasis to lymph nodes in vivo. This study supports further investigations using soy and tea combinations as effective nutritional regimens for prevention of prostate cancer. According to authors, studies of tea polyphenols suggest that epigallocatechin gallate (EGCG) is the major bioactive component in green tea and less is present in black tea. Black tea also contains other tea polyphenols such as theaflavins and thearubigins. They also affirm that chemopreventive properties of the soy isoflavone genistein have been the subject of extensive in vitro and in vivo.

Lambert and Yang [23] affirm that although numerous health benefits have been proposed for the consumption of tea, the effectiveness of tea as a cancer preventive agent in humans remains unclear. Animal models of carcinogenesis may be different from the human situation (e.g., the doses of tea and tea components used in animal studies are often much higher than those consumed by humans), and many confounding factors are involved in epidemiological studies. Interindividual variation in biotransformation and bioavailability may also affect the efficacy of tea as a cancer preventive agent. For them further studies on definitive mechanisms of cancer preventive activities of tea in animal models are needed. Although many possible mechanisms have been proposed, their relevance in vivo needs to be demonstrated. With some exceptions, the concentrations of catechins or theaflavins used in cell culture systems exceed the plasma concentrations obtained in animal studies by 10- to 100-fold. Mechanisms based on the use of such high concentrations may be relevant for cancers of the gastrointestinal tract but not for sites such as the lung, prostate and breast, which depend on systemic bioavailability. In spite of many in vitro and in vivo studies, the molecular mechanisms for the cancer preventive actions of these compounds are not clearly known. The relationship between tea consumption and cancer risk has not been conclusively demonstrated, and the relationship may become clearer if we consider the effects of specific types of tea, at defined doses, in populations with certain dietary patterns or genetic polymorphisms. Human intervention trials and large prospective studies are needed to further assess cancer preventive activities of tea constituents [24]. For the National Cancer Institute [25] more than 50 epidemiologic studies of the association between tea consumption and cancer risk have been published since 2006. The results of these studies have often been inconsistent, but some have linked tea consumption to reduced risks of cancers of the colon, breast, ovary, prostate, and lung. They also believe that the inconsistent results may be due to variables such as differences in tea preparation and consumption, the types of tea studied (green, black, or both), the methods of tea production, the bioavailability of tea compounds, genetic variation in how people respond to tea consumption, the concomitant use of tobacco and alcohol, and other lifestyle factors that may influence a person's risk of developing cancer, such as physical activity or weight status.

A double-blind intervention trial conducted in patients with oral mucosa leukoplakia using a mixed tea showed some direct evidence on the protective effects of tea on oral cancer. In this study developed by Li et al. [26] fifty-nine oral mucosa leukoplakia patients, diagnosed by established clinical and pathological criteria, were randomly divided into a treated group (3 g mixed tea oral administration and topical treatment) and a control group (placebo and glycerin treatment). After the 6-month trial, the size of oral lesion was decreased in 37.9% of the 29 treated patients and increased in 3.4%; whereas the oral lesion was decreased in 10.0% of the 30 control patients and increased in 6.7%.

3.2. Vitamins and micronutrients

Natural inhibitors of oxidizing agents that are found in the diet are important in preventing cancer and typically do not have the undesirable side effects of many xenobiotic compounds. Some vitamins, such as the antioxidant Vitamins A, E, and C, demonstrate these protective effects. The daily ingestion of antioxidants has the potential of not only protecting against cancer, but also cardiovascular disorders and neurological degenerative diseases [28]. Antioxidants nutrients such as vitamin E, vitamin C, vitamin A, and Beta-carotene are involved in detoxification of the Reactive oxygen species (ROS). Vitamin E, A, and Beta-carotene are lipophilic antioxidants whereas vitamin C is hydrophilic antioxidant. Vitamin E function as a free radical chain breaker particularly it interferes with the propagation step of lipid peroxidation. Vitamin A and Beta-carotene have actions by quenching both singlet oxygen and other free radicals generated by photochemical reactions [28].

The changes in the DNA by a deficiency of some micronutrients (folic acid, vitamin B12, vitamin B6, niacin, vitamin C, vitamin E, iron and zinc) are considered as the most likely cause of some types of cancer [29].

Studies investigating the interactions between dietary exposure and genetic polymorphisms have the potential to clarify mechanisms and identify susceptible subgroups so that preventative strategies can be focused on the subgroups for maximum benefit. Red meat or meat cooking methods such as frying and doneness levels have been associated with the increased risk of colorectal and other cancers [30]. It is not clear whether it is red meat intake or the way meat is cooked that is involved in the etiology of colorectal cancer, as stated above. Both cooking methods and doneness level of red meat are thought to be surrogates for heterocyclic amines (HCA) consumption [31]. Sinha and Caporaso [31] affirm that genetics polymorphisms may interact with various dietary components and thus define subgroups of individuals who may be at a higher risk of getting cancer. For them there are also other polymorphic enzymes that may interact with various dietary components and play a role in human carcinogenesis. The authors describe categories of susceptibility genes, potential dietary carcinogens and anticarcinogens, and cancer sites in which they may be involved (see Table 4). Many studies are currently investigating the role of circulating vitamin D metabolites and dietary calcium. Because the vitamin D receptor is involved in vitamin D and calcium metabolism, the vitamin D receptor polymorphisms may also be important for colorectal cancers. Martinez et al. [32] investigated the associations between the intake of calcium and vitamin D and the occurrence of colorectal cancer. They found that vitamin D is suggestive of an inverse association, particularly for total vitamin D in relation to rectal cancer. However, since most of the support for this protective effect was seen for total vitamin D. They not rule out the possibility that something other than vitamin D in multivitamin supplements contributes to this apparent effect. The relation between vitamin D and colorectal cancer may be better elucidated with additional dietary measurements and further follow-up. They conclude that available evidence does not warrant an increase in calcium intake to prevent colon cancer, but longer-term studies of both calcium and especially vitamin D in relation to colorectal cancer risk are needed.

Carotenoids are the pigments that give fruits and vegetables such as carrots, cantaloupe, sweet potato, and kale their vibrant orange, yellow, and green colors. Beta-carotene, lycopene, and lutein are all different varieties of carotenoids. They all act as antioxidants with strong cancer-fighting properties. Preclinical studies have shown that some carotenoids have potent antitumor effects both in vitro and in vivo, suggesting potential preventive and/or therapeutic roles for the compounds. Since chemoprevention is one of the most important strategies in the control of cancer development, molecular mechanism-based cancer chemoprevention using carotenoids seems to be an attractive approach [33]. Epidemiologic studies have shown an

Dietary component	Polymorphic gene/phenotype[1]	Cancer site
Carcinogens		
Heterocyclic amines	NAT2, (NAT1), CYP1A2 (CYP1A1)	Colorectal, breast, other sites
Polycyclic hydrocarbons	CYP1A1, GSTM1	Gastrointestinal tract Nasophyrangeal, stomach
Nitrosamines	CYP2E1	
Aflatoxins	GSTM1, EPHX	Liver
Alcohol	ADH (ALDH, CYP2E1)	Colorectal, oral
Anticarcinogens		
Cruciferous vegetables	CYP1A2, GST	Colorectal, other sites
Fruits and vegetables	CYP1A2, GST	Many sites
Calcium/vitamin D	Vitamin D receptor	Colorectal, prostate
Retinoids	Retinoic acid receptor Variant	Acute promylocytic Leukemia, skin, Head and neck, breast
Folate, methionine	MTHFR, Methionine Synthase	Colorectal, cervix

1 Abbreviations used: NAT, N-acetyltminsferase; CYP, cytochrome p450; GST, glutathione-S-transferase; EPHX, epoxide hydrolase; ADH, alcohol dehydrogenase; MTHFR, metheylenetetrahydrofolate reductase. Adapted from reference [31].

Table 4. Polymorphic genes, dietary components and cancer: possible candidates

inverse relationship between the presence of various cancers and dietary or blood carotenoid levels. According to Tanaka, Shnimizu and Moriwaki [33] the epidemiologic observations of the possible protective effects of high dietary (not supplemental) β-carotene intakes against cancer, along with what is known about carotenoid biochemical functions, has led to further study of the effect of β-carotene on cancer risk. Long-term large randomized intervention trials were designed to test the efficacy of high doses of β-carotene (20–30 mg/day) in the prevention of cancer. These results are summarized in Table 5.

Studies	Population	Study Designs		
		Intervention	Duration	Cancer outcome
ATBC	29,133 Finish male smokers (50–69 years of age)	β-carotene, 20 mg/day; vitamin E, 50 mg/day	5–8 years	18% increase in lung cancer; 8% increase in mortality
CARET	18,314 men and women and asbestoss workers (45–74 years of age)	β-carotene, 30 mg/day; vitamin A, 25,000 IU	<4 years	28% increase in lung cancer; 17% increase in deaths
PHS	22,071 male physicians (40–84 years of age)	β-carotene, 50 mg on alternate days	12 years	No effect of supplementation in incidence of cancer
Linxian	29,584 men and women, vitamin and mineral deficient (40–69 years of age)	β-carotene, 15 mg/day; selenium, 50 mg/day; α-tocopherol, 30 mg/day	5 years	13% decrease in total cancers; 9% decrease in overall deaths
Women's Health Study	39,876 female health professionals (over 45 years of age)	β-carotene, 50 mg on alternate days	4.1 years (2.1 years' treatment and 2.0 years' follow-up)	No effect of supplementation in incidence of cancer

Data adapted from reference [33].
CARET, Beta-Carotene and Retinol Efficacy Trial; ATBC, Alpha Tocopherol and Beta-Carotene Cancer Prevention; PHS, Physicians' Health Study.

Table 5. β-Carotene supplementation trials.

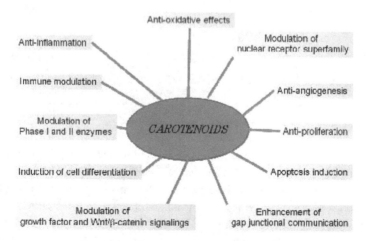

Figure 4. Proposed mechanisms by which certain carotenoids suppress carcinogenesis. Adapted from reference [33].

The authors [33] wrote an important review which showed a table (Table 6) about cancer prevention by means of carotenoids with dietary sources, function e effects. According to these authors the mechanisms underlying the anticancer and/or cancer chemopreventive activities of carotenoids may involve changes in pathways leading to cell growth or cell death. These include immune modulation, hormone and growth factor signaling, regulatory mechanisms of cell cycle progression, cell differentiation and apoptosis. In this sense the authors also showed an interesting figure proposing possible mechanisms by which certain carotenoids suppress carcinogenesis (see Figure 4 on the left).

Studies involving the use of vitamin C in cancer prevention are the most contradictory. Vitamin C is an essential vitamin the human body needs to function well. It is a water-soluble vitamin that cannot be made by the body, and must be obtained from foods or other sources. Vitamin C is found in abundance in citrus fruits such as oranges, grapefruit, and lemons, and in green leafy vegetables, potatoes, strawberries, bell peppers, and cantaloupe. American Cancer Society [34] wrote that many studies have shown a connection between eating foods rich in vitamin C, such as fruits and vegetables, and a reduced risk of cancer. On the other hand, evidence indicates that vitamin C supplements do not reduce cancer risk. This suggests that the activity of fruits and vegetables in preventing cancer is due to a combination of many vitamins and other phytochemicals and not to vitamin C alone. Clinical trials of high doses vitamin C as a treatment for cancer have not shown any benefit. High doses of vitamin C can cause a number of side effects.

According to Block [35] epidemiologic evidence of a protective effect of vitamin C for non-hormone-dependent cancers is strong. Of the 46 such studies in which a dietary vitamin C index was calculated, 33 found statistically significant protection, with high intake conferring approximately a twofold protective effect compared with low intake. 0f 29 additional studies that assessed fruit intake, 2 1 found significant protection. For cancers of the esophagus, larynx, oral cavity, and pancreas, evidence for a protective effect of vitamin C or some component in fruit is strong and consistent. For cancers of the stomach, rectum, breast, and cervix there is also strong evidence. Several recent lung cancer studies found significant protective effects of vitamin C or of foods that are better sources of vitamin C than of /3-carotene. It is likely that ascorbic acid, carotenoids, and other factors in fruits and vegetables act jointly.

Several lines of evidence suggest that vitamin C is a powerful antioxidant in biological systems in vitro. However, its antioxidant role in humans has not been supported by currently available clinical studies. Diets high in fruits and vegetables protect against cardiovascular disease and cancer, but such a protective effect cannot as yet be ascribed to vitamin C. In vivo markers of oxidative damage are being developed, and these have yet not shown major changes with vitamin C intake in humans [36]. The most important problem about vitamin C is that it can exert a pro-oxidant activity under certain conditions, particularly in the presence of transition metal ions or alkali. Thus, vitamin C *in vitro* reduces free ferric iron that generates hydrogen peroxide in the Fenton reaction and results in the production of hydroxyl radicals. The reactive hydroxyl radical quickly reacts with critical cellular macromolecules, including DNA, which may lead to mutagenesis and the initiation of cancer [37]. According to authors, the high

Carotenoids	Dietary Sources	Function	Effects
α-Carotene	Yellow-orange vegetables (carrots, sweet totatoes, pumpkin) and Dark-green vegetables (broccoli, green beans, spinach)	Provitamin A activity; Anti-oxidant	Immune- enhancement; Stimulate cell to cell communication; Decreases risk of some cancers
β-Carotene	Green leafy vegetables and orange and yellow fruits and vegetables (carrots, apricots, spinach, sweet potetoes, pumpkin, pepper, kale, cantaloupe)	Provitamin A activity; Antioxidant	Immune-enhancement; Decreases risk of some cancers and some cardiovascular events; high-dose supplementation may increase the risk of lung cancer among smokers
Lycopene	Tomatoes, water melon, apricot, peaches	Anti-oxidant	Decreases risk of some cancers and some cardiovascular events, diabetes, and osteoporosis
β-Cyptoxanthin	Orange fruits (mandarin orange and papaya, etc.), corn, peas, and egg yolks	Provitamin A activity; Anti-oxidant	Anti-inflammatory effects; Inhibits risks of some cancer and cardiovascular events; Immune enhancemen
Lutein/Zeaxanthin	Dark green leafy vegetables (spinach, kale), red peppers, maize, tomatoes, corn, and egg yolks	Anti-photosensitizing agent and photosynthetic pigment; Acts as antioxidants and blue light filters	Decrease age-related macular degeneration, cataract, and risk of cardiovascular disease and certain cancers
Astaxanthin	Green algae, salmon, trout, Crustacean	Antioxidant; Coloration	Prevent certain cancers, cataract, diabetes, and inflammatory neurodegenerative and cardiovascular diseases
Canthaxanthin	Salmon, crustacean	Antioxidant; Coloration	Immune enhancement; Decreases risk of some cancers
Focoxanthin	Brown algae, heterokonts	Antioxidant	Anti-cancer, anti-allergic, anti-obese, anti-inflammatory, and anti-osteoporotic activities

Adapted from reference [33].

Table 6. Sources, function, and effects of different carotenoids.

consumption of vitamin C–rich fruit and vegetables is not likely to be harmful. In general, data from in vitro and in vivo experiments and population-based studies do not indicate that high doses of vitamin C are linked to increased oxidative DNA damage or an elevated risk of cancer.

Lee et al. [37] believe that the cancer preventive effects of vegetables and fruit may result from multiple combined effects of various phenolic phytochemicals, vitamins, dietary fibers, indoles, allium compounds, and selenium rather than from the effect of a single active ingredient. For them, many dietary phenolic phytochemicals may have stronger antioxidant and antitumor promotion effects than do antioxidant vitamins, which may contribute to the chemopreventive effects of the phytochemicals in carcinogenesis. However, these authors suggest that the chemopreventive effects of vitamin C in carcinogenesis may be linked to the protective effects of vitamin C against epigenetic mechanisms, such as the inflammation and inhibition of gap junction intercellular communication (GJIC), as well as to antioxidant activities (see Figure 5).

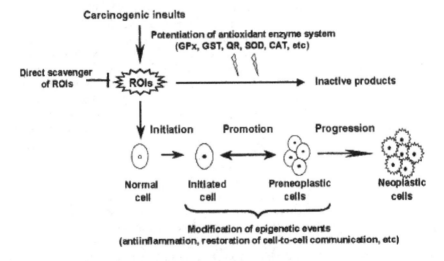

Figure 5. Possible chemopreventive mechanisms of vitamin C in carcinogenesis. ROIs, reactive oxygen intermediates; GPx, glutathione peroxidase; GST, glutathione S-transferase; QR, quinone oxidoreductase; SOD, superoxide dismutase; CAT, catalase. Adapted from reference [37].

Regarding the use of vitamin C in cancer patient the results were not promising. In a double-blind study 100 patients with advanced colorectal cancer were randomly assigned to treatment with either high-dose vitamin C (10 g daily) or placebo. Overall, these patients were in very good general condition, with minimal symptoms. None had received any previous treatment with cytotoxic drugs. Vitamin C therapy showed no advantage over placebo therapy with regard to either the interval between the beginning of treatment and disease progression or patient survival. Among patients with measurable disease, none had objective improvement. On the basis of this and our previous randomized study, it can be concluded that high-dose vitamin C therapy is not effective against advanced malignant disease regardless of whether the patient has had any prior chemotherapy [38].

The terms folic acid and folate are often used interchangeably for this water-soluble B-complex vitamin. Folic acid, the more stable form, occurs rarely in foods or the human body but is the form most often used in vitamin supplements and fortified foods. Folic acid is essential to numerous bodily functions ranging from nucleotide biosynthesis to the remethylation of homocysteine. The human body needs folate to synthesize DNA, repair DNA, and methylate DNA as well as to act as a cofactor in biological reactions involving folate.

Considerable epidemiological evidence suggests that a low-folate diet is associated with an increased risk of colorectal neoplasia. Much animal data support an antineoplastic effect of folate. However, in some animal studies, folate deficiency protects against, and supplementation increases, experimental carcinogenesis. Cole et al. [39] developed a double-blind, placebo-controlled, 2-factor, phase 3, randomized clinical trial conducted at 9 clinical centers between July 6, 1994, and October 1, 2004. Participants included 1021 men and women with a recent history of colorectal adenomas and no previous invasive large intestine carcinoma. Participants were randomly assigned in a 1:1 ratio to receive 1 mg/d of folic acid (n=516) or placebo (n=505), and were separately randomized to receive aspirin (81 or 325 mg/d) or placebo. Follow-up consisted of 2 colonoscopic surveillance cycles (the first interval was at 3 years and the second at 3 or 5 years later). In this double-blind, placebo-controlled, randomized clinical trial, was found that folic acid supplementation did not decrease the risk of adenoma occurrence among participants with a recent history of adenomas. The authors concluded that folate, when administered as folic acid for up to 6 years, does not decrease the risk of adenoma formation in the large intestine among individuals with previously removed adenomas. For them, the evidence for an increased risk of adenomas is equivocal and requires further research.

In March of 1996, the U.S. Food and Drug Administration mandated that all enriched flour and uncooked cereal grains sold in the United States should be fortified with 140 µg folic acid/100 g of flour no later than January of 1998. Following the institution of fortification population-based studies showed the effectiveness of this measure: plasma levels of folate in the adult population increased ~2-fold as a result and the incidence of births complicated by neural tube defects was variously reported to decline by 20% to 50%. However, analyses of several cereal grains that were purchased after the institution of fortification showed that in many instances the actual amount of folate was 150% to 300% greater than the mandate, suggesting that in this early era of fortification, manufacturers often included "overage" to ensure that they were meeting the minimal level of mandated fortification [40]. Thus, the authors hypothesize, by means of an epidemiological study, that the institution of folic acid fortification may have been wholly or partly responsible for the observed increase in colorectal cancer rates in the mid-1990s. The authors affirm that wish to highlight the potential complexity of the response to this nutrient and emphasize prior observations that have been made in both preclinical and clinical studies that indicate that administering high doses of folic acid to susceptible individuals or in an inappropriate time frame may accelerate the growth of existing neoplasms.

Vitamin C, also known as ascorbic acid, is a water-soluble vitamin. Unlike most mammals and other animals, humans do not have the ability to make their own vitamin C. Therefore, we must obtain vitamin C through our diet. Vitamin C is required for the synthesis of collagen, an important structural component of blood vessels, tendons, ligaments, and bone. Vitamin C also plays an important role in the synthesis of the neurotransmitter, norepinephrine. Neurotransmitters are critical to brain function and are known to affect mood. Vitamin C is also a highly effective antioxidant. Even in small amounts vitamin C can protect indispensable molecules in the body, such as proteins, lipids (fats), carbohydrates, and nucleic acids (DNA and RNA), from damage by free radicals and reactive oxygen species that can be generated during normal metabolism as well as through exposure to toxins and pollutants (e.g., cigarette smoke). In the U.S., the recommended dietary allowance (RDA) for vitamin C was revised in 2000 upward from the previous recommendation of 60 mg daily for men and women. The RDA continues to be based primarily on the prevention of deficiency disease, rather than the prevention of chronic disease and the promotion of optimum health. The recommended intake for smokers is 35 mg/day higher than for non-smokers, because smokers are under increased oxidative stress from the toxins in cigarette smoke and generally have lower blood levels of vitamin C (see Table 7 – reference [41]).

Life Stage	Age	Males (mg/day)	Females (mg/day)
Infants	0-6 months	40 (AI)	40 (AI)
Infants	7-12 months	50 (AI)	50 (AI)
Children	1-3 years	15	15
Children	4-8 years	25	25
Children	9-13 years	45	45
Adolescents	14-18 years	75	65
Adults	19 years and older	90	75
Smokers	19 years and older	125	110
Pregnancy	18 years and younger	-	80
Pregnancy	19 years and older	-	85
Breast-feeding	18 years and younger	-	115
Breast-feeding	19 years and older	-	120

Data from reference [41].

Table 7. Recommended Dietary Allowance (RDA) for Vitamin C

The relations between the intake of beta-carotene, vitamin C, selenium, and 25-yr mortality from lung cancer and total cancer were analyzed within the Zutphen Study, a cohort study on diet and chronic diseases [42]. The Zutphen Study is a prospective study on the relations between diet, other risk factors, and the incidence of chronic diseases. The results of this study suggest that vitamin C intake may be more important for prevention of lung cancer than beta-carotene. It can, however, not be ruled out that substances present in fruit other than vitamin C (eg, phenols, flavones, and terpenes) may also be of importance in lung cancer prevention. The results suggest that a vitamin C intake of ≥ 70 mg/d may be of importance in lung cancer prevention. Due to the role of vitamin C in the formation of N-nitrosocompounds, this may also be of importance for stomach cancer prevention. Another hand, 8 prospective studies does not suggest that intakes of vitamins A, C and E and folate reduce the risk of lung cancer. The results were similar with different analytic approaches and across studies, sex, smoking status and lung cancer cell type [43].

Data on intake of specific carotenoids and breast cancer risk are limited. Furthermore, studies of vitamins A, C, and E in relation to breast cancer risk are inconclusive. Zhang et al. [44] were made studies, using multivariate analysis, demonstrated associations between intakes of specific carotenoids, vitamins A, C, and E, consumption of fruits and vegetables, and breast cancer risk in a cohort of 83,234 women (aged 33-60 years in 1980). Through 1994, they identified 2,697 incident cases of invasive breast cancer (784 premenopausal and 1913 post-menopausal). The results demonstrated that intakes of beta-carotene from food and supplements, lutein/zeaxanthin, and vitamin A from foods were weakly inversely associated with breast cancer risk in premenopausal women. Strong inverse associations were found for increasing quintiles of alpha-carotene, beta-carotene, lutein/zeaxanthin, total vitamin C from foods, and total vitamin A among premenopausal women with a positive family history of breast cancer. An inverse association was also found for increasing quintiles of beta-carotene among premenopausal women who consumed 15 g or more of alcohol per day. Premenopausal women who consumed five or more servings per day of fruits and vegetables had modestly lower risk of breast cancer than those who had less than two servings per day (relative risk [RR] = 0.77; 95% confidence interval [CI] = 0.58-1.02); this association was stronger among premenopausal women who had a positive family history of breast cancer (RR = 0.29; 95% CI = 0.13-0.62) or those who consumed 15 g or more of alcohol per day (RR = 0.53; 95% CI = 0.27-1.04). The author concluded that consumption of fruits and vegetables high in specific carotenoids and vitamins may reduce premenopausal breast cancer risk [44].

In recent years, the intake of vitamins, minerals and herbs as a dietary supplement has increased dramatically. The supplementation with vitamins and minerals are used more often than the herbs. The most common supplements among users in the U.S. are multivitamins (75%), followed by vitamin C (38%), and iron (38%) [45]. Food supplementation with vitamins is a polemic question and it differs among authors. There are evidences that dietary supplementation with vitamin C may reduce the incidence of gastric cancer in certain populations, but it is unclear whether it was the antioxidant, vitamin or other property, responsible for this action [46]. However, the author states that it does not justify, in terms of cancer prevention to make a diet supplemented with vitamin C if the person has a good diet. Claycombe and Meydani [47] were made a review reporting the protective effect of vitamin E against chromosomal alterations induced by oxidation of DNA. However, the authors call attention to the careful supplementation, simultaneous with C vitamin E, considering a possible genotoxicity in the association of the two vitamins. Although most animal studies have shown cancer-preventive effects, a few recent studies suggest that soy phytoestrogens may stimulate breast cancer cell growth under certain circumstances. Before recommendations regarding phytoestrogen supplements can be safely made, we must have more information on the effects of the extracts on bone, heart and breast health. Until safety with respect to breast cancer is established, phytoestrogen supplements should not be recommended, particularly for women at high risk of breast cancer [48].

Cancer prevention can be done with a diet rich in vegetables, fruits, and low in red meat, saturated fats, salt and sugar. Carbohydrates should be consumed in the form of cereals - wheat bread and brown rice. The addition of fats should be in the form of fats dehydrogenated [49]. The types of vegetables or fruit that most often appear to be protective against cancer are allium vegetables, carrots, green vegetables, cruciferous vegetables, and tomatoes. Substances present in some vegetable and fruit may help cancer prevention and they include dithiolthiones, isothiocyanates, indole-3-carbinol, allium compounds, isoflavones, protease inhibitors, saponins, phytosterols, inositol hexaphosphate, vitamin C, D-limonene, lutein, folic acid, beta carotene, lycopene, selenium, vitamin E, flavonoids, and dietary fiber. Current US vegetable and fruit intake, which averages about 3.4 servings per day, is discussed, as are possible non-cancer-related effects of increased vegetable and fruit consumption, including benefits against cardiovascular disease, diabetes, stroke, obesity, diverticulosis, and cataracts [50].

4. Conclusion

Cancer incidence is projected to increase in the future and an effectual preventive strategy is required to face this challenge. Alteration of dietary habits is potentially an effective approach for reducing cancer risk. Assessment of biological effects of a specific food or bioactive component that is linked to cancer and prediction of individual susceptibility as a function of nutrient-nutrient interactions and genetics is an essential element to evaluate the beneficiaries of dietary interventions [51]. We know that diet is an important factor both to minimize, as to increase the risk of cancer development. But diet is not the only factor. There are several risk factors that can trigger a process of tumor formation. Sedentary life, environmental issues, viruses, smoking, alcohol in excess, are factors that contribute to and are also strategic points that should be worked in cancer prevention.

Author details

Júlio César Nepomuceno

Universidade Federal de Uberlândia/ Instituto de Genética e Bioquímica; Centro Universitário de Patos de Minas /Laboratório de Citogenética e Mutagênese, Brazil

References

[1] Pitot HC, Goldsworthy T., Moran S. The natural history of carcinogenesis: Implications of experimental carcinogenesis in the genesis of human cancer. Journal of Supramolecular Structure and Cellular Biochemistry. 2004;17: 133-146.

[2] Setlow RB. Human cancer: etiologic agents/dose responses/DNA repair/cellular and animal models. Mutat Res 2001;477(1-2): 1-6.

[3] Fujii T.M.M., Medeiros R. and Yamada R. Nutrigenomics and nutrigenetics: importante concepts for the nutrition science. J Brazilian Soc Food Nutr 2010;35(1): 149-166.

[4] Fogg-Johnson N and Kaput J. Nutrigenomics: An Emerging Scientific Discipline. Foodtechnology 2003;57(4): 60-67.

[5] Gabory A, Attig L and Junien C. Epigenetic mechanisms involved in developmental nutritional programming. World J Diabetes 2011;15; 2(10): 64-175.

[6] Phillips T. The role of methylation in gene expression; 2008 Nature Education http://www.nature.com/scitable/topicpage/the-role-of-methylation-in-gene-expression-107 (accessed 215 August 2012).

[7] Choi, Sang-Woon and Friso S. Epigenetics: A New Bridge between Nutritionand Health. Adv Nutr 2010;1: 8–16.

[8] Viré E, Brenner C, Deplus R, Blanchon L, Fraga M, Didelot C, Morey L, Van Eynde A, Bernard D, Vanderwinden JM, Bollen M, Esteller M, Di Croce L, de Launoit Y, Fuks F. The Polycomb group protein EZH2 directly controls DNA methylation. NATURE 2007;446(7137):824.

[9] Robertson KD. DNA methylation and human disease. Nat Rev Genet 2005;6(8): 597-610.

[10] Kucharski R, Maleszka J, Foret S, Maleszka R. Nutritional Control of Reproductive Status in Honeybees via DNA Methylation. Science 2008;319: 1827-1830.

[11] Scaplehorn N. Genome Instability, Cell 2011;145: 5-7.

[12] Ames BN and Wakimoto P. Are micronutrient deficiencies a major cancer risk? Nature Reviews Cancer 2002;2:694–704.

[13] Heydari AR, Unnikrishnan A, Lucente LV and Richardson A. Caloric restriction and genomic stability. Nucleic Acids Research 2007;35(22): 7485–7496.

[14] Fenech M and Ferguson LR. Vitamins/minerals and genomic stability in humans. Mutation Research/Fundamental and Molecular Mechanisms of Mutagenesis 2001;475:1-6

[15] Milner JA and Romagnolo DF. Nutrition and Health: Bioactive Compounds and Cancer, Edited by: J.A. Milner, D.F. Romagnolo, DOI 10.1007/978-1-60761-627-6_2, Humana Press. 824p., 2010.

[16] Berrino F, Krogh V and Riboli E. Epidemiology studies on diet and cancer. Tumori 2003;89: 581-585.

[17] Kushi LH, Byers T, Doyle C, Bandera EV, McCullough M, McTiernan A, Gansler T, Andrews KS and Thun MJ. Nutrition and Physical Activity Guidelines Advisory

Committee. American Cancer Society Guidelines on Nutrition and Physical Activity for Cancer Prevention Reducing the Risk of Cancer With Healthy Food Choices and Physical Activity. CA Cancer J Clin 2012;62:30–67.

[18] Davis CD. Nutritional Interactions: Credentialing of Molecular Targets for Cancer Prevention. Exp Biol Med 2007;232(2): 176-183.

[19] Scalbert A, Manach C, Morand C, Rémésy C, Jiménez L. Dietary Polyphenols and the Prevention of Diseases. Crit Rev Food Sci Nutr 2005;45(4): 287-306.

[20] He S, Sun C and Pan Y. Red Wine Polyphenols for Cancer Prevention. Int J Mol Sci 2008;9: 842-853.

[21] Dashwood RH. Frontiers in Polyphenols and Cancer Prevention. J Nutr 2007;137: 267S–269S.

[22] Zhou Jin-Rong, Yu L, Zhong Y and Blackburn GL. Soy Phytochemicals and Tea Bio-active Components Synergistically Inhibit Androgen-Sensitive Human Prostate Tumors in Mice. J Nutr 2003;133(2): 516-521.

[23] Lambert JD and Yang CS. Mechanisms of Cancer Prevention by Tea Constituents. Proceedings of the Third International Scientific Symposium on Tea and Human Health: Role of Flavonoids in the Diet. J Nutr 2003;133(10): 3262S-3267S.

[24] Yang, C S, Ju J, Lu G, Xiao H, Hao X, Sang S and Lambert JD (). Cancer prevention by tea and tea polyphenols. Asia Pac J Clin Nutr 2008;17(S1): 245-248.

[25] National Cancer Institute (2010) Tea and Cancer Prevention: Strengths and Limits of the Evidence. http://www.cancer.gov/cancertopics/factsheet/prevention/tea#r13 (accessed 20 August 2012).

[26] Li N, Sun Z, Han C, Chen J. The chemopreventive effects of tea on human oral pre-cancerous mucosa lesions. Proceedings from the Society of Experimental Biology and Medicine 1999;220(4):218–224.

[27] Costa WF and Nepomuceno JC. Protective Effects of a Mixture of Antioxidant Vitamins and Minerals on the Genotoxicity of Doxorubicin in Somatic Cells of Drosophila melanogaster. Environmental and MolecularMutagenesis 2005;47(1):18-24.

[28] Nepomuceno, JC. Antioxidants in Cancer Treatment, Current Cancer Treatment: Intech, 2011. http://www.intechopen.com/books/current-cancer-treatment-novel-be-yond-conventional-approaches/antioxidants-in-cancer-treatment (accessed 20 August 2012).

[29] Ames BN. DNA damage from micronutrient deficiencies is likely to be a major cause of cancer. Mutation Res 2001;475: 7-20.

[30] Glade MJ. Food, Nutrition and the Prevention of Cancer: A Global Perspective. American Institute for Cancer Research, Washington, DC, Nutrition 1997;15(6): 523-6.

[31] Sinha R and Caporaso N. Diet, Genetic Susceptibility and Human Cancer Etiology Symposium: Interactions of Diet and Nutrition with Genetic Susceptibility in Cancer. J Nutr 1999;129(2): 556S-559S.

[32] Martinez M, Giovannucci EL, Colditz GA, Stampfer M, Hunter DJ, Speizer FE, Wing A and Willet WC. Calcium, Vitamin D, and the Occurrence of Colorectal Cancer Among Women. J Natl Cancer Inst 1996;88:1375-82.

[33] Tanaka T, Shnimizu M and Moriwaki H. Cancer Chemoprevention by Carotenoids, Molecules 2012;17: 3202-3242.

[34] American Cancer Society. Vitamin C. http://www.cancer.org/Treatment/TreatmentsandSideEffects/ComplementaryandAlternativeMedicine/HerbsVitaminsandMinerals/vitamin-c (accessed 215 August 2012).

[35] Block G. Vitamin C and cancer prevention: the epidemiologic evidence. Am J Clin Nutr 1991;53: 270S-82S.

[36] Padayatty, S.J., Katz, A., Wang, Y., Eck, P., Kwon, O., Lee, J.H., Chen, S., Corpe, C., Dutta, A., Dutta, S.K. & Levine, M. (2003). Vitamin C as an Antioxidant: Evaluation of Its Role in Disease Prevention, J Am Coll Nutr 22(1):18-35.

[37] Lee KW, Lee HJ, Surh YJ and Lee CY. Vitamin C and cancer chemoprevention: reappraisal, Am J Clin Nutr 2003;78: 1074–8.

[38] Moertel CG, Fleming TR, Creagan ET, Rubin J, O'Connell MJ and Ames MM. High-Dose Vitamin C versus Placebo in the Treatment of Patients with Advanced Cancer Who Have Had No Prior Chemotherapy — A Randomized Double-Blind Comparison. N Engl J Med 1985;312:137-141

[39] Cole BF, Baron JA, Sandler RS, Haile RW, Ahnen DJ, Bresalier RS, McKeown-Eyssen G, Summers RW, Rothstein RI, Burke CA, Snover DC, Church TR, Allen JI, Robertson DJ, Beck GJ, Bond JH, Byers T, Mandel JS, Mott LA, Pearson LH, Barry EL, Rees JR, Marcon N, Saibil F, Ueland PM and Greenberg ER; Polyp Prevention Study Group. Folic Acid for the Prevention of Colorectal Adenomas - A Randomized Clinical Trial. JAMA 2007;297: 2351-2359.

[40] Mason JB, Dickstein A, Jacques PF, Haggarty P, Selhub J, Dallal G and Rosenberg IH. A Temporal Association between Folic Acid Fortification and an Increase in Colorectal Cancer Rates May Be Illuminating Important Biological Principles: A Hypothesis. Cancer Epidemiol Biomarkers Prev 2007;16: 1325-1329.

[41] Linus Pauling Institute. Micronutrient Information Center; Vitamin C. http://lpi.oregonstate.edu/infocenter/vitamins/vitaminC/ (accessed 12 September 2012).

[42] Kromhout D. Essential micronutrients in relation to carcinogenesis. Am J Clin Nutr May 1987;45(5):1361-1367.

[43] Cho E, Hunter DJ, Spiegelman D, Albanes D, Beeson WL, van den Brandt PA, Colditz GA, Feskanich D, Folsom AR, Fraser GE, Freudenheim JL, Giovannucci E, Gold-

bohm RA, Graham S, Miller AB, Rohan TE, Sellers TA, Virtamo J, Willett WC, Smith-Warner SA. Intakes of vitamins A, C and E and folate and multivitamins and lung cancer: a pooled analysis of 8 prospective studies. Int J Cancer 2006;118(4):970-8.

[44] Zhang S, Hunter DJ, Forman MR, Rosner BA, Speizer FE, Colditz GA, Manson JE, Hankinson SE, Willett WC. Dietary carotenoids and vitamins A, C, and E and risk of breast cancer. J Natl Cancer Inst 1999;91(6):547-56.

[45] Yu C. Contribution of Dietary Supplements to the Nutritional Status of College Students. (2011). Honors Scholar Theses. Paper 180. http://digitalcommons.uconn.edu/srhonors_theses/180

[46] Halliwell B. Vitamin C and genomic stability. Mutation Res 2001;475: 29-35.

[47] Claycombe KJ, Meydani SN. Vitamin E and genome stability. Mutat Res 2001;475(1-2):37-44.

[48] Kurzer MS. Phytoestrogen Supplement Use by Women. J Nutr 2003;133(6): 1983S-1986S.

[49] Willett WC. Diet and Cancer An Evolving Picture. JAMA 2005;293(2): 233-234.

[50] Steinmetz KA, Potter JD. Vegetables, fruit, and cancer prevention: a review. J Am Diet Assoc. 1996;96(10):1027-39.

[51] Ardekani AM and Jabbari S. Nutrigenomics and Cancer. Avicenna J Med Biotech 2009;1(1): 9-17.

Chapter 3

The Treatment of Cancer: A Comprehensive Therapeutic Model Entailing a Complex of Interaction Modalities

R. Saggini and M. Calvani

Additional information is available at the end of the chapter

1. Introduction

Although an overall rise in cancer incidence has been observed over the past 300 years concomitantly with the industrial revolution, a more prominent increase has been recorded since the '30s, with a further acceleration during the last 2 decades.

Genetic factors are thought to account for 5-10% of all malignant neoplasms, even though hereditary susceptibility will be variably relevant depending on histotype, anatomic site, and epidemiologic context; additionally, a key role is played by environmental factors. Socioeconomic improvements have resulted in an increase in food availability as well as significant changes in lifestyle habits; with new technologies allowing for automation of manual work, an overall physical activity reduction has been observed leading to unbalances between caloric intake and energy expenditure.

Cancer is no longer a rapidly lethal disease for an increasing number of patients. Knowledge of the main risk factors for cancer development is essential for establishing a comprehensive and integrated treatment plan (tab 1).

Cancer patients receiving treatment combinations of surgery, radiation therapy and chemotherapy are prone to developing several treatment-related diseases.

Pain, heightened risk of infection, neural deficits, lymphedema, fatigue, nausea and vomiting, loss of flexibility, myopathies, muscle weakness, cachexia, dehydration, emotional distress, shortness of breath are common side-effects capable of negatively affecting patients' lifestyle and physical activities. Any combination of surgical treatments, chemotherapy, and radiotherapy must be integrated within a global therapeutic plan aimed to reduce the above-

1. Obesity and overweight
2. Low fruit and vegetable intake
3. Physical inactivity
4. Smoking
5. Alcohol consumption
6. Unprotected sex
7. Urban air pollution
8. Indoor air pollution due to household use of solid fuels
9. Spread of bacterial and viral infections through unsafe health care procedures

Table 1. The 9 modifiable risk factors responsible for a third of all cancer deaths in the world

mentioned negative effects that may become apparent immediately as well as after several months or years.

Mullan (1985) classified the life of cancer survivors into three stages: 1) Acute Stage, spanning from diagnosis to the first year after primary treatment; 2) Extended Stage, until the 5th year after primary treatment; 3) Permanent Stage, from the 5th year after primary treatment onwards.

The first year after primary treatment should be considered just as the "tip of the iceberg", and it is crucial that any approach to cancer treatment is holistic and comprehensive, based on the assumption that cancer is a chronic illness rather than an acute condition.

The aim of this chapter is not to describe the specifics of early management of patients diagnosed with cancer; however, the authors' view is that such approach should be as integrative and comprehensive as possible.

It is essential that physicians in the process of planning specific therapeutic interventions (either actions specifically aimed to the primary disease or supportive therapies) extensively profile patients according to their physical status in order to establish an individual patient-tailored strategy.

The integrative management approach relies on a number of basic interventions, including:

1. Therapeutic changes of lifestyle habits and daily diet;

2. Specific physical exercises and walking prescriptions;

3. Physical therapies coupled with psychophysical techniques.

2. Therapeutic changes of lifestyle habits and daily diet

2.1. What do you know?

Up to 30-40% of all malignant cancers could be prevented by interventions on diet, physical activities, and daily lifestyle.

Calories intake directly correlates with risk of developing obesity as well as cancer.

Obesity *per se* is considered to be to blame for up to 14% and 20% of all men and women deaths.

Approximately 50% of all primary malignant cancers arise in tissues with a primary involvement in obesity physiopatology.

Cancer is responsible of approximately 25% of all deaths in the US.

According to recent predictions, by 2020 the global world population will have reached 7,5 billion, with a cancer incidence and disease-specific mortality of 15 million per year and 12 million per year, respectively.

At present the total US cancer survivors population is made of 5-y cancer survivors for up to 66%, and by 2020 it has been estimated that cancer survivors aged at least 65 years will have been increased by 42% compared to now.

The diet is responsible for approximately 30-35 % of total mortality in the US, with its impact on cancer development depending on histotype and anatomic location; nutrition may play a key role in up to 70% of colorectal cancer-related deaths.

Nowadays, men and women in Occidental countries are progressively increasing in body size, with average body-mass indexes (BMI, i.e. the ratio between weight and squared height) relentlessly soaring beyond the normal range (18.5-24.9); conversely, an increasing number of individuals is falling into the overweight range (25-29.9) as well as the overt obesity range (> 30).

Obesity is easily diagnosed by assessing the increase in horizontal body dimensions compared to height.

One method for measuring such imbalance is the BMI, i.e. the ratio between weight (kilograms) and squared height (centimeters^2). BMI ranges identifying malnutrition, normal weight, overweight and different obesity degrees (mild and severe) have been defined.

BMI, however, being frequently used in epidemiological studies to assess the effect of diet as a risk factor, may become a confounding factor; indeed, BMI is less reliable in elderly patients, with height being gradually reduced due to spinal degenerative processes. Likewise, children BMI measurements may be biased by different growth rates in different body areas. Additionally, BMI fail to provide any definite information regarding body composition, i.e. the percentage of lean body mass versus fat mass, bone mineralization status, and total body water, just to name a few examples.

The value of lean body mass is critical because it is the body component consuming higher energy values per weight unit, being therefore critical for any estimations of appropriate caloric intakes.

Any diet based on caloric restriction alone would be ineffective as well as potentially dangerous if no caloric intake assessment were to be calculated according to body composition and estimated energy requirements for performing daily physical activity (including walking, writing, or accomplishing ordinary housework actions).

Obesity plays a critical role in cancer promotion, progression, and therapy resistance; obesity oncogenic actions are thought to be mediated by dysregulation of hormonal networks (i.e., circulating insuline, IGF-1, testosterone, and estrogens levels) as well as through pro-inflammatory effects due to adipose tissues cytokines.

Increased BMI values correlate with circulating inflammatory cytokines levels, that appear to be related to insulin resistance.

A positive correlation between high BMI values (>30) and cancer risk is being observed in different areas worldwide, with significant increases in cancer risk being recorded for every 5 Kg/m^2-gain in BMI.

Obesity directly promotes tissue inflammation. Lipids intake should be proportional to that of other nutrients in order to reach an adequate energy balance; in this regard, it should be remembered that 1g of fat provides approximately 9 Kcal of energy, while 1g of carbohydrates or proteins only provides 4.5 Kcal. However, specific lipids significantly differ in their chemical structure and will result in different metabolic responses when given at equal calories levels. Increased amounts of fat per portion, a phenomenon commonly occurring in restaurant and cafèteria, leads to significant inflammatory response spikes, that can be quantified by assessing increases of circulating inflammatory factors; the latter are capable of inducing insulin resistance and free radicals production, resulting in oxidation of cell structures such as nucleic acids, proteins, and membrane lipids. Other lipids possess an anti-inflammatory activity. There is plenty of literature addressing the beneficial administration of omega-3 unsaturated lipids for lessening the inflammatory consequences of several chronic diseases. Omega-3 unsaturated lipids are available either as dedicated over-the-counter preparations or through several common foods, more prominently fish and dried fruit. Omega-3 lipids are unsaturated lipids, i.e. they are in liquid form at room temperature (oils); they can easily undergo oxidation if not protected by intrinsic animals antioxidant systems or by vitamin E addition in commercially available preparations. Their content in fish meat changes according to the species, the fishing site, temperature, type of feeding (algae or other kinds of food for livestock); these features make difficult to calculate the omega-3 unsaturated lipids daily dose. Many public health authorities have been encouraging increases in diet fish intake, but it is important to know diet fish origins because of the risk related to heavy metals; it is therefore necessary to avoid eating exceedingly large amounts fish. Of course, such details are hardly specified, if ever, in epidemiological studies assessing the effects of fish-based diets. Obesity results in a status of enduring subclinical inflammation within fat tissues. In obese individuals both visceral and subcutaneous adipose tissues are infiltrated by macrophages surrounding necrotic adipocytes forming the so-called crown-like structures (CLS). The infiltrating macrophages release inflammatory cytokines whose plasma levels in post-menopausal breast cancer patients were shown to correlate with cancer progression and disease-specific mortality. In both experimental animals and humans the CLS number is directly related to BMI values.

Diets with high concentration in saturated fatty acids (cafeteria food, sausages, dairy products, red meat) are becoming more and more frequent worldwide, leading to a global escalation in overnutrition-related diseases.

Diets rich in saturated fatty acids closely correlate with metabolic syndrome and inflammation, especially inflammation of the white adipose tissue, which is not only a storage organ for lipids but also an endocrine organ.

It has been known since 1885 that hyperglycemia is more frequent among cancer patients than in the healthy population.

Warburg in 1930 highlighted the abnormal glucidic metabolism occurring in cancer cells, i.e. the so-called aerobic glycolysis, defined as the tendency of the cancer tissues to produce lactic acid even in the presence of sufficient oxygen to sustain Krebs cycle and mitochondrial membrane oxidation processes.

Glucose intolerance is an established risk factor for several cancers (including colorectal, breast, prostatic, pancreatic, and gastric cancer). Obesity and glucose intolerance are part of the metabolic syndrome, a condition characterized by increased insulin levels both during fasting and after glucose load. Metabolic syndrome, first described by Reaven in 1988, is defined by the presence of at least three of the following components: intra-abdominal or visceral obesity, glucose intolerance, hypertension, low HDL blood levels, and high triglyceride levels. In 2001, the National Cholesterol Education Program developed an alternative definition, which required the presence of at least 3 of the following 5 factors: increased waist circumference, hypertriglyceridemia, low HDL cholesterol, hypertension, and high levels of fasting glycemic levels. At the roots of metabolic syndrome there are increase in visceral fat, excessive caloric intake, and low physical activity.

The prevalence of metabolic syndrome is steadily increasing all over the world together with the increase in several types of cancer.

In subjects with glucose intolerance (IGT), both the levels of glycemia and fasting insulin are increased. The latter are coupled until glycemia reaches the concentration of 7-8 mM, a level beyond which insulin does not show further increases and may even begin to decline as a result of functional failure of pancreatic β-cells (De Fronzo 1992). This is paralleled by the gradual increase in glycemia, starting with postprandial glycemia.

Many people with newly diagnosed cancer are obese, with further changes in body structure being induced by chemotherapy, surgery, and therapy-related physical inactivity.

Chemotherapy often changes, even a year later, body composition, increasing fat mass and reducing muscle mass, creating a phenotype that could be defined as post-cancer sarcopenic obesity; the latter appears to correlate with a high risk of cancer recurrence.

Modifications in body composition in cancer patients imply that many studies conducted through questionnaires, perhaps using only one scale, were affected by significant biases. The reduction in caloric intake as a strategy to reduce obesity should be assessed on a case by case basis, followed over time, and maintained proportional with nutritional needs of the whole body in order to prevent secondary nutritional deficiencies.

The caloric intake, however, should be calibrated according to the composition of energy sources (carbohydrates, lipids, proteins); the latter, in a typical Mediterranean diet, should be in the ratio of 60%, 25%, 15%, respectively.

The American Cancer Society guidelines suggests that carbohydrates should be in the ratio of 40-65% of the energy pool, the same as for healthy population, lipids in the ratio of 20-35%, of which <10% saturated fats, and proteins should be 10-35%.

Daily protein intake should not be less than 0.8-1 grams per Kg of body weight.

Nutrition does not mean only caloric intake, but also replenishment of the very primary elements that the body uses to live. Nutritionists from different countries define the optimal daily replenishment levels of micronutrients depending on gender, age, and functional status (i.e., pregnancy, sporting activities, etc.). However, patients suffering from cancer will be almost always exhibiting to nutritional deficiencies.

Obesity itself is a malnutrition disease characterized by several deficiencies, including vitamin D deficiency. Many other deficits can be induced by specific therapies (i.e., those impairing renal tubular reabsorption through tubular damage, or intestinal absorption through mucositis, anorexia, and vomiting) and by treatments for related comorbidities (cholesterol-lowering agents, diuretics, anti-hypertensive drugs, etc...) resulting in minerals and antioxidants loss. These events may worsen the peroxidation phenomena of several biological structures, that will have been already compromised by metabolic syndrome and administration of chemotherapy.

Obesity is also associated with insulin resistance, i.e. the insulin inability, despite being available in physiological concentrations, of exerting its metabolic tasks in different body districts.

Insulin resistance assessment is performed in specialized centers, at times requiring expensive and complex methods. Such assessment could be easier by evaluation of blood glucose levels and fasting insulin levels according to the HOMA-IR algorithm, with values above 2.5 being indicative of insulin resistance.

Diet should not cause any further increase in insulin levels, either basal or food-induced.

The daily intake of carbohydrates (i.e., glycemic load) should be proportional with the body composition, the energy percentage (calculated in relation with other energy sources), and the degree of physical activity (including daily activities as well as activities planned by the rehabilitation system to reduce overweight and improve muscular function).

Carbohydrates intake should be progressively reduced throughout the day in light of the circadian increase in insulin resistance, more prominently observed during the last day hours.

Last but not least, it is necessary to avoid foods with high glycemic index (GI). The GI is determined by comparing the post prandial glycemic response of a food with the postprandial glycemic response to the same amount of available carbohydrate from a standard food in the same individual.

Baseline plasma levels of cytokines in obese people return to normal values after weight loss.

3. Diet, caloric restriction and cooking: A therapeutic way

The nutritional sources of food themselves are different from those used by our ancestors. The production doesn't respect the proximity criteria (0 km), seasonality criteria, or crop rotation criteria, resulting in a loss of micro-elements in soil. Fruits and vegetables generally meet more the preservation criteria instead of those of maturation with the result of the unpredictability of their content in terms of micronutrients.

The taste for food has been gradually changing giving priority to a rapid food intake (fast food), high levels of fat, flour and refined sugar. The large use of sweetened drinks contributes to increase the excessive energy introduction.

As for oxygen free radicals (ROS) production, it is related to inflammation during oxidative stress.

In obese patients and in those with cancer the ROS problem has a special role; supplements or diets with high content of vegetables with antioxidant activity have been given. The use of fruits and vegetables showed positive results in reducing the risk for cancer and recurrences.

Data, however, are not univocal. Each vegetable contains many different compounds, their availability is not always in relation with their content (it is a typical example for Beta carotene of carrot), the contents of a type of antioxidant may differ for the production site, stage of maturation to collection, preservation, and preparation methods (tomato sauce contains more available lycopene than raw tomato). The availability of a substance may change in different individuals according to the integrity of the intestinal mucosa (often damaged by chemotherapy) or to the kind of intestinal flora (1-1,5 kg of bacteria). This condition can also modify the food chemical structure, producing harmful or healthy substances for our health as in the case of soy isoflavones transformed into the much more active Equol only in subjects with suitable bacteria. In our blood and urine there's a large amount of products of bacterial metabolism which may influence our health; it may differ depending on the breed, gender, functional states (pregnancy) and dietary habits: there's much more complexity in epidemiological studies with the use of the food or nutritional supplements than expected in the research protocol.

The real availability (absorption) of substances in food or in supplements has a good chance to be different from that hypothesized and calculated with questionnaires or bromatological tables.

Diet should not cause any further increase in insulin levels, either basal or food-induced.

The daily intake of carbohydrates (i.e., glycemic load) should be in proportional with the body composition, the energy percentage (calculated in relation with other energy sources), and the degree of physical activity (including daily activities as well as activities planned by the rehabilitation system to reduce overweight and improve muscular function).

Carbohydrates intake should be progressively reduced throughout the day according to the circadian increase in insulin resistance, more prominently observed during the last day hours.

Last but not least, it is necessary to avoid foods with high glycemic index (GI). The GI is determined by comparing the postprandial glycemic response of a food with the postprandial glycemic response to the same amount of available carbohydrate from a standard food in the same individual.

Often using fruit we take more attention to the amount (5 servings a day) and to the concentration in antioxidants rather than the sugar content, which brings us back to the problem of calories and metabolic syndrome (fructose plugged to lead to a lower insulin response, is indeed much more dangerous than glucose for the pathogenesis of metabolic syndrome).

Diet is often unbalanced, not respecting the right proportions between carbohydrates (60%), lipids (25%) and proteins (15%).

The use of processed foods induces a higher salt intake, with effects on blood pressure and 10 on the integrity of structures such as the gastric mucosa with possible susceptibility to cancer.

The use of sweetened drinks and refined flour, without fibers, which are characteristics of white bread and pasta, causes a rapid absorption of carbohydrates and a rapid elevation of blood glucose, followed by a massive insulin response. Insulin is a hormone with multiple activities involved in the regulation of blood glucose, the transport of amino acids, the mobilization of fat from their deposits, the monitoring of urine output and of cell proliferation.

Persistent high levels of insulin indicate a loss of activity of the hormone (insulin resistance) that goes together with obesity, dyslipidemia (low HDL cholesterol, high triglycerides), high blood pressure and, according to data, even the cancer.

Fast food diets, also known with the term "Cafeteria Diet", are often characterized by an excessive fat content, often saturated, (those who melt at higher temperatures) contained in marbled meat, so defined because at a thin shear it shows impregnation of lipids within the muscle structure, typical of those animals kept under movement restriction.

A high-fatty acids diet an altered ratio between saturated and unsaturated fats, an alteration in the ratio of unsaturated omega-6 (those that have a double bond in position 6 from terminal COOH) and omega-3 (those that have the double bond in position 3, typical of fish, nuts, etc.) causes increase in blood inflammatory markers. In a state of inflammation it leads to resistance to insulin receptors, which is the first step for obesity and metabolic syndrome.

Foods with sugar and refined flour should be reduced or abolished. Bread and pasta should be made with whole grain flours, that give them a distinctive dark color, rice should be strictly integral.

As for pasta it should be investigated whether the product is integral outset or if fibers have been added to starch in a second time. The difference is huge because the slow release of the starch in an originally integral flour can give an IG <40% than the refined flour = 75%. Rice and pasta should never be overcooked.

It is absolutely necessary to avoid using fructose as an alternative to sucrose.

Salt is an important part in the preparation and storage of food. It is blamed for stomach cancer, but may be also critical for its action on blood pressure and, indirectly, on the metabolic and inflammatory situation. Very often it is not calculated in nutritional epidemiological studies in oncology.

During the cooking process an improper use of heat can turn food into a non-profit element, even dangerous for health. The use of high temperatures for long periods can produce carcinogenic substances. The use of cooking helps the extraction of carotenoids from tomatoes and carrots, but degrades the antioxidants in cruciferous vegetables, often investigated for their anticancer properties. The problem regarding the cooking should be extended to the used instruments types (oven, microwave, fry, steam, etc.).

All food should be cooked with adequate methods, tools and cooking times. A typical example may be that of the french fries, for which the interest in compositional characteristics of nutritional caused a controversy about their potential toxicity, related to frying due to the formation of acrylamide.

4. Caloric restriction

Caloric restriction is an integral part of religion requirements in several countries (Islamic Ramadan, Orthodox Church abstinence during Christmas, Easter, Assumption, the Jewish tradition of Daniel's fasting, etc.).

Over the past 30 years there have been more and more studies addressing health benefits related to caloric intake reduction in animal models and in humans.

Data seem to show that maximum benefits may be achieved by applying the highest possible calory reduction without resulting in overt malnutrition, and by prolonging this status as long as possible.

In animal models, caloric reduction of not more than 10-40% of the normal calories intake exerts an anticancer effect which is directly related to its duration.

Caloric restriction induces changes in metabolic and hormonal status in a similar way among animals and humans.

Caloric restriction improves sensitivity to insulin and improves glucose metabolism.

Caloric restriction can reduce oxidative stress.

Caloric restriction can increase life expectancy in animals; however, the restriction of carbo-hydrates or lipids alone does not seem to influence this result, which instead appears to be related to the reduction in methionine intake by lowering consumption of animal proteins. One year-long caloric restriction alone, even without physical activity, can reduce several markers of inflammation in obese postmenopausal women, including C-reactive protein, serum amyloid, and IL-6.

Accordingly, the excess of caloric intake induces obesity and represents a risk factor for cancer.

From rodents to primates, including humans, caloric restriction has been shown to be one of the most powerful tools in the prevention of carcinogenesis.

However, epidemiological data deriving from forced restrictions during the events of II World War showed conflicting results.

Conversely, Norwegians with a mean caloric intake reduction of about 50%, maintaining a balanced diet, showed a reduction in the incidence of breast cancer compared to controls.

In the Netherlands, a caloric intake reduction (70% in adults, 50% children) was paralleled by an increase in breast cancer but not in other forms of cancer.

The survivors of German and Russian concentration camps showed a sharp increase in all forms of cancer.

This apparent inconsistency of results can be due, in our opinion, to the distinction between caloric restriction and forced malnutrition characterized by the presence of other factors such as emotional stress, infections, etc.

5. Physical exercise and walking prescriptions

5.1. What do you know?

About the component of physical exercise, the American Cancer Society recommends the exercise like part of a continuum of cancer survival care.

The physical exercise is able to reduce the risk to develop the breast cancer and colon on 25% and pulmonary cancer on 30%, uterine cancer and ovary cancer about on 20% and on 9% about the prostate cancer.

After the diagnosis and the treatment there is a reduction from 26 to 40% of recruitment of Brest cancer and of colon cancer with daily physical exercise and also good quality of life.

Also during the prostate cancer the aerobic and endurance physical activity can reduce the fatigue and improve the life's quality.

During the hematological cancer especially in non-Hodgkin lymphoma and multiple myeloma, the physical exercise can improve the quality of life with reduction of fatigue and also the aerobic capability in bone marrow transplantation.

The general benefits of physical exercise in cancer treatment are numerous and include: improved cardiac output, increased ventilation, improved flexibility and range of motion; increased muscular strength and endurance; decreased resting heart rate; improved stroke volume, vasodilatation, perfusion; improved metabolic efficiency; improved blood counts; improved psychological attitude to resist to the cancer disease. The cancer-specific benefits are related to cancer treatment toxicity especially to muscular degeneration with 1) fatigue and weakness, 2) neurotoxicity, 3) cardiotoxicity, 4) pulmonary toxicity.

Our therapeutic approach using the physical exercise and walking prescriptions is divided in 3 phases to: 1) recovery of residual capacity; 2) sensory-motor and functional recovery capacity; 3) the quality of life improvement.

The recovery of residual capacity is designed to recovery joint mobility and to increase the uninjured muscle tone after reprogram of flexibility.

In the cancer patient there is usually a marked reduction of the flexibility.

Flexibility is one of the physiological parameters involved in almost all forms of the human movement and is similar to aerobic capacity, strength, and neuromuscular endurance in being a trainable fitness parameter.

Flexibility has been defined as mobility compliance and, alternatively, as the reciprocal counterpart of stiffness. Most of the authors define flexibility either as range of motion at or about a joint. Another definition represents flexibility like the ability of a joint to move throughout its potential range of motion. Those definitions confuse the property of flexibility with the criterion able to measure the range of motion and using hardly synonymous; since potential range of motion is a variable factor among others in deterring flexibility, flexibility cannot be understood simple as relative to it.

We define flexibility like the disposition of body tissues to allow, without injury, excursions at a joint or set of joints. This property is measured by, but not equivalent to, range of motion. Both joint tissues and the surrounding soft tissues contribute to flexibility, although only the latter should be modified in order to enhance flexibility.

To increase this capability is possible to use yoga, slow / static and dynamic stretching techniques, Pilates method; in our experience we prefer anyway Elispheric Imoove method (fig. 5) and exercises deriving from proprioceptive neuromuscular facilitation (PNF). This last technique is designed as a manual, partner-assisted stretching; a partner is needed to provide the fixed resistance against which the lengthened agonist isometrical contracted at or near maximum (to use spindle facilitation).

Some factors that affect flexibility are modifiable, subject to voluntary control to some or large extent, others are not modifiable.

Flexibility decreases with age. In cancer patients, it suggests that regular activities, in order to maintain elasticity, or to do specific stretching programs, are important for aging.

Gender is another factor that influences flexibility. Females are generally more flexible than males especially during the same stretching program; probably women have a larger percentage of elastin in their miofascia.

Flexibility varies during the course of the day. There is greater flexibility of cervical spine during the late afternoon and evening hours and about the lower lumbar spine data show an improvement during daytime later hours.

About the anatomical constraints, the excessive fatty tissue limits range of motion related to the tightness of soft tissue structures. This problem is connected with some conditions of diseases like arthritis, diabetes mellitus, hemophilia and finally the cancer but also is correlated to bad posture in orthostasis or with seated flexed posture.

Other ways to improve flexibility: massage, warm-up and stretching are three basic techniques used to increase flexibility but neither massage or warm-up is as efficient as a proper stretching regimen in increasing flexibility.

The best method to realize stretching involves a series of less than maximal isometric contractions of the agonist muscles in a pre-lengthened state (to set up the stretch), followed by concentric contractions of the antagonist muscle group (to lengthen the agonist) in conjunction with light pressure from a partner when needed and with an instrumentation like sensorized postural bench system (TecnoBody, Italy).Though this mode the objectives are to alleviate muscle tension, to facilitate healing by increasing blood flow, to decrease muscle pain by reducing vasoconstriction. This work is to applied day by day using at the cancer patients home a specific personalized postural bench like Fleximat postural bench (fig. 1 DeltaDue, Italy).

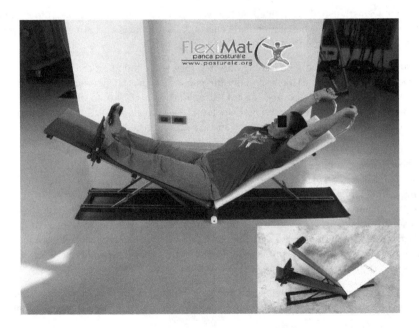

Figure 1. Fleximat

When it is not possible to get a flexibility increase in cancer treatment: there are specific contraindications, due to time and circumstances, where stretching should not be performed to get flexibility improvement. Especially when there are reduced joint receptor and pain sensation, when mobilization of tissue is not possible, for example in post-acute cancer surgical treatment or when stretching or tension in tissue elicits pain.

After the recovery the joint mobility with the flexibility replanning, the improvement of the uninjured muscle tone and strength should be possible using before focused vibratory acoustic stimulation at high intensity with Vissone (fig. 4 Vissman, Italy) and after anaerobic work with TRX system. Vibrations are able to induce muscular adaptions to the recovery of muscle tone at the 300 Hz, of frequency and to stimulate the upper motors centers in order to obtain a better performance of controls, responsible for the muscle recruitment. Is noted that so is possible to 1) activate the aerobic metabolism; 2) determine an analgesic effect; 3) increase local circulation and bone density; 4) finally increase the contractile capacity and elasticity of the muscle treated.

6. Walking prescriptions

To elicit the sensory-motor and functional recovery we need to get acceptable walking.

Human movement usually is defined by the walk and is not limited to bipedal locomotion; however, such locomotion is a fundamental part of daily life and is a prominent focus of public health physical activity guidelines.

The human gait is more complex; going one step forward, although it can start from the hip flexors of the Deep Frontal Line, especially the psoas and iliacus, afterwards, it involves the hip flexion, the knee extension, and the ankle dorsiflexion necessary to step forward, thanks to the myofascia of the Superficial Frontal Line. As the leg travels forward, the entire myofascia prepares to receive the weight of the body and the ground reaction.

Once the heel places on the ground and the step begins, the Superficial Back Line takes over as the back of leg engages into hip extension and plantar flexion. The abductors of Lateral Line, Ischio-Tibial-Tract, and the lateral compartment of the lower leg provide stability that prevents the hip adduction, while the adductor group and the other tissues of the Deep Frontal Line assist the flexion- extension motions and provide stability to the inner arch of the foot and up the inside of the leg. In the upper body, the common contralateral walking pattern involves the Functional Lines bringing the right shoulder forward to counterbalance the left leg when it swings forward and vice versa. Therefore the gist of walking capability is to improve the miofascial flexibility.

The walking objective monitoring evolution, using pedometer and accelerometer technology, offers an opportunity to perform guidelines, including recommendations for cancer patients.

All the studies in literature have used a variety of objective parameters using instruments that have been previously validated. The Yamax pedometer is considered a criterion research quality pedometer (Schneider et al., 2004), the Lifecorder's validity is well documented (Crouter et al., 2003; Schneider et al., 2004), and the ActiGraph has been adopted by national surveillance strategies (Troiano et al., 2008) and is probably the most utilized accelerometer in research today.

Therefore is possible to define with the pedometer the sedentary level into < 2,500 steps/ day (basally active) and into < 2,500 to 4,999 steps/day (limited activity); but using an established step-defined physical activity scale is possible to establish a level one for sedentary < 5,000 steps/day ; a level two >5,000 <7,499 steps/day for low active; a level three >7,500 <9,999 steps/day for somewhat active ; a level four >10,000 <12,499 steps/day for active; and a level five ≥ 12,500 steps/day for highly active.

We also noticed that healthy adults can perform between approximately 4,000 and 18,000 steps/day, and, in our opinion, also 7,500-9,9990 steps / day, resulting in between 50/ 85 steps /minute. That would be a reasonable target for the cancer patients in the first Mullan phase.

In order to get a better walking performance in the first phase of Mullan, and also in the second phase, we adopt two integrate procedures: 1) normalization of the foot-ground reaction forces using a personalized viscoelastic insoles to control vertical and shear forces on the foot during the stance phase without the obligatory use of athletic shoes; 2) use of the microgravitary system S.P.A.D (fig. 2) that determine the sensory-motor and functional recovery of the posture during the walking in combination to the development of proprioceptive information from the periphery to the cortical central system.

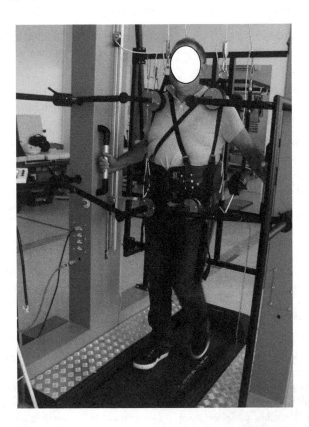

Figure 2. SPAD

7. Physical therapies connected with psychophysical techniques

During the first year after the cancer treatment the immune system shows some specific changes in patient with cancer especially in some specific T-cell populations.

There is no scientific evidence that physical therapies, like magnetic fields, are effective in the treatment of cancer itself. Global physics community perfectly knows what the extreme low frequencies and intensity of magnetic fields are. They also know how they provoke the resonance of ions (Ion Cyclotron Resonance), with the exact frequency in order to remove an ion from its orbit of rotation in order to escape.

Only in the last decades the studies in biophysics have shown that with the ion cyclotron resonance is possible to stimulate the passage of ions through the membranes of the cells of the living beings changing their permeability and therefore improving the ion exchange on both sides of the membrane itself. The increase of the bioavailability of the essential ions, makes better the efficiency of the cell itself to achieve its correct metabolism.

The role of electromagnetic fields for control of cancer pain and chemotherapy nausea-induced symptoms remains controversial but this theory is to be correlate to water coherence domains' theory (G. Preparata, E. Del Giudice, G. Talpo 1999).

The activities and the exchanges of the molecules in the body doesn't happen by chance, but they follow an "order" dictated by the magnetic field produced by the water, where all the elements fluctuate in phase in the those regions called coherence domains.

Only the molecules which react to the frequency of this magnetic field, interact with each other, starting in ordered way the correct chemical reactions necessary for life of the cell and the organism. An imbalance of this 'order' jeopardizes the functioning of the cell, with the consequence of the manifestations of the diseases.

The 40% of the water is coherent and it can receive and deliver electromagnetic information, while the remaining 60% is not coherent, equally essential for life; it represents the solvent of the ions and of the fundamental elements to the cellular economy.

Also Montagnier L. in 2009 has recognized the validity of the coherence domains, stating how the water is not an inert substance, but may take special configurations emitting electromagnetic waves that can become an not pharmacological instrument of the therapy and the adjustment, but always deeply medical care.

The cells' DNA emits extremely low frequency waves, from zero to a few hundred of Hertz. The studies were published on the unbalance of this "range" that disturbs the harmony of the cell, with the onset of the manifestations of diseases. Some chronic diseases such as Alzheimer's, Parkinson's, multiple sclerosis, rheumatoid arthritis, and the viral diseases such as HIV -AIDS, influenza A and hepatitis C, "inform" the water of our body (biological water) of their presence issuing a special electromagnetic signals that can then be "read and decoded".

With Ion Cyclotron Resonance we have the possibility to intervene in a not invasive, natural and precise adjustment mechanisms of the body's homeostasis, where the only pharmacological support can be not complete.

Therefore you get the possibility:

1. To rebalance subjective metabolism

2. To adjust the enzyme functions, the ion channels and the body pH

3. To strengthen the immune system

4. To encourage the bioavailability and absorption of nutrients for cell metabolism

5. To treat neuralgia, headaches and migraines

6. To stimulate healing in all kinds of wounds, even after surgery.

7. To balance the water retention

8. To enhance the effect of drugs and supplements

9. To detoxify and to allow antioxidant function against free radicals, metabolites, toxins

10. To stimulate a pain-killer function (acute and chronic)

11. To get muscle relaxation, from anxiety and stress

12. To improve the homeostasis recovery under stress (physiological micro trauma and muscle protein catabolism)

13. To improve the quality of life for cancer patients.

In a preliminary observational study of 43 cancer patient group, they were divided into 3 groups of 14 patients, using also the Ion Cyclotron Resonance with QUEC PHISIS QPS1 (fig. 3) we observed the initial and final values of d-ROMs Test.

The first group only used the QUEC PHISIS QPS1

The second group used the QUEC PHISIS QPS1 and the antioxidants.

The third group only used the antioxidants.

The study shows a significant improvement after 90 minutes before the beginning of the first treatment. The values are improved and consolidated in the time after a month about the end of the cycle of treatments with the values well below average.

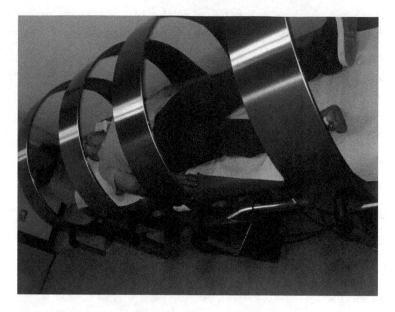

Figure 3. Qps 1

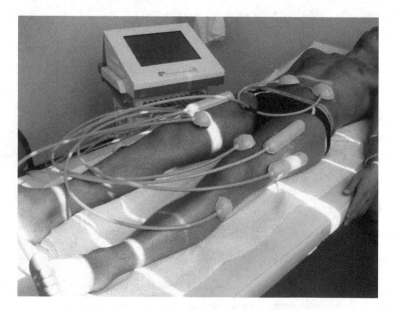

Figure 4. Viss

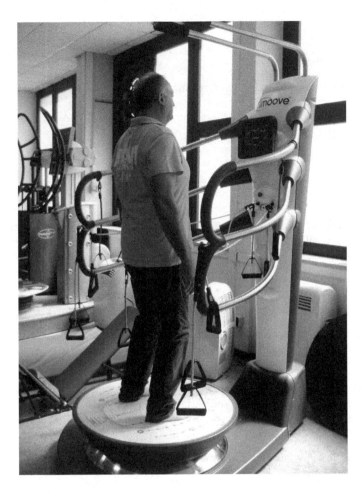

Figure 5. Imoove

8. Conclusion

The integration between the pharmacology, the biochemistry, the biophysics and the lifestyle
with energetic modulation using therapeutic diet through the use of the information and the
signals, probably will be able to restore a robust immune response in the tumor-bearing host
or to promote by adoptive transfer of activated effector cells or tumor-specific antibodies into
the tumor-bearing host.

Author details

R. Saggini[1,2] and M. Calvani[1,2]

1 Dept. of Neuroscience and Imaging, "G. d'Annunzio" University, Chieti, Italy

2 Specialitation school of Physical Medicine and Rehabilitation, "G. d'Annunzio" University, Chieti, Italy

References

[1] Amin Esfahani,, Julia M. W. Wong, Arash Mirrahimi, Korbua Srichaikul, David J. A. Jenkins, Cyril W. C. Kendall, Glycemic Index: Physiological Significance Journal of the American College of Nutrition, Vol. 28, No. 4, 439S–445S (2009).

[2] Amin Esfahani,, Julia M. W. Wong, Arash Mirrahimi, Korbua Srichaikul, David J. A. Jenkins, Cyril W. C. Kendall, Glycemic Index: Physiological Significance Journal of the American College of Nutrition, Vol. 28, No. 4, 439S–445S (2009).

[3] Arvidsson E, Viguerie N, Andersson I, Verdich C, Langin D, and Arner P. Effects of different hypocaloric diets on protein secretion from adipose tissue of obese women. *Diabetes* 53: 1966–1971, 2004.

[4] Bachelot T, Ray-Coquard I, Menetrier-Caux C, et al. Prognostic value of serum levels of interleukin 6 and of serum and plasmalevels of vascular endothelial growth factor in hormonerefractory metastatic breast cancer patients. *Br J Cancer.* 2003; 88:1721-1726.

[5] Balkau B, Barrett-Connor E, Eschwege E, et al. Diabetes and pancreatic carcinoma. Diabete Metab 1993;19:458–62.

[6] Bastard JP, Jardel C, Bruckert E, Blondy P, Capeau J, Laville M, Vidal H, and Hainque B. Elevated levels of interleukin 6 are reduced in serum and subcutaneous adipose tissue of obese women after weight loss. *J Clin Endocrinol Metab* 85: 3338–3342, 2000

[7] Bellomo R.G., Iodice P., Savoia V., Saggini A., Vermiglio G., Saggini R. (2009). Balance and posture in the elderly: an analysis of a sensorimotor rehabilitation protocol. *International journal of immunopathology and pharmacology,* vol. 22 No 3 (S), p. 37-44, ISSN: 0394-6320

[8] Bianchini F, Kaaks R, Vainio H. Overweight, obesity and cancer risk. Lancet Oncol 2002;3:565–74; Bray GA. The underlying basis for obesity: relationship to cancer. J Nutr 2002;132:3451S–5S)

[9]   Caan B, Sternfeld B, Gunderson E, et al. Life After Cancer Epidemiology (LACE) Study: a cohort of early stage breast cancer survivors (United States). Cancer Causes Control 2005;16:545–556.

[10] Calle EE, Kaaks R. Overweight, obesity and cancer: epidemiological evidence and proposed mechanisms. Nat Rev Cancer 2004;4:579 –91.

[11] Calle EE, Rodriguez C, Walker-Thurmond K, Thun MJ. Overweight, obesity, and mortality from cancer in a prospectively studied cohort of U.S. adults. N Engl J Med 2003;348:1625–1638.

[12] Calle EE, Rodriguez C, Walker-Thurmond K, Thun MJ: Overweight,obesity, and mortality from cancer in a prospectively studied cohort of U.S. adults. *N Engl J Med* 2003, 348:1625-1638.)

[13] Camoriano JK, Loprinzi CL, Ingle JN, et al.Weight change in women treated with adjuvant therapy or observed following mastectomy for node-positive breast cancer. J Clin Oncol 1990; 8:1327–1334.

[14] Cancello R, Henegar C, Viguerie N, et al. Reduction of macrophage infiltration and chemoattractant gene expression changes in white adipose tissue of morbidly obese subjects after surgeryinduced weight loss. *Diabetes*. 2005;54:2277-2286

[15] Chao A, Connell CJ, Jacobs EJ, McCullough ML, Patel AV, Calle EE, Cokkinides VE, Thun MJ. Amount, type, and timing of recreational physical activity in relation to colon and rectal cancer in older adults: the Cancer Prevention Study II Nutrition Cohort. *Cancer Epidemiol Biomarkers Prev*. 2004 Dec;13(12):2187-2195.

[16] Chia-Ming Chang, Chien-Liang Wu and Yen-Ta Lu (2012). Cancer-associated immune deficiency: A form of accelerated immunosenescence? in Mohan R. (ed.) Topics in cancer survivorship pag 95-108. InTech Croatia isbn 978-953-307-894-6.

[17] Clement K, Viguerie N, Poitou C, Carette C, Pelloux V, Curat CA, Sicard A, Rome S, Benis A, Zucker JD, Vidal H, Laville M, Barsh GS, Basdevant A, Stich V, Cancello R, and Langin D. Weight loss regulates inflammation-related genes in white adipose tissue of obese subjects. *FASEB J* 18: 1657–1669, 2004

[18] Cnop M. Fatty acids and glucolipotoxicity in the pathogenesis of Type 2diabetes. Biochem Soc Trans. 2008;36:348–52.

[19] Coleman EA, Coon S, Hall-Barrow J, et al. Feasibility of exercise during treatment for multiple myeloma. Cancer Nurs 2003;26:410–419.

[20] Colleen Doyl; Lawrence H. Kushi; Tim Byers; Kerry S. Courneya; Wendy Demark-Wahnefried; Barbara Grant; Anne McTiernan; Cheryl L. Rock; Cyndi Thompson; Ted Gansler; Kimberly S. Andrews; for The 2006 Nutrition, Physical Activity and Cancer Survivorship Advisory Committee, Nutrition and Physical ActivityDuring and After Cancer Treatment: An American Cancer Society Guidefor Informed Choices CA Cancer J Clin 2006;56:323–353.

[21] Colman,R.J. et al. (2009) Caloric restriction delays disease onset and mortality in rhesus monkeys. Science, 325, 201–204.

[22] Courneya KS, Friedenreich CM, Arthur K, Bobick TM. Physical exercise and quality of life in postsurgical colorectal cancer patients. Psychology, Health and Medicine 1999;4:181–187.

[23] Courneya KS, Friedenreich CM, Quinney HA, et al. A randomized trial of exercise and quality of life in colorectal cancer survivors. Eur J Cancer Care (Engl) 2003;12:347–357.

[24] Courneya KS, Friedenreich CM. Relationship between exercise pattern across the cancer experience and current quality of life in colorectal cancer sur vivors. J Altern Complement Med 1997;3:215–226.

[25] Courneya KS. Exercise in cancer survivors: an overview of research. Med Sci Sports Exerc 2003;35:1846–1852.

[26] Cust AE (2011) Physical activity and gynecologic cancer prevention. In: Courneya KS, Friedenreich CM (eds) Physical activity and cancer: Recent results in cancer research, vol 186. *Springer*, Berlin Heidelberg.

[27] D.L. Roberts, C.Dive, A.G Renehan Biological mechanisms linking obesity and cancer risk: new perspectives, Annu Rev Med. 2010;61:301-16.

[28] Dandona P, Mohanty P, Ghanim H, Aljada A, Browne R, Hamouda W,Prabhala A, Afzal A, Garg R: The suppressive effect of dietary restriction and weight loss in the obese on the generation of reactive oxygen species by leukocytes, lipid peroxidation, and protein carbonylation. JClin Endocrinol Metab 2001, 86:355-362.

[29] Dandona P, Weinstock R, Thusu K, et al. Tumor necrosis factor alpha in sera of obese patients: fall with weight loss. *J Clin Endocrinol Metab*. 1998;83:2907-2910.

[30] Devesa SS, Blot WJ, Stone BJ, Miller BA, Tarone RE, Fraumeni JF Jr. Recent cancer trends in the United States. J Natl Cancer Inst 1995;87:175–82.

[31] Dimeo F, Bertz H, Finke J, et al. An aerobic exercise program for patients with haematological malignancies after bone marrow transplantation. Bone Marrow Transplant 1996;18:1157–1160.

[32] Dimeo FC, Tilmann MH, Bertz H, et al. Aerobic exercise in the rehabilitation of cancer patients after high dose chemotherapy and autologous peripheral stem cell transplantation. Cancer 1997;79:1717–1722.

[33] Elias S.G. et al. (2005) The 1944–1945 Dutch famine and subsequent overall cancer incidence. Cancer Epidemiol. Biomarkers Prev., 14, 1981–1985.

[34] Emaus A, Thune I (2011) Physical activity and lung cancer prevention. In: Courneya KS, Friedenreich CM (eds) Physical activity and cancer: Recent results in cancer research, vol 186. *Springer*, Berlin Heidelberg.

[35] Enger SM, Bernstein L. Exercise activity, body size and premenopausal breast cancer survival. Br J Cancer 2004;90:2138–2141.

[36] Enger SM, Bernstein L. Exercise activity, body size and premenopausal breast cancer survival. Br J Cancer 2004;90:2138–2141.

[37] Enger SM, Greif JM, Polikoff J, Press M. Body weight correlates with mortality in ear-lystage breast cancer. Arch Surg 2004;139:954–958; discussion 58–60.

[38] F. Brayand, and B. Moller. Predicting the future burden ofcancer. Nat. Rev. Cancer. 6:63–74 (2006))

[39] Flegal KM, Carroll MD, Ogden CL, Curtin LR. 2010. Prevalence and trends in obesity among US adults, 1999–2008. *JAMA* 303:235–41; World Cancer Res. Fund/Am. Inst. Cancer Res. 2007. *Food, Nutrition, Physical Activity, and the Prevention of Cancer: A Global Perspective.* Washington, DC: Am. Inst. Cancer Res.

[40] Freund E. Diagnosis des Carcinomas. Wiener Medizinische 1885; B1:268–268

[41] Friedenreich CM (eds) Physical activity and cancer: Recent results in cancer research. *Springer,* Berlin Heidelberg

[42] G. Danaei, S. Vander Hoorn, A. D Lopez, C. J L Murray, M. Ezzati, and the Compara-tive Risk Assessment collaborating group (Cancers), Causes of cancer in the world: comparative risk assessment of nine behavioural and environmental risk factors. Lancet 2005; 366: 1784–93.

[43] Galassetti PR, Nemet D, Pescatello A, Rose-Gottron C, Larson J, Cooper DM: Exer-cise, caloric restriction, and systemic oxidative stress. J Investig Med 2006, 54:67-75.

[44] Gapstur SM, Gann PH, Colangelo LA, et al. Postload plasmaglucose concentration and 27-year prostate cancer mortality (United States). Cancer Causes Control 2001;12:763–72.

[45] Gerber M, Corpet D. Energy balance and cancers. Eur J Cancer Prev1999;8:77– 89.

[46] Harvie MN, Campbell IT, Baildam A, Howell A. Energy balance in early breast can-cer patients receiving adjuvant chemotherapy. Breast Cancer Res Treat 2004;83:201–210

[47] Haydon AM, Macinnis RJ, English DR, Giles GG. Effect of physical activity and body size on survival after diagnosis with colorectal cancer. Gut 2006;55:62–67.

[48] Hayes S, Davies PS, Parker T, et al. Quality of life changes following peripheral blood stem cell transplantation and participation in a mixedtype, moderate-intensity, exer-cise program. Bone Marrow Transplant 2004;33:553–558.

[49] Hayes SC, Rowbottom D, Davies PS, et al Immunological changes after cancer treat-ment and participation in an exercise program. Med Sci Sports Exerc 2003;35:2–9.

[50] Heilbronn L.K. et al. (2006) Effect of 6-month calorie restriction on biomarkers of lon-
      gevity, metabolic adaptation, and oxidative stress in overweight individuals: a
      randomized controlled trial. JAMA, 295, 1539–1548.

[51] Holmes MD, Chen WY, Feskanich D, et al. Physical activity and survival after breast
      cancer diagnosis. JAMA 2005;293:2479–2486.

[52] Holmes MD, Chen WY, Feskanich D, et al. Physical activity and survival after breast
      cancer diagnosis. JAMA 2005;293:2479–2486

[53] Holt LE, Pelham TW, Campagna PD. Hemodynamics during a series of machine-aid-
      ed and intensity-controlled proprioceptive neuromuscular facilitations. Can J Appl
      Physiol. 1995;20:407–416.

[54] Howell,A. et al. (2009) Energy restriction for breast cancer prevention. Recent Results
      Cancer Res., 181, 97–111

[55] Huntington MO 1985 Weight gain in patients receiving adjuvant chemotherapy for
      carcinoma of the breast. Cancer 56:472–474.

[56] Hursting SD, Berger NA. 2010. Energy balance, host-related factors, and cancer pro-
      gression. J. Clin. Oncol. 28:4058–65.

[57] Hursting SD, Sarah M.Smith, LauraM.Lashinger, Alison E.Harvey and Susan N.Per-
      kins; Calories and carcinogenesis: lessons learned from 30 years of calorie restriction.
      Research Carcinogenesis vol.31 no.1 pp.83–89, 2010.

[58] Hursting,S.D. et al. (2007) Energy balance and carcinogenesis: underlying pathways
      and targets for intervention. Curr. Cancer Drug Targets, 7, 484–491.

[59] I.Imayama, C. M. Ulrich, C.M. Alfano, C.Wang, L. Xiao, M. H. Wener, K. L. Camp-
      bell, C. Duggan, K. E. Foster-Schubert, A. Kong, C. E. Mason, C. Wang, G. L. Black-
      burn, C. E. Bain, H. J. Thompson, and A. McTiernan, Effects of a Caloric Restriction
      Weight Loss Diet and Exercise on Inflammatory Biomarkers in Overweight/Obese
      Postmenopausal Women: A Randomized Controlled Trial Cancer Res May 1, 2012 72;
      2314

[60] Institute of Medicine. Dietary Reference Intakes for Energy, Carbohydrate, Fiber, Fat,
      Fatty ,Acids ,Cholesterol, Protein, and Amino Acids (Macronutrients). Washington,
      DC: National Academy Press; 2002

[61] Iodice Pierpaolo, Bellomo Rosa Grazia, Gialluca Glauco, Fanò Giorgio, Saggini Raoul
      (2011). Acute and cumulative effects of focused high-frequency vibrations on the en-
      docrine system and muscle strength. EUROPEAN JOURNAL OF APPLIED PHYSI-
      OLOGY, vol. 111(6), p. 897-904, ISSN: 1439-6319

[62] J. F Trepanowski, R. E Canale, K. E Marshall, M. M Kabir and R. J Bloomer. Impact of
      caloric and dietary restriction regimen on markers of health and longevity in humans
      and animals: a summary of available findings. Nutrition Journal 2011, 10:107-120

[63] Jemal R., Siegel E., Ward T., Murray J., Xu and M. J. Thun. Cancer statistics, 2007. CA Cancer J. Clin. 57:43–66 (2007).

[64] Jenkins DJ, Wolever TM, Taylor RH, Barker H, Fielden H, Baldwin JM, Bowling AC, Newman HC, Jenkins AL, Goff DV: Glycemic index of foods: a physiological basis for carbohydrate exchange. Am J C.

[65] Jenkins DJ, Wolever TM, Taylor RH, Barker H, Fielden H, Baldwin JM, Bowling AC, Newman HC, Jenkins AL, Goff DV: Glycemic index of foods: a physiological basis for carbohydrate exchange. Am J C.

[66] Johnson L, Mander A, Jones L, Emmett P, Jebb S. Energy-dense, lowfiber, high-fat dietary pattern is associated with increased fatness in childhood. Am J Clin Nutr. 2008;87:846–54.

[67] Jones LW, Courneya KS, Vallance JK, et al. Association between exercise and quality of life in multiple myeloma cancer survivors. Support Care Cancer 2004;12:780–788.

[68] K. M. Huffman, L. M. Redman, L. R. Landerman, C. F. Pieper, R. D. Stevens,M. J. Muehlbauer, B. R. Wenner, J. R. Bain, V. B. Kraus, C. B. Newgard, E. Ravussin, W. E. Kraus; Caloric Restriction Alters the Metabolic Response to Mixed-Meal: Results from a Randomized, Controlled Trial. PLoS ONE April 2012, Vol 7, Iss. 4.

[69] Kagawa,Y. (1978) Impact of Westernization on the nutrition of Japanese: changes in physique, cancer, longevity and centenarians. Prev. Med., 7, 205–217.

[70] Keinan-Boker,L. et al. (2009) Cancer incidence in Israeli Jewish survivors of World War II. J. Natl Cancer Inst., 101, 1489–1500.

[71] Kien CL, Bunn JY, Ugrasbul F. Increasing dietary palmitic acid decreases fat oxidation and daily energy expenditure. Am J Clin Nutr. 2005;82:320–6.

[72] Kim DJ, Gallagher RP, Hislop TG, et al. Premorbid diet in relation to survival from prostate cancer (Canada). Cancer Causes Control 2000;11: 65–77.

[73] Kim YI. Diet, lifestyle, and colorectal cancer: is hyperinsulinemia the missing link? Nutr Rev 1998;56:275–9.

[74] Knols R, Aaronson NK, Uebelhart D, et al. Physical exercise in cancer patients during and after medical treatment: a systematic review of randomized and controlled clinical trials. J Clin Oncol 2005;23:

[75] Koupil,I. et al. (2009) Cancer mortality in women and men who survived the siege of Leningrad (1941–1944). Int. J. Cancer, 124, 1416–

[76] Kroenke CH, Chen WY, Rosner B, Holmes MD. Weight, weight gain, and survival after breast cancer diagnosis. J Clin Oncol 2005;23:1370.

[77] L. S. A. Augustin, S. Gallus, E. Negri & C. La Vecchia, Glycemic index, glycemic load and risk of gastric cancer *Annals of Oncology* 15: 581–584, 2004

[78] Loi S, Milne RL, Friedlander ML, et al. Obesity and outcomes in premenopausal and postmenopausal breast cancer. Cancer EpidemiolBiomarkers Prev 2005;14:1686–1691.

[79] Lundman P, Boquist S, Samnega°rd A, Bennermo M, Held C, Ericsson CG, Silveira A, Hamsten A, Tornvall PA. high-fat meal is accompanied by increased plasma interleukin-6 concentrations. Nutr Metab Cardiovasc Dis. 2007;17:195–202.

[80] Lynch BM, Neilson HK, Friedenreich C (2011) Physical activity and breast cancer prevention. In: Courneya KS, Friedenreich CM (eds) Physical activity and cancer: Recent results in cancer research, vol 186. *Springer*, Berlin Heidelberg.

[81] McCarty MF, Barroso-Aranda J, Contreras F: The low-methionine content of vegan diets may make methionine restriction feasible as a life extension strategy. Med Hypotheses 2009, 72:125-128.

[82] Megna M., Amico A.P., Cristella G., Saggini R., Jirillo E., Ranieri M. (2012). *Effects of herbal supplements on the immune system in relation to exercise. International journal of immunopathology and pharmacology*, vol. 25, p. 43-50, ISSN: 0394-6320

[83] Meloni G, Proia A, Capria S, et al. Obesity and autologous stem cell transplantation in acute myeloid leukemia. Bone Marrow Transplant 2001;28:365–367.

[84] Meyerhardt JA, Giovannucci EL, Holmes MD, et al. Physical activity and survival after colorectal cancer diagnosis. J Clin Oncol 2006;24:3527–3534.

[85] Meyerhardt JA, Heseltine D, Niedzwiecki D, et al. Impact of physical activity on cancer recurrence and survival in patients with stage III colon cancer: findings from CALGB 89803. J Clin Oncol 2006;24:3535–3541.

[86] Michels,K.B. et al. (2004) Caloric restriction and incidence of breast cancer. JAMA, 291, 1226–1230.

[87] Miller RA, Buehner G, Chang Y, Harper JM, Sigler R, Smith-Wheelock M: Methionine-deficient diet extends mouse lifespan, slows immune and lens aging, alters glucose, T4, IGF-I and insulin levels, and increases hepatocyte MIF levels and stress resistance. Aging Cell 2005, 4:119-125.

[88] Morris PG, Hudis CA, Giri D, et al. Inflammation and increased aromatase expression occur in the breast tissue of obese women with breast cancer. *Cancer Prev Res (Phila)*. 2011;4:1021-1029.

[89] Mullan F. (1985).Seasons of Survival: Reflections of a Physician with Cancer N Engl J Med 1985; 313:270-273 July 25, 1985.

[90] Myers T.W. (2001). Anatomy Trains. Churchill Livingstone isbn 0-443-06351-6.

[91] N. Parekh, U. Chandranand E. V. Bandera. Obesity in Cancer Survival Annu. Rev. Nutr. 2012.32:311-342.

[92] Olefsky JM, Glass CK. Macrophages, inflammation, and insulin resistance. *Annu Rev Physiol.* 2010;72:219-246.

[93] Pan SY, Morrison H (2011) Physical activity and hematologic cancer prevention. In: Courneya KS, Friedenreich CM (eds) Physical activity and cancer: Recent results in cancer research, vol 186. *Springer*, Berlin Heidelberg.

[94] Parry C, Kent EE, Mariotto AB,AlfanoCM,Rowland JH. 2011. Cancer survivors: a booming population. *Cancer Epidemiol. Biomarkers Prev.* 20:1996–2005; Cancer Soc. 2011. *Cancer Facts & Figures 2011.* Atlanta, GA: Am. Cancer Soc. http://www.cancer.org/acs/groups/content/@epidemiologysurveilance/documents/document/acspc-029771)

[95] Patrick G. Morris, MD, MSc, Kotha Subbaramaiah, PhD,Andrew J. Dannenberg, MD, and Clifford A. Hudis, MD; Inflammation in the Pathogenesis and Progression of Breast Cancer educational summaries ?

[96] Pietrangelo T, Mancinelli R, Toniolo L, Cancellara L, Paoli A, Puglielli C, Iodice P, Doria C, Bosco G, D'Amelio L, di Tano G, Fulle S, Saggini R, Fanò G, Reggiani C. (2009). Effects of local vibrations on skeletal muscle trophism in elderly people: mechanical, cellular, and molecular events. International journal of molecular medicine, vol. 24, p. 503-512, ISSN: 1107-3756.

[97] R. A. De Fronzo, R C. Bonadonna, E. Ferrannini, Pathogenesis of NIDDM. A Balanced Overview. 1992 , Diabetes Care, 15:318-368.

[98] R. A. De Fronzo, R C. Bonadonna, E. Ferrannini, Pathogenesis of NIDDM. A Balanced Overview. 1992 , Diabetes Care, 15:318-368.

[99] R. Doll, and R. Peto. The causes of cancer: quantitative estimates of avoidable risks of cancer in the United States today. J. Natl. Cancer Inst. 66:1191–308 (1981); W. C. Willett. Diet and cancer. Oncologist. 5:393–404 (2000).

[100] R. J. Freedman, N. Aziz, D. Albanes, T. Hartman, D. Danforth, S. Hill, N. Sebring, J. C. Reynolds, And J. A. Yanovski Weight and Body Composition Changes during and after Adjuvant Chemotherapy in Women with Breast Cancer, The Journal of Clinical Endocrinology & Metabolism 89(5):2248–2253

[101] Reaven GM. Banting lecture 1988. Role of insulin resistance in human disease. Diabetes 1988;37:1595– 607.

[102] Redman,L.M. et al. (2009) Metabolic and behavioral compensations in response to caloric restriction: implications for the maintenance of weight loss. PLoS One, 4, e4377.

[103] Rise'rus U. Fatty acids and insulin sensitivity. Curr Opin Clin Nutr Metab Care. 2008;11:100–5.

[104] S. H. Saydah, C. M. Loria, M. S. Eberhardt, and F. L. Brancati. Abnormal Glucose Tolerance and the Risk of Cancer Death in the United State Am J Epidemiol 2003;157:1092–1100s.

[105] Saggini R. and Calvani M. (2012). Rehabilitation in cancer survivors: interaction between lifestyle and physical activity in Mohan R. (ed.) Topics in cancer survivorship pag 177-194. InTech Croatia isbn 978-953-307-894-6.

[106] Saggini R., Bellomo R.G., Iodice P., Lessiani G. (2009). Venous insufficiency and foot dysmorphism: effectiveness of visco-elastic rehabilitation systems on veno-muscle system of the foot and of the calf. *International journal of immunopathology and pharmacology*, vol. 22, No 3 (S), p. 1-8. ISSN: 0394-6320.

[107] Saggini R., Bellomo R.G., Saggini A., Iodice P., Toniato E. (2009). Rehabilitative treatment for lock pain with external pulsed electromagnetic fields. *International journal of immunopathology and pharmacology*, vol. 22 No 3 (S), p. 25-28, ISSN: 0394-6320

[108] Saggini R., Calvani M., Bellomo Rosa Grazia, Saggini Andrea (2008). Rehabilitation in cancer survivors: interaction between lifestyle and physical activity. *European journal of inflammation*, vol. 6, p. 99-104, ISSN: 1721-727.

[109] Schmitz KH, Holtzman J, Courneya KS, et al. Controlled physical activity trials in cancer survivors: a systematic review and meta-analysis. Cancer Epidemiol Biomarkers Prev 2005;14:1588–1595.

[110] Schoen RE, Tangen CM, Kuller LH, et al. Increased blood glucose and insulin, body size, and incident colorectal cancer. J Natl Cancer Inst 1999;91:1147–54.

[111] Segal RJ, Reid RD, Courneya KS, et al. Resistance exercise in men receiving androgen deprivation therapy for prostate cancer. J Clin Oncol 2003;21:1653–1659.

[112] Shaw JE, Hodge AM, de Courten M, et al. Isolated post-challenge hyperglycaemia confirmed as a risk factor for mortality. Diabetologia 1999;42:1050–4.

[113] Siegel R, Ward E, Brawley O, Jemal A. 2011. Cancer statistics, 2011: the impact of eliminating socioeconomic and racial disparities on premature cancer deaths. *CA Cancer J. Clin.* 61:212–36).

[114] Skrha J, Kunesova M, Hilgertova J, Weiserova H, Krizova J, Kotrlikova E: Short-term very low calorie diet reduces oxidative stress in obese type 2 diabetic patients. Physiol Res 2005, 54:33-39.

[115] Stoll BA. Western nutrition and the insulin resistance syndrome: a link to breast cancer. Eur J Clin Nutr 1999;53:83–7.

[116] Tretli,S. et al. (1996) Lifestyle changes during adolescence and risk of breast cancer: an ecologic study of the effect of World War II in Norway. Cancer Causes Control, 7, 507–512.

[117] Vallance JK, Courneya KS, Jones LW, Reiman T. Differences in quality of life between non- Hodgkin's lymphoma survivors meeting and not meeting public health exercise guidelines. Psychooncology 2005;14:979–991.

[118] Vallejo,E.A. (1957) [Hunger diet on alternate days in the nutrition of the aged.]. Prensa Med. Argent., 44, 119–120.

[119] van Kruijsdijk RC, van der Wall E, Visseren FL. Obesity and cancer: the role of dysfunctional adipose tissue. *Cancer Epidemiol Biomarkers Prev*. 2009;18:2569-2578.

[120] Vanio H, Bianchini F. IARC Handbooks of Cancer Prevention. Volume 6: Weight Control and Physical Activity. Lyon, France: International Agency for Research on Cancer; 2002.

[121] Vanio H, Bianchini F. IARC Handbooks of Cancer Prevention. Volume 6: Weight Control and Physical Activity. Lyon, France: International Agency for Research on Cancer; 2002.

[122] Vastag B: Obesity Is Now on Everyone's Plate. *Jama* 2004,291:1186-1188)

[123] Vozarova B, Weyer C, Hanson K, et al. Circulating interleukin-6 in relation to adiposity, insulin action, and insulin secretion. *Obes Res*. 2001;9:414-417).

[124] Walford RL, Mock D, MacCallum T, Laseter JL: Physiologic changes in humans subjected to severe, selective calorie restriction for two years in biosphere 2: health, aging, and toxicological perspectives. Toxicol Sci 1999, 52:61-65.

[125] Walford RL, Mock D, Verdery R, MacCallum T: Calorie restriction inbiosphere 2: alterations in physiologic, hematologic, hormonal, and biochemical parameters in humans restricted for a 2-year period. J Gerontol A Biol Sci Med Sci 2002, 57:B211-24.

[126] Warburg O. The metabolism of tumors. London, United Kingdom: Constable Press, 1930.

[127] WCRF/AICR: Food, nutrition and the prevention of cancer: aglobal perspective:. World Cancer Research Fund / American Institute for Cancer Research 1997.

[128] Weiss EP, Racette SB, Villareal DT, Fontana L, Steger-May K, Schechtman KB,Klein S, Holloszy JO, Washington University School of Medicine CALERIE Group: Improvements in glucose tolerance and insulin action induced by increasing energy expenditure or decreasing energy intake: a randomized controlled trial. Am J Clin Nutr 2006, 84:1033-1042.

[129] White E, Lee CY, Kristal AR. Evaluation of the increase in breast cancer incidence in relation to mammography use. J Natl Cancer Inst 1990;82:1546 –52.

[130] Windsor PM, Nicol KF, Potter J. A randomized, controlled tr ial of aerobic exercise for treatment-related fatigue in men receiving radical external beam radiotherapy for localized prostate carcinoma. Cancer 2004;101:

[131] Wolin KY, Tuchman H (2011) Physical activity and gastrointestinal cancer prevention. In: Courneya KS.

Supportive Care for Cancer Patients

Impact of Cancer Treatment on Reproductive Health and Options for Fertility Preservation

Kenny A. Rodriguez-Wallberg

Additional information is available at the end of the chapter

1. Introduction

1.1. Cancer in patients of reproductive age

Cancer is in general regarded as a disease of elderly people. Nevertheless, although age is the most significant risk factor for cancer in both sexes, young adults and children may also develop cancer diseases. Overall, men have a 45% risk of developing cancer at some time during their lives. For women, this risk is a bit lower, approximately 37% [1] and thus, in many cases, male and female cancer patients would be young and may not have been started building their families at the time of diagnosis. In people younger than 39 years, the risk of cancer is of about 1/72 for men and 1/51 for women. This risk increases with aging and between 40-59 years, 1/12 men and 1/11 women will develop cancer [1].

The majority of children, adolescents, and young adults diagnosed with cancer today will become long-term survivors. One primary concern of cancer survivors will be the ability to reproduce and have children. Detrimental effects on the reproductive system following cancer treatment have shown to negatively affect quality of life[2], [3]. Large studies of women and men with cancer have reported that the risk of infertility related to their treatments may be an important issue for those who have not yet started or completed their family size [2], [4].

2. Cancer treatment modalities with impact in reproductive health

Cancer surgery may have impact in fertility by removing reproductive organs or damaging structures needed for reproduction. Chemotherapy and radiotherapy have toxic effects on the gonads and may in certain cases induce ovarian and testicular failure, affecting thus all aspects of reproductive health, including pubertal development, impairment of hormone production and sexual function in adults. Effects of cancer biological therapy on gametes and reproductive organs are not yet established.

3. Cancer surgery may cause infertility

Surgery is currently the most effective treatment for cancer and eventually up to 100% of patients may be cured when complete removal of the tumor is achieved. Surgery may also be indicated for cancer prophylaxis, such as the case of premalignant disease of the cervix in female patients. In those very early stages of cervix cancer, the conization of a significant part of the cervix, may offer to patients a complete disease-free survival. However, in case of loop excisions, even if they are small, surgery of the cervix may induce subfertility by affecting the normal functioning of the cervix and its glandular secretion. Infertility induced by those interventions may be overcomed by using assisted reproductive technologies, such as treating the patient with intrauterine insemination or performing In Vitro Fertilization, IVF.

Surgery may also affect future fertility if there is removal or damage of the reproductive organs. In male patients, surgery for pelvic cancer such as for prostate, bladder or colon cancer may damage nerves and affect potency or ejaculation. Further on, surgical adjuvant treatment by removing the gonads may be indicated in female and male patients with hormone sensitive tumors.

In case of large tumors, neo-adjuvant chemotherapy and radiation may be indicated as first line treatment aiming to a reduction of tumor size and control of subclinical metastatic disease before surgical treatment. Neo-adjuvant therapy is usually planned before surgery in female patients with stage III breast cancer and young male cancer patients with bulky testicular cancer.

3.1. Cancer surgery aiming at preserving fertility

Fertility-sparing surgery may be an option for selected patients who wish to retain the ability to achieve a pregnancy. In many cases, pregnancies will occur spontaneously, nevertheless, causes of subfertility may be present in some patients, and a number of those may further require assisted reproduction treatments [5]. In gynecologic and urologic oncologic surgery, there has been a gradual development of fertility-sparing surgery aiming at preserving reproductive organs without compromising survival. Indications for fertility-sparing surgery include, in general, a well-differentiated low-grade tumor in its early stages or with low malignant potential.

3.2. Fertility sparing surgery in female patients

Table 1 presents a compilation of current data on fertility sparing surgery for young female patients with gynaecological cancer. In cases of selected ovarian tumors i.e. borderline tumors, young female patients may be offered a single oophorectomy aiming at preserving the uterus and the contralateral ovary[6].

Diagnosis	Type of surgery	Description	Obstetric outcome	Oncologic outcome
Cervical cancer stage IA1,1A2,1B1	Radical vaginal trachelectomy	Laparoscopic pelvic lymphadenectomy. Vaginal resection of the cervix and surrounding parametria keeping the corpus of the uterus and the ovaries intact	Spontaneous pregnancies described in up to 70%. Risk of second trimester pregnancy loss and preterm delivery	Rates of recurrence and mortality are comparable to those described for similar cases treated by means of radical hysterectomy or radiation therapy
Borderline ovarian tumors FIGO stage I	Unilateral oophorectomy	Removal of the affected ovary only, keeping in place the unaffected one and the uterus	Pregnancies have been reported and favorable obstetric outcome	Oncologic outcome is comparable with the more radical approach of removing both ovaries and the uterus. Recurrence 0-20% vs 12-58% when only cystectomy was performed
Ovarian epithelial cancer stage I, grade 1	Unilateral oophorectomy	Removal of the affected ovary only, keeping in place the unaffected one and the uterus	Pregnancies have been reported and favorable obstetric outcome	7% recurrence of the ovarian malignancy and 5% deaths
Malignant ovarian germ cell tumors/sex cord stromal tumors	Unilateral oophorectomy	Removal of the affected ovary only	Pregnancies have been reported and favorable obstetric outcome	Risk of recurrence similar to historical controls
Endometrial adenocarcinoma Grade 1, stage 1A (without myometrial or cervical invasion)	Hormonal treatment with progestational agents for 6 months	Follow-up with endometrial biopsies every 3 months	Pregnancies have been reported	Recurrence rate 30-40%. Five percent recurrence during progesterone treatment

Table 1. Fertility-sparing interventions in female patients. Reprinted, with permission from Rodriguez-Macias Wallberg et al, *J Pediatric Blood & Cancer, 2009*, Ref [6].

The most established surgical procedure for fertility preservation of women is the radical trachelectomy described first by Dargent in 1994 [7]. It is currently offered in cases of invasive cervical cancer in early stages to patients interested in preserving fertility. About 500 cases have been reported worldwide, most of them in European countries, Japan, U.S.A, Canada and China [8-12].

The global utilization of fertility-sparing surgery in female patients is currently unknown. A recent European study collecting data from several countries demonstrated a low incidence of those procedures and it raised concerns on the need to centralize fertility sparing treatments of gynaecological cancer at accredited units, to ensure a sufficient number of patients at each center aiming at maintaining thus healthcare quality [13].

3.3. Cervical cancer and fertility sparing surgery during pregnancy

In pregnant women, the gynaecological cancer most commonly diagnosed is also the cancer of the cervix, usually detected at an early stage in those patients. The treatment of pregnant women should be established in the same way as in non-pregnant patients, based on the stage of the disease according to the International Federation of Gynecology (FIGO). Nevertheless, individualization of the treatment should be considered based on the desire to continue the pregnancy, the gestational age and the risks of modifying or delaying cancer treatment during the pregnancy. Clinical practice guidelines by the European Society for Medical Oncology ESMO are available on this respect [14]. Both abdominal radical trachelectomy [15] and vaginal trachelectomy [16] with lymphadenectomies have been reported during pregnancy to preserve an ongoing pregnancy and female fertility.

3.4. Fertility sparing surgery in males

In men, a partial orchidectomy has become an established method to preserve hormonal and sperm production in carefully selected patients. This method, originally developed for treatment of benign teratomas in prepubertal patients, has shown good results when adopted for treatment of testicular malignancies in adults [17]. Data from The German Testicular Cancer Study Group reported a 98.6% disease-free survival rate at 7 years follow-up after conservative surgery of tumors <2 cm [18].

4. Radiotherapy treatments and their impact in reproductive health

Radiation therapy is a component of curative therapy for a number of diseases, including those presenting frequently in young patients such as breast cancer, Hodgkin's disease, head and neck cancer and gynecologic cancers. It is often indicated for the treatment of prostate cancer as well.

It is known that cancer cells present with defects in their ability to repair sub-lethal DNA whereas normal cells have the ability to recover. Although radiation therapy is aimed to a loco-regional application and although cancer cells are the target, radiation may also induce damage to normal cells in the tissues.

The response to radiation therapy depends on various factors such as the phase of cell cycle the cells are (cells in late G1 and S are more resistant), the degree of cell ability to repair the DNA damage and other factors such as hypoxia (hypoxic cells are more resistant), tumor mass and growth fraction. Non-dividing cells are more resistant than dividing cells.

Except for the bone marrow, the most sensitive organs to radiation therapy in the body are the gonads, both the male testis and the female ovary. The extent of damage in the female and male gonads depends on the dose, fractionation schedule and irradiation field [19] [20]. Radiation therapy can be administered as teletherapy, which aims at treating a large volume of tissue. For small volumes of tissue, such as in the case of cervix cancer in the female, radiation therapy can be administered in encapsulated sources of radiation that can be implanted directly into or adjacent to tumor tissue.

Whenever female reproductive organs are involved in the irradiated field, i.e., the ovaries, the uterus and the vagina may be compromised and damaged by direct irradiation. Scattered radiation may also damage reproductive organs. In the female, radiation therapy results in dose-related damage of the gonads by the destruction of primordial follicles, which constitute the nonrenewable follicle pool. In women, the degree and persistence of the damage is also influenced by age at the time of exposure to radiotherapy and due to a reduced reserve of primordial follicles in older women, the number of follicles remaining may be also be reduced at older ages [21]. Table 2 presents a compilation of current knowledge on the impact of radiation doses and age at radiotherapy in male and female gonadal function [22]. In general, a dose of about 2 Gy applied to the gonadal area destroys up to 50 % of the ovarian follicle reserve. In pediatric patients, failure in pubertal development may be the first sign of gonadal failure in both sexes. Total body irradiation (TBI) given in conjunction with myeloablative conditioning prior to bone marrow transplantation is one of the most toxic treatments for the gonads and it is highly related to gonadal failure in both sexes [23] [24].

High risk of prolonged azoospermia in men or amenorrhea in women
Total Body Irradiation (TBI) for bone marrow transplant/stem cell transplant (9,15,16)
Testicular radiation dose "/>2.5 Gy in adult men (9,17)
Testicular radiation dose ≥ 6 Gy in pre-pubertal boys (18,19)
Pelvic or whole abdominal radiation dose ≥ 6 Gy in adult women (20,21,22)
Pelvic or whole abdominal radiation dose ≥ 10 Gy in post-pubertal girls (21,22,23,24)
Pelvic radiation or whole abdominal dose ≥ 15 Gy in pre-pubertal girls (21,22,23,24)
Intermediate risk
Testicular radiation dose 1-6 Gy from scattered pelvic or abdominal radiation (13,16)
Pelvic or whole abdominal radiation dose 5-10 Gy in post-pubertal girls (21,24)
Pelvic or whole abdominal radiation dose 10-15 Gy in pre-pubertal girls (21,22,24)
Craniospinal radiotherapy dose ≥ 25 Gy (14)

Table 2. Radiotherapy protocols with high or intermediate impact on ovarian and testicular function. Reprinted, with permission from Rodriguez-Wallberg and Oktay, *J Ped Hematol Oncol*, 2010, Ref [22].

In men, the gonadal stem cells responsible for the continual differentiation and production of mature spermatozoa, the spermatogoniae, are extremely sensitive to radiation. The Leydig cells, which are responsible for the hormonal production of testosterone, are on the contrary more resistant to radiotherapy and adult patients may thus preserve hormonal production although becoming infertile. In prepubertal boys, the sensitivity to radiation therapy of Leydig cells is greater than that of older males at very high doses [25]. Prepubertal patients may retain Leydig cell function after radiation therapy during childhood and in those cases they will present with normal pubertal development and well-preserved sexual function later in life. Nevertheless, most of those patients present at adulthood with reduced testicular size, impaired spermatogenesis and infertility.

4.1. Gonadal shielding and ovarian transposition

The standard medical procedure currently offered to reduce scatter radiation to reproductive organs and preserve fertility in male and female patients, both adult and prepubertal, is the use of shielding. When shielding of the gonadal area is not possible, the surgical fixation of the ovaries in females far from the radiation field known as oophoropexy (ovarian transposition) may be considered. It is estimated that this procedure significantly reduces the risk of ovarian failure by about 50% and those patients may retain some menstrual function and fertility [26]. Scattered radiation and damage of the blood vessels that supply the ovaries are related to the failure of this procedure [26].

4.2. Radiotherapy of the uterus

Radiotherapy of the uterus in young women and girls has shown to induce tissue fibrosis, restricted uterine capacity, restricted blood flow and impaired uterine growth during pregnancy, as shown by follow-up of cancer survivors [27] [28]. The uterine damage seems to be more pronounced in the youngest patients at the time of radiotherapy. As a consequence, radiotherapy-treated female patients present with a high risk of unfavorable pregnancy outcomes such as spontaneous abortion, premature labor and low birth weight offspring [27] [28]. Irradiation of the vagina is related to fertility and sexual issues due to loss of lubrication, anatomical impairments and in some cases vaginal stenosis.

4.3. Cranial irradiation and hormonal dysfunction

Cranial irradiation may induce disruption of the hypothalamic-pituitary-gonadal axis, which is a recognized potential complication that can lead to infertility in both female and male patients. Follow-up of female patients treated for brain tumors with cranial irradiation post- and pre-pubertally has evidenced a high incidence of primary hypothalamic and pituitary dysfunction with consecuent disturbance in gonadotropin secretion. In some cases, precocious puberty may also be induced by cranial irradiation in childhood, which has been attributed to cortical disruption and loss of inhibition by the hypothalamus.

5. Impact of chemotherapy in reproductive health

Chemotherapy given as only treatment may be curative for a series of cancer presenting in young adults and children. In a vast majority of cancer treatments, chemotherapy protocols combine several agents and there is a possibility of a synergistic gonadotoxic effect[29]. In the female, primordial ovarian follicles including their oocytes and granulosa cells are particularly sensitive to alkylating agents, which induce apoptosis, as demonstrated in vitro [26], and in vivo using human ovarian tissue xenotransplanted in SCID mouse [30]. Ovarian failure is thus common after alkylating treatment [22].

Because of a high ovarian reserve with high numbers of follicles in young women, the risk of developing ovarian failure and permanent infertility after a cancer treatment is lower in younger than in older women [21]. Younger patients at the time of cancer treatment have thus a higher chance of recovering ovarian function following chemotherapy, nevertheless their fertility window might be reduced, and they should be recommended not to delay childbearing for too long [31].

5.1. Clinical evaluation of ovarian reserve

The development of amenorrhea should be considered unfavorable as it may be due to permanent gonadal failure. On the other hand, the presence of cycles should not be interpreted as proof of fertility. In the clinical setting, a gynecological examination including ultrasonography and estimation of antral follicle counts together with the determination of hormones such as follicle-stimulating hormone (FSH) and estradiol, inhibin and anti-mullerian hormone (AMH), may help the clinician in evaluating patient's remaining ovarian reserve after a cancer treatment and providing counseling on her chances to obtain a pregnancy.

5.2. Conception following chemotherapy

Due to toxicity of cancer treatments on growing oocytes, patients should be advised to avoid conception in the 6 -12 month period immediately following completion of chemotherapy treatment [32]. There is a high risk of teratogenesis during or immediately following chemotherapy, nevertheless DNA integrity has shown to return over time after a cancer treatment and thus no increase in childhood malignancies or genetic malformations have been shown in a large follow-up of more than 4000 children of cancer survivors [33].

5.3. Chemotherapy in males

In male patients, prepubertal status does not provide protection from gonadal damage and alkylating agents at high doses induce germ cell injury although Leydig cell function is commonly preserved [29]. Because most chemotherapy agents are given as part of a combination regimen, it has been difficult to quantify the gonadotoxicty of individual drugs.

Table 3 summarizes the gonadotoxic impact of chemotherapy agents on the female ovary and male testis.

High risk of prolonged azoospermia in men or amenorrhea in women
Cyclophosphamide
Ifosphamide
Melphalan
Busulfan
Nitrogen mustard
Procarbazine
Chlorambucil
Intermediate risk
Cisplatin with low cumulative dose
Carboplatin with low cumulative dose
Adriamycin
Low risk
Treatment protocols for Hodgkin lymphoma without alkylating agents
Bleomycin
Actinomycin D
Vincristine
Methotrexate
5 fluorouracil

Table 3. Chemotherapy agents with high or intermediate gonadotoxic impact in women and men

6. Options to preserve fertility by using cryopreservation methods

In 2006, an expert panel commissioned by the American Society of Clinical Oncology ASCO published guidelines for fertility preservation for male and female patients [26]. Established cryopreservation methods for fertility preservation available for adult female and male cancer patients before starting cancer treatments included sperm freezing for male patients and embryo cryopreservation following ovarian stimulation with gonadotropins and In Vitro Fertilization, IVF for females. All remaining options were still considered experimental at that time and they included the freezing of unfertilized oocytes for adult women and the cryopreservation of gonadal tissue, ovarian or testicular, both methods still under development which constitute the only options that can be offered to pre-pubertal children (Figure 1).

Recently, by the end of 2012, the methods for cryopreservation of oocytes by vitrification techniques have markedly improved and thus freezing of unfertilized eggs is currently becoming an established clinical option for female patients.

Strategies for fertility preservation in males and females

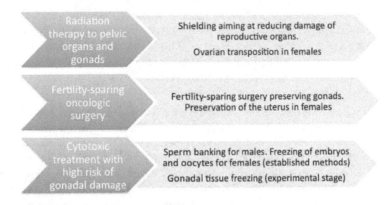

Radiation therapy to pelvic organs and gonads — Shielding aiming at reducing damage of reproductive organs.
Ovarian transposition in females

Fertility-sparing oncologic surgery — Fertility-sparing surgery preserving gonads.
Preservation of the uterus in females

Cytotoxic treatment with high risk of gonadal damage — Sperm banking for males. Freezing of embryos and oocytes for females (established methods)
Gonadal tissue freezing (experimental stage)

Rodriguez-Wallberg, 2013

Figure 1. Strategies for fertility preservation in males and females

6.1. Sperm banking for male patients

As many children are born after fertility treatments using frozen-thawed sperm, the cryopreservation of ejaculated semen is regarded as an established fertility preservation method in adult patients and pubertal boys. Although spermatogenesis starts in the pre-pubertal period and mature spermatozoa can be found at a Tanner III stage with a testis volume above 5 ml, spermatozoa production is generally effective only at the age of 13-14 years [33]. Sperm cryopreservation has been reported in adolescent patients from the age of 13 years with a high prevalence of normal sperm counts and semen volumes [34] [35]. Traditionally, sperm banking by cryopreservation of at least three semen samples with an abstinence period of at least 48 hours in between the samples has been recommended for adult males desiring to preserve their fertility [36].

In the situation of ejaculation failure, the search for spermatozoa in a urine sample could be proposed. When failure in obtaining a semen sample in young men and adolescents, a testicular sperm extraction TESE can be performed to retrieve spermatozoa [35]. Other methods described to retrieve spermatozoa in adolescents include penile vibratory stimulation and electro ejaculation.

6.2. Cryopreservation of embryos or oocytes after controlled ovarian stimulation in females

Adult women wishing to preserve fertility may undergo controlled ovulation stimulation with gonadotropins, for retrieval of matured oocytes and egg freezing, or, if the woman wishes, for in vitro fertilization (IVF) of the retrieved eggs and freezing of embryos. In general, controlled ovarian stimulation with gonadotropins for IVF may require only two weeks to achieve, as it has been shown that a random-start in the stimulation cycle, independently of cycle day, does not have a negative impact on the number and quality of oocytes retrieved.

Oocyte retrieval is undertaken usually by vaginal ultrasound assistance under sedation or general anaesthesia. Fertilization of the oocytes for embryo cryopreservation has traditionally been offered to woman having a partner. Transfer of frozen/thawed embryos today is a clinical routine in fertility clinics worldwide and it has been used for over 25 years. Intact embryos after thawing have similar implantation potential as fresh embryos and this treatment can lead to a 59% pregnancy rate and a 26% live birth rate [37].

Freezing unfertilized oocytes aiming at later thawing and fertilizing them by IVF is also a promising option to preserve fertility today. As the methods for cryopreservation of eggs have notably developed in recent years with the development of vitrification techniques, improving success in oocyte survival and fertilization rates has been achieved, approaching that of fresh oocytes. Worldwide, an increasing number of pregnancies and children born after fertilization of frozen-thaw noocytes has been reported and although overall pregnancy rates are still relatively lower than those with embryo freezing [38-40], pregnancy rates and livebirths after thawing and fertilizing frozen eggs are currently reaching those obtained after embryo cryopreservation [41].

6.3. Ovarian stimulation using aromatase inhibitors to maintain low systemic estradiol levels in case of breast cancer

Ovarian stimulation with gonadotropins before egg retrieval aims at obtaining more than one oocyte per cycle and it is a key component of the success of IVF.

In women with an estrogen-sensitive tumor, the elevation of circulating estradiol levels during ovulation stimulation is undesirable and it has been regarded as potentially harmful. Therefore, hormone positive breast cancer patients have been largely excluded of the option to preserve fertility aiming at freezing eggs or embryos [42].

Alternative protocols, including natural cycle IVF (without hormone stimulation) or inducing ovulation by using Selective Estrogen Receptor Modulators (SERMs) and aromatase inhibitors alone or in combination with gonadotropins have been proposed, as they might be potentially safer. Natural cycle IVF gives only one oocyte or embryo per cycle and this treatment protocol has a high rate of cycle cancellation.

Both tamoxifen and letrozole can be administered alone or alongside with gonadotropins to increase the number of oocytes yielded for cryopreservation. Stimulation protocols using letrozole alongside with gonadotropins have shown to be most effective resulting in higher number of oocytes obtained and fertilized when compared to tamoxifen protocols [43]. The short-term follow-up of breast cancer patients having undergone ovarian stimulation with letrozole for fertility preservation has not shown any detrimental effects on survival [44].

Although aromatase inhibitors are contraindicated during pregnancy, data indicate that fertility treatments with letrozole are safe and the use of letrozole before conception does not induce any increased risks for the fetus [45]. Letrozole is currently used in the treatment of anovulatory infertility in many countries.

6.4. Cryopreservation of immature oocytes obtained without hormonal stimulation

Freezing immature oocytes is also an option for female fertility preservation in case of patients having a contraindication for hormonal stimulation or when there is not time available for stimulation. The oocytes are retrieved in the natural cycle and frozen at an immature stage or after maturation *in vitro* (IVM) [46]. Immature oocytes survive cryopreservation better than mature metaphase II oocytes [47]. After thawing they can be matured in vitro and fertilized. In vitro maturation of oocytes is at an experimental stage and needs further development. Only few fertility centers worldwide offer treatments using this technique.

6.5. Ovarian tissue freezing for prepubertal and adult patients

As the vast majority of eggs making up the ovarian reserve are within primordial follicles in the ovarian cortex, small cortical ovarian biopsies may provide a high number of eggs to be preserved. This procedure is usually performed by laparoscopy, can be planned immediately after the diagnosis of malignant disease and does not require hormonal stimulation. In cases when the patient needs to undergo abdominal surgery for the treatment of cancer, the ovarian tissue can be harvested during the same surgical procedure. Although it is preferable to carry out cryopreservation of ovarian tissue before a gonadotoxic treatment, young women, adolescents and girls have normally an abundant number of primordial follicles in their ovaries and attempts to harvest ovarian tissue for cryopreservation may still be worthwhile after the first courses of chemotherapy, if the procedure was not possible before [6].

Cryopreservation of ovarian tissue is the only option in prepubertal girls, as sexual maturity is not required. As this procedure does not cause any significant delay to initiation of cancer treatment and it does not require ovarian stimulation, some adult female patients also prefer to preserve fertility by this method.

6.6. Ovarian tissue transplantation

Transplantation of frozen-thawn ovarian cortex has shown to be a new promising method for recovery of ovarian function [48] and in some cases sufficient to restore fertility [49-51]. Ovarian tissue can be transplanted orthotopically, i.e. at the anatomical intrapelvic ovarian site or heterotopically, i.e. at other places including extrapelvic sites [52, 53].

There have been hundreds of patients undergoing ovarian tissue freezing but only a small percentage of these have returned for ovarian transplantation.

Autotransplantation is only possible if absence of malignant cells in the graft is confirmed. Methods for detection of cancer cells in the ovarian tissue of patients having suffered from hematological malignancies are under development including immunohistochemistry or the polymerase chain reaction applied to the tissue [54]. The investigation of residual malignant cells in the ovarian tissue may also be performed by xeno-transplantation to immunodeficient SCID mouse. Autotransplantation of ovarian tissue in patients having suffered from systemic hematological malignancies is not recommended due to the high risk of retransmission of malignancy and only patients with cancer diagnosis associated with a negligible or no risk of ovarian compromise should be considered for future autotransplantation [55]. Ovarian tissue cryopreservation and transplantation has shown not to interfere with proper genomic imprinting in mice pups [56] but additional studies in other animal models are needed.

6.7. In vitro culture of ovarian follicles

Although many improvements have been reported on the in vitro culture of follicles at early stages aiming at developing them into competent mature follicles, those methods are still on development [57-59]. Follicles cultured isolated or within a piece of thawed tissue will be the option for patients with hematological and ovarian malignancies. The normality of imprinted genes of cryobanked oocytes cultured and matured in vitro has yet to be verified experimentally.

6.8. Testicular tissue cryopreservation

This technique involves removal of testicular tissue from the male patient before cytotoxic therapy is initiated. In prepubertal boys, as there is absence of spermatozoa and spermatids, studies have been going on to cryopreserve the testicular totipotent precursors, i.e. the spermatogonial stem cells. Success has been reported in cryopreservation methods of testicular tissue [60] but more research is still needed in how to use the frozen-thawed tissue and obtain mature spermatozoa in vitro. Research suggests that in vitro spermatogenesis is likely to be the safest option for boys suffering from haematological malignancies, which might be re-transmitted by retransplantation, but this technique is still to be fully developed [61]. Although there are promising results in experimental animal studies of autologous retransplantation of spermatogonial stem cells showing re-colonization of seminiferous tubules generating complete spermatogenesis and mature germ cells and thus restoring natural fertility, the technique is still experimental in humans [61].

Cryopreservation of gonadal tissue offers hope to childhood cancer survivors, however it also raises several medical and ethical questions. Experimental methods for fertility preservation should only be offered to patients at specialized centers working with ethics board-approved research protocols and only in case when the recognized risks associated to the procedure are minimal.

6.9. Ovarian suppression to prevent gonadal damage

It has been hypothesized that suppressing the gonadal function transiently during chemo-therapy could prevent ovarian follicle destruction in female patients by maintaining the follicles dormant. However, the pool of primordial follicles is normally non-proliferating. Those follicles lack FSH receptors [62] and their initial recruitment is not controlled by gonadotropins [63], therefore hormonal manipulation by suppressing gonadotropin release is not likely to affect them [64]. The vast majority of available studies having investigating gonadal protection by gonadotropin-releasing hormone analogues (GnRHa) agonists or antagonists during chemotherapy in females have been small, retrospective and uncontrolled. A significant number of those studies had used resumption of menses as a surrogate marker for fertility and many of them had reported higher frequency of resumption of menses in women having received GnRHa but none has demonstrated a beneficial effect regarding fertility recovery. Although data indicate that infertility is increased after a chemotherapy treatment, even if menstrual cycles are resumed [65], studies suggesting a beneficial effect of GnRHa co-treatment on preserving menstruation have had a great impact in the medical community and the empirical use of GnRHa for ovarian protection during chemotherapy is currently widely spread [26].

7. Counseling and prompt referal increase the chances to preserve fertility

Despite the fact that fertility issues are recognized in young people with cancer, health care professionals still report never referring cancer patients of reproductive age to a reproductive specialists for fertility preservation, indicating that many patients still do not receive adequate and timely information [66] [67]. This contrasts to data indicating that approximately three out of four cancer patients younger than 35 years and childless at the time of cancer treatment may be interested in having children in the future [2]. Because incidence of most cancers increases with age, the trend of delaying childbearing in Western societies will naturally result in more female cancer patients interested in fertility preservation.

In despite of this, recent data indicate that female cancer patients are still poorly informed on fertility threats of cancer treatment and options to preserve fertility in comparison with their gender counterparts. A recent Swedish survey found that less than half of female patients recalled having received appropriate information on reproductive threats of cancer therapy whereas 80% of male patients recalled having had an appropriate discussion [67]. Only a small number of female patients used fertility preservation methods compared to a rate >70% of sperm freezing in male patients in that study. Urgency to start cancer treatment and lack of appropriate time, lack of knowledge on fertility preservation and awareness of the costs of assisted reproduction methods are recognized barriers to counseling and referring patients to fertility preservation [68].

8. Conclusion

Infertility due to gonadal failure is one of the major consequences of cancer therapy, particularly in patients who receive aggressive chemotherapy and/or radiotherapy treatment. Many surveys of cancer survivors have found that those patients are at increased risk of emotional distress if they become infertile as a result of their treatment. Evidence suggests that long-term survival after treatment for cancer during childhood is associated with increased risk of impaired quality of life and higher frequency of psychosocial problems often related to infertility issues. Adolescent cancer survivors have increased anxieties about body image and dating, and pediatric cancer survivors are less likely to marry than matched controls. Although cancer survivors can become parents by adoption or gamete donation, most would prefer to have biological parenthood and biologically related children.

Oncologists should thus be prepared to discuss the negative impact of cancer therapy on reproductive potential with their patients in the same way as any other risks of cancer treatment are discussed. Furthermore, patients interested in fertility preservation should be promptly referred to a reproductive medicine expert to offer timely and appropriate counseling and improve success of fertility preservation. Close collaboration between the oncology team and the reproductive endocrinologists should be encouraged.

Author details

Kenny A. Rodriguez-Wallberg[1,2,3]

Address all correspondence to: kenny.rodriguez-wallberg@karolinska.se

1 Clinical Responsible of Fertility Preservation Programme, Karolinska University Hospital, Stockholm, Sweden

2 Karolinska Institutet, Department of Clinical Science, Intervention and Technology, Division of Obstetrics and Gynecology, Sweden

3 Karolinska University Hospital Huddinge, Fertility Unit, Stockholm, Sweden

References

[1] SEER Cancer Statistics Review 1975-2007, N.C.I., updated January 7, 2011 2011.

[2] Schover, L.R., et al., *Having children after cancer. A pilot survey of survivors' attitudes and experiences.* Cancer, 1999. 86(4): p. 697-709.

[3] Rosen, A., K.A. Rodriguez-Wallberg, and L. Rosenzweig, *Psychosocial distress in young cancer survivors.* Semin Oncol Nurs, 2009. 25(4): p. 268-77.

[4] Schover, L.R., et al., *Knowledge and experience regarding cancer, infertility, and sperm banking in younger male survivors.* Journal of clinical oncology : official journal of the American Society of Clinical Oncology, 2002. 20(7): p. 1880-9.

[5] Wong, I., et al., *Assisted conception following radical trachelectomy.* Human reproduction (Oxford, England), 2009. 24(4): p. 876-9.

[6] Wallberg, K.A., V. Keros, and O. Hovatta, *Clinical aspects of fertility preservation in female patients.* Pediatr Blood Cancer, 2009. 53(2): p. 254-60.

[7] Dargent, D., et al., *La trachelectomie elargie(te), une alternative a l'hysterectomie radicale dans le traitement des cancer infiltrants developpes sur la face externe du col uterin.* 1994. 2: p. 285-292.

[8]   Morice, P., et al., *[Effects of radiotherapy (external and/or internal) and chemotherapy on female fertility].* Bull Acad Natl Med, 2010. 194(3): p. 481-92; discussion 492-4, 529-30.

[9]   Liou, W.S., et al., *Innovations in fertility preservation for patients with gynecologic cancers.* Fertil Steril, 2005. 84(6): p. 1561-73.

[10] Abu-Rustum, N.R. and Y. Sonoda, *Fertility-sparing surgery in early-stage cervical cancer: indications and applications.* J Natl Compr Canc Netw, 2010. 8(12): p. 1435-8.

[11] Plante, M., et al., *The vaginal radical trachelectomy: An update of a series of 125 cases and 106 pregnancies.* Gynecologic oncology, 2011. 121(2): p. 290-7.

[12] Li, J., et al., *Radical abdominal trachelectomy for cervical malignancies: Surgical, oncological and fertility outcomes in 62 patients.* Gynecologic oncology, 2011. 121(3): p. 565-70.

[13] Kesic, V., et al., *Fertility Preserving Management in Gynecologic Cancer Patients: The Need for Centralization.* International Journal of Gynecological Cancer, 2010. 20(9): p. 1613-9.

[14] Pentheroudakis, G., et al., *Cancer, fertility and pregnancy: ESMO Clinical Practice Guidelines for diagnosis, treatment and follow-up.* Ann Oncol, 2010. 21 Suppl 5: p. v266-73.

[15] Ungar, L., et al., *Abdominal radical trachelectomy during pregnancy to preserve pregnancy and fertility.* Obstet Gynecol, 2006. 108(3 Pt 2): p. 811-4.

[16] Sioutas, A., et al., *Three cases of vaginal radical trachelectomy during pregnancy.* Gynecologic oncology, 2011. 121(2): p. 420-1.

[17] Sabanegh, E.S. and A.M. Ragheb, *Male fertility after cancer.* Urology, 2009. 73(2): p. 225-31.

[18] Heidenreich, A., et al., *Organ sparing surgery for malignant germ cell tumor of the testis.* The Journal of urology, 2001. 166(6): p. 2161-5.

[19] Gosden, R.G., et al., *Impact of congenital or experimental hypogonadotrophism on the radiation sensitivity of the mouse ovary.* Human reproduction (Oxford, England), 1997. 12(11): p. 2483-8.

[20] Speiser, B., P. Rubin, and G. Casarett, *Aspermia following lower truncal irradiation in Hodgkin's disease.* Cancer, 1973. 32(3): p. 692-8.

[21] Wallace, W.H.B., R.A. Anderson, and D.S. Irvine, *Fertility preservation for young patients with cancer: who is at risk and what can be offered?* The lancet oncology, 2005. 6(4): p. 209-18.

[22] Rodriguez-Wallberg, K.A. and K. Oktay, *Fertility preservation medicine: options for young adults and children with cancer.* Journal of pediatric hematology/oncology : official journal of the American Society of Pediatric Hematology/Oncology, 2010. 32(5): p. 390-6.

[23] Sklar, C., *Growth and endocrine disturbances after bone marrow transplantation in child-hood.* Acta paediatrica (Oslo, Norway : 1992) Supplement, 1995. 411: p. 57-61; discussion 62.

[24] Thibaud, E., et al., *Ovarian function after bone marrow transplantation during childhood.* Bone marrow transplantation, 1998. 21(3): p. 287-90.

[25] Shalet, S.M., et al., *Vulnerability of the human Leydig cell to radiation damage is dependent upon age.* The Journal of endocrinology, 1989. 120(1): p. 161-5.

[26] Lee, S.J., et al., *American Society of Clinical Oncology recommendations on fertility preservation in cancer patients.* Journal of clinical oncology : official journal of the American Society of Clinical Oncology, 2006. 24(18): p. 2917-31.

[27] Wo, J.Y. and A.N. Viswanathan, *Impact of radiotherapy on fertility, pregnancy, and neonatal outcomes in female cancer patients.* International journal of radiation oncology, biology, physics, 2009. 73(5): p. 1304-12.

[28] Green, D.M., et al., *Ovarian failure and reproductive outcomes after childhood cancer treatment: results from the Childhood Cancer Survivor Study.* Journal of clinical oncology : official journal of the American Society of Clinical Oncology, 2009. 27(14): p. 2374-81.

[29] Hudson, M.M., *Reproductive outcomes for survivors of childhood cancer.* Obstetrics and gynecology, 2010. 116(5): p. 1171-83.

[30] Oktem, O. and K. Oktay, *A novel ovarian xenografting model to characterize the impact of chemotherapy agents on human primordial follicle reserve.* Cancer research, 2007. 67(21): p. 10159-62.

[31] Wallberg, K.A.R.-M., V. Keros, and O. Hovatta, *Clinical aspects of fertility preservation in female patients.* Pediatric blood & cancer, 2009. 53(2): p. 254-60.

[32] Meirow, D., et al., *Administration of cyclophosphamide at different stages of follicular maturation in mice: effects on reproductive performance and fetal malformations.* Human reproduction (Oxford, England), 2001. 16(4): p. 632-7.

[33] Guerin, J.F., *[Testicular tissue cryoconservation for prepubertal boy: indications and feasibility].* Gynecol Obstet Fertil, 2005. 33(10): p. 804-8.

[34] Bahadur, G., et al., *Semen quality and cryopreservation in adolescent cancer patients.* Hum Reprod, 2002. 17(12): p. 3157-61.

[35] Menon, S., et al., *Fertility preservation in adolescent males: experience over 22 years at Rouen University Hospital.* Hum Reprod, 2009. 24(1): p. 37-44.

[36] Meseguer, M., et al., *Sperm cryopreservation in oncological patients: a 14-year follow-up study.* Fertil Steril, 2006. 85(3): p. 640-5.

[37] Marrs, R.P., J. Greene, and B.A. Stone, *Potential factors affecting embryo survival and clinical outcome with cryopreserved pronuclear human embryos*. Am J Obstet Gynecol, 2004. 190(6): p. 1766-71; discussion 1771-2.

[38] Oktay, K., A.P. Cil, and H. Bang, *Efficiency of oocyte cryopreservation: a meta-analysis*. Fertility and sterility, 2006. 86(1): p. 70-80.

[39] Practice Committee of the American Society for Reproductive Medicine, P.C.o.t.S.f.A.R.T., *Ovarian tissue and oocyte cryopreservation*. Fertil Steril, 2008. 90: p. 134-5.

[40] Medicine, P.C.o.t.A.S.f.R., *ASRM Practice Committee response to Rybak and Lieman: elective self-donation of oocytes*. Fertil Steril, 2009. 92(5): p. 1513-14.

[41] Noyes, N., E. Porcu, and A. Borini, *Over 900 oocyte cryopreservation babies born with no apparent increase in congenital anomalies*. Reprod Biomed Online, 2009. 18(6): p. 769-76.

[42] Rodriguez-Wallberg, K.A. and K. Oktay, *Fertility preservation in women with breast cancer*. Clinical obstetrics and gynecology, 2010. 53(4): p. 753-62.

[43] Oktay, K., et al., *Fertility preservation in breast cancer patients: a prospective controlled comparison of ovarian stimulation with tamoxifen and letrozole for embryo cryopreservation*. Journal of clinical oncology : official journal of the American Society of Clinical Oncology, 2005. 23(19): p. 4347-53.

[44] Azim, A.A., M. Costantini-Ferrando, and K. Oktay, *Safety of fertility preservation by ovarian stimulation with letrozole and gonadotropins in patients with breast cancer: a prospective controlled study*. Journal of clinical oncology : official journal of the American Society of Clinical Oncology, 2008. 26(16): p. 2630-5.

[45] Tulandi, T., et al., *Congenital malformations among 911 newborns conceived after infertility treatment with letrozole or clomiphene citrate*. Fertil Steril, 2006. 85(6): p. 1761-5.

[46] Chian, R.C., et al., *Live birth after vitrification of in vitro matured human oocytes*. Fertil Steril, 2009. 91(2): p. 372-6.

[47] Boiso, I., et al., *A confocal microscopy analysis of the spindle and chromosome configurations of human oocytes cryopreserved at the germinal vesicle and metaphase II stage*. Hum Reprod, 2002. 17(7): p. 1885-91.

[48] Oktay, K. and G. Karlikaya, *Ovarian function after transplantation of frozen, banked autologous ovarian tissue*. The New England journal of medicine, 2000. 342(25): p. 1919.

[49] Andersen, C.Y., et al., *Two successful pregnancies following autotransplantation of frozen/thawed ovarian tissue*. Hum Reprod, 2008. 23(10): p. 2266-72.

[50] von Wolff, M., et al., *Cryopreservation and autotransplantation of human ovarian tissue prior to cytotoxic therapy--a technique in its infancy but already successful in fertility preservation*. European journal of cancer (Oxford, England : 1990), 2009. 45(9): p. 1547-53.

[51] Oktay, K., I. Turkcuoglu, and K.A. Rodriguez-Wallberg, *Four spontaneous pregnancies and three live births following subcutaneous transplantation of frozen banked ovarian tissue: what is the explanation?* Fertility and sterility, 2011. 95(2): p. 804 e7-10.

[52] Oktay, K., et al., *Embryo development after heterotopic transplantation of cryopreserved ovarian tissue.* Lancet, 2004. 363(9412): p. 837-40.

[53] Sonmezer, M. and K. Oktay, *Orthotopic and heterotopic ovarian tissue transplantation.* Best Pract Res Clin Obstet Gynaecol, 2010. 24(1): p. 113-26.

[54] Meirow, D., et al., *Searching for evidence of disease and malignant cell contamination in ovarian tissue stored from hematologic cancer patients.* Hum Reprod, 2008. 23(5): p. 1007-13.

[55] Ajala, T., et al., *Fertility preservation for cancer patients: a review.* Obstet Gynecol Int, 2010. 2010: p. 160386.

[56] al, S.e., *Immature cryopreserved ovary restores puberty and fertility in mice without alteration of epigenetic marks.* PLoS One, 2008.

[57] Telfer, E.E., et al., *A two-step serum-free culture system supports development of human oocytes from primordial follicles in the presence of activin.* Hum Reprod, 2008. 23(5): p. 1151-8.

[58] Smitz, J., et al., *Current achievements and future research directions in ovarian tissue culture, in vitro follicle development and transplantation: implications for fertility preservation.* Hum Reprod Update, 2010. 16(4): p. 395-414.

[59] Telfer, E.E. and M. McLaughlin, *In vitro development of ovarian follicles.* Semin Reprod Med, 2011. 29(1): p. 15-23.

[60] Keros, V., et al., *Methods of cryopreservation of testicular tissue with viable spermatogonia in pre-pubertal boys undergoing gonadotoxic cancer treatment.* Hum Reprod, 2007. 22(5): p. 1384-95.

[61] Jahnukainen, K., et al., *Intratesticular transplantation of testicular cells from leukemic rats causes transmission of leukemia.* Cancer Res, 2001. 61(2): p. 706-10.

[62] Rice, S., et al., *Stage-specific expression of androgen receptor, follicle-stimulating hormone receptor, and anti-Mullerian hormone type II receptor in single, isolated, human preantral follicles: relevance to polycystic ovaries.* J Clin Endocrinol Metab, 2007. 92(3): p. 1034-40.

[63] McGee, E.A. and A.J. Hsueh, *Initial and cyclic recruitment of ovarian follicles.* Endocr Rev, 2000. 21(2): p. 200-14.

[64] Oktay, K., D. Briggs, and R.G. Gosden, *Ontogeny of follicle-stimulating hormone receptor gene expression in isolated human ovarian follicles.* The Journal of clinical endocrinology and metabolism, 1997. 82(11): p. 3748-51.

[65] Letourneau, J.M., et al., *The prevalence of self-reported reproductive impairment in young female cancer survivors throuhgout California.* Fertil Steril, 2010. 94(4): p. 510 (Abstract).

[66] Forman, E.J., C.K. Anders, and M.A. Behera, *Pilot survey of oncologists regarding treatment-related infertility and fertility preservation in female cancer patients.* J Reprod Med, 2009. 54(4): p. 203-7.

[67] Armuand, G.M., Rodriguez-Wallberg K.A. et al., *Sex differences in fertility-related information received by young adult cancer survivors.* J Clin Oncol, 2012. 30(17): p. 2147-53.

[68] Quinn, G.P., et al., *Patient-physician communication barriers regarding fertility preservation among newly diagnosed cancer patients.* Soc Sci Med, 2008. 66(3): p. 784-9.

Chapter 5

Supportive and Palliative Care in Solid Cancer Patients

Bassam Abdul Rasool Hassan,
Zuraidah Binti Mohd Yusoff,
Mohamed Azmi Hassali and Saad Bin Othman

Additional information is available at the end of the chapter

1. Introduction

1.1. Cancer background

During this century, cancer has become one of the major problem and diseases which has caused predominant death and it will even surpass heart diseases. Many of the researchers begin to use the term lifetime risk for cancer patients which refer to the time that cancer will progress and developed or the time that the patient will die because of cancer. There are many problems (i.e., side effects) associated with cancer diseases either solid type or hematological type such as nausea, vomiting, diarrhea, constipation, hypercalcemia, pain, lost of appetite, anemia, fatigue, cachexia, leucopenia, neutropenia and thrombocytopenia. However the major problems are nausea and vomiting, neutropenia, anemia, thrombocytopenia and hypercalcemia. Hence due to these reasons cancer is consider as one of the major diseases that will effect on the quality of life for human [1-6].

1.2. Chemotherapy background

Chemotherapy was developed and used since the Word War I from the chemical weapon program of the United State of America (USA). Since then chemotherapy has became as one of the most important and significant treatment of cancer. Its main mechanism of action is by destroying the cancer cells which are characterized by their high multiplication and growth speed. However when comparing chemotherapy with other types of treatments, it still remain potentially high risk with many side effects which are difficult to manage. Chemotherapy used required the involvement of various clinical professionals during its various stages of administration and enormous patient health care is needed to overcome its side effects [7-8].

1.3. Chemotherapy side effects

The goal of chemotherapy is to be as effective as possible with tolerable side effects, since the dose of chemotherapy will be toxic to the cancer cells as well as to the normal cells. A proportion of the cancer patients suffer from only mild side effects whereas others may suffer from serious side effects. These side effects are classified as:

1. Acute, which develop within 24 hours after chemotherapy administration.

2. Delayed, which developed after 24 hours and up to 6 to 8 weeks after chemotherapy treatments.

3. Short term, combination of both acute and delayed effect.

4. Late/ long term, which developed after months or years of chemotherapy treatment.

5. Expected, which developed among 75% of the patients.

6. Common, occurred in 25%-75% of the patients.

7. Uncommon, happened is less than 15% of the patients.

8. Rare, occur in only 5% of the patients.

9. Very rare, occur with less than 1% of the patients.

Occurrence of specific side effects will vary according to the chemotherapy or medications used. The most common side effects experienced are nausea and vomiting, anemia, hair lost, bleeding (thrombocytopenia), hyperuricemia, neurotoxicity, cardiotoxicity, bone marrow depression, alopecia, nephrotoxicity, pulmonary toxicity, dehydration, cystitis and mucositis. So different parameters must be taken into consideration to prevent, reduce and overcome these side effects [8-10]. This chapter will focus on the main side effects caused by cancer disease and/ or chemotherapy.

2. Main problems caused by cancer disease itself and/ or chemotherapy treatment

2.1. Nausea and vomiting

Both nausea and vomiting are recognized as two separate and distinct conditions. Nausea is an unpleasant sensation of being vomit or urge to vomit which may or may not result in vomiting. While, vomiting or emesis is the process of expelling of undigested food through the mouth. Nausea and vomiting can arises from different or wide spectrum of etiologies which are either directly associated to cancer disease itself or to its treatment. According to the new ranking of chemotherapy side effects, nausea is the number one or the most disturbing side effect while vomiting is the third and sometimes the fifth disturbing chemotherapy side effects. Even so, not all cancer patients suffer from nausea and/ or vomiting because not all of them were treated with emetogenic chemotherapy [11-17].

2.1.1. Nausea and vomiting in solid cancer patients

Nausea and vomiting are two of the major problems that are associated with cancer patients and 50%-55% of cancer patients suffer from both nausea and vomiting even with the use of antiemetic drugs. The main causes for this are either due to the chemotherapy or because of the cancer progression. Some of the cancer patients who were treated with chemotherapy did not suffer from nausea or vomiting because the chemotherapy used were not significantly emetogenic. Nausea and vomiting still remain the major side effects that occur and are associated with chemotherapy and cancer diseases [11, 18-20].

2.1.2. Understanding nausea and vomiting in advanced solid cancer

Both nausea and vomiting are very common problems especially with advanced stages of solid cancer diseases like breast cancer and stomach cancer where 50 to 60% of the patients are mainly female under 65 years of age [21]. In this situation, nausea and vomiting occur because of the advanced stages of solid cancer diseases characterized by more severe complications than that caused by chemoradiotherapy or other treatments. The main causes for those problems are gastric stasis, obstruction of the intestine, opioid use, constipation caused by morphine uses, hypercalcemia, brain metastasis, renal failure, hyponatremia, increases in the intracranial pressure and tumor burden [21].

2.1.3. Pathophysiology of chemotherapy-induced nausea and vomiting

Chemotherapy cause nausea by stimulating the autonomic nervous system (ANS), while vomiting is triggered when afferent impulses from chemoreceptor trigger zone (CTZ), pharynx, cerebral cortex and vagal afferent fiber stimulate the vomiting center (VC) located in the medulla. The stimulation of the VC leads to contraction of muscles of abdomen, chest wall and diaphragm, so this will lead to an expulsion of stomach and intestine contents [11-20]. The main mechanism of chemotherapy induced vomiting is the stimulation of the entrochromaffin cells lining the wall of the gastrointestinal tract (GIT) hence causes the release of the serotonin. The serotonin will then bind to the vagal afferent 5-HT_3 receptors in the GIT which will send impulses to the CTZ and VC. Vomiting will be triggered when afferent impulses from CTZ, pharynx, cerebral cortex and vagal afferent fiber transfer impulses to the VC [22].

2.1.4. Major patients risk factors related with nausea and vomiting

1- Gender, 2-Age, 3- History of motion sickness and history of vomiting during pregnancy, 4-History of drinking alcohol, 5-Patient anxiety [11, 16, 18, 23-25]

2.1.5. Major chemotherapy factors responsible for incidence of nausea and vomiting

There are several chemotherapeutics factors that play a major role in the incidence and severity of both nausea and vomiting which are:

1- Emetogenic potential of the drug, 2- Dosage level, 3- Schedule of administration, 4- Route of administration, 5- History of previous chemotherapy, 6- Rate of I.V infusion [11, 16, 18, 23, 26].

2.1.6. Classification of chemotherapy induced nausea and vomiting

This classification is based on the emetogenic potential of the chemotherapeutic drug.

1. Severe (90% of the patients will experience nausea and vomiting) Example: Carmustine I.V $\geq$ 250 mg/ m^2, Cisplatin I.V $\geq$ 50 mg/ m^2, Cyclophosphamide I.V > 1500 mg/ m^2, Dacarbazine, Mechlorethamine, Nitrogen mustard and Streptozocin.

2. High (60%-90%) Example: Carboplatin, Carmustine I.V $\leq$ 250 mg/ m^2, Cisplatin I.V < 50 mg/ m^2, Cyclophosphamide I.V 750 mg/ m^2 to 1500 mg/ m^2, Cytarabine I.V > 1gm/ m^2, Dactinomycin, Daunorubicin, Doxorubicin I.V > 60 mg/ m^2, Irinotecan, Methotrexate I.V > 1 gm/ m^2 and Procarbazine PO dose.

3. Moderate (30%-60%) Example: Altretamine I.V PO dose, Asparginase, Cyclophospha-mide (I.V) $\leq$ 750 mg/ m^2, Cyclophosphamide PO dose, Doxorubicin (I.V) 20 to 60 mg/ m^2, Epirubicin I.V, Idarubicin, Ifosfamide, Lomustine PO dose, Methotrexate (I.V) 250-1000 mg/ m^2, Mitoxantrone (I.V) < 15 mg/ m^2, Pemetrexed, Raltitrexed, Temozalamide and Topotecan.

4. Low (10%-30%) Example: Aldesleukin, Amsacrine, Bortezomib, Capecitabine, PO dose, Docetaxel, Doxorubicin liposomal, Etoposide all dose I.V or PO, Erlotrinib PO dose, Fluorouracil, Gefitinib PO dose, Gemcitabine, Methotrexate (I.V) 50-250 mg/ m^2, Mito-mycin, Paclitaxel, Porfimer, Teniposide and Trastuzumab.

5. Very low (less than 10%) Example: Bleomycin, Busulfan PO dose, Chlorambucil PO dose, Cladribine, Fludaradine, Hydroxyurea PO dose, Interferon, Levamisole, Melphalan PO dose, Methotrexate < 50mg/ m^2, Rituximab, Thalidomide, Thioguanine, Thiotepa, Vin-blastine, Vincristine, Vinorelbine and Vindesine [25, 27].

2.1.7. Classification and incidence of chemotherapy induced nausea and vomiting

CINV are clinically classified as:

1- Acute chemotherapy related nausea and vomiting, 2- Delayed emesis, 3- Anticipatory emesis [11, 16, 18, 28].

2.1.8. Nausea and vomiting treatment options

The main goal of the antiemetic treatment is to abolish nausea and vomiting which in the last twenty years consider as an inevitable chemotherapy side effect. This prevention is focused on the entire period of emetic risk which is 4 days for patients who received highly or moderately emetogenic chemotherapy [22, 29]. This could be perfectly achieved by understanding the mechanisms of these antiemetic drugs either alone or in combination so as to get their maximum benefit [30]. Modern antiemetic treatments help in preventing 70%-80% of nausea and vomiting problems. Combination antiemetic treatment becomes the standard regimen used for the control of nausea and vomiting caused by chemotherapy [30]. The different types of treatments are as follows: Serotonin-receptor antagonists (5-HT_3), Dopamine-2-receptor antagonists, Corticosteroids, Neurokinin-1-recptor antagonists, Cannabinoids & Benzodiazepines [29].

2.1.9. Genetic polymorphism and incidence of nausea and vomiting

Interindividual diversity in drug metabolism is caused by many factors including environmental factors, cultural factors related with type of diet, concomitant drug therapy as well as genetic factors i.e., ethnic variation. All of these variations play an important role in changing pharmacokinetic and pharmacodynamic properties, volume of distribution, elimination, disposition and clinical effect for many drugs [31, 32]. Much of this distinction has shown to be caused by genetic polymorphisms of the human cytochrome P450 enzymes (CYP) [32]. CYP is the most vital enzymatic system concerned with drug metabolism. Approximately 65% of common drugs used are metabolized by cytochrome P450 enzymes and half of them are mediated by the CYP3A subfamily [32].

2.2. Anemia

This is a condition characterized by lack of blood or in other word a reduction of total quantity of erythrocyte (red blood cells, RBC) or hemoglobin in the circulation which are necessary for normal function. This is caused by the inability of the bone marrow to replace the erythrocyte lost. The normal level of RBC for the male is 5.4×10^6 cell/ µl and for female is 4.8×10^6 cell/ µl [11, 33-35]. It is considered as one of the most frequent hematological demonstration of malignant diseases, which will lead to momentous impairment in every tissues and organs of cancer patients and put them under serious stress. This major problem may arise because of the underlining diseases (i.e., cancer diseases) or radiotherapy or chemotherapy treatment received [36, 37].

2.2.1. Red blood cell (RBC) and iron

The large proportion of body iron (20 mg per day) is used in the synthesis of erythrocyte cells. The body absorbed about 1 mg of iron per day from the gut to compensate the amount of daily iron lost. After the transition from erythroblast to reticulocyte, it will then remain for 3 to 4 days in the bone marrow after which being released into the blood circulation and circulate for about 100-120 days. Red blood cell (RBC) has no mitochondria so are totally dependent on ATP generated during glycolysis process. In the circulation RBC loss about 20% of its hemoglobin and shows physiological steps of aging. They will be phagocytes by the macrophage leading to destruction of the erythrocyte and the removal of the iron from the hemoglobin (Hb) which will be released into the plasma and redistributed again [38].

2.2.2. Types of anemia

There are different types of anemia as follows:

1- Iron deficiency anemia, 2- Folic acid deficiency anemia, 3- Vitamin (Vit) B_{12} deficiency anemia, 4- Vit C deficiency anemia, 5- Hemolytic anemia. It is an acquired type of anemia, 6- Thalassemias, 7- Sickle cell anemia, 8- Anemia of chronic diseases (ACD) [36, 37].

2.2.3. Erythropoietin (EPO) description and action

EPO is a glycoprotein hormone consists of 165 amino acid with a peptide mass of 18.2 kDa. It is mainly produce by the liver during fetal stage but after birth the kidneys become the primary production sites. It has been realized that most of EPO in the circulation comes and produce from the cortex of the kidney [39]. EPO production is mainly controlled by the feedback system between kidney and bone marrow. The kidneys mainly depend on the renal oxygen sensor for EPO production. Kidney cells response greatly towards hypoxia by increasing the EPO production. Serum level of EPO ranges between 10 to 20 mU/ mL and for normal situation the observed EPO concentration/ predictive EPO concentration (O/P) ratio must range between 0.8-1.2 [41]. EPO maintain erythropoiesis is by preventing the colony forming unit-erythroid (CFU-E) from death by apoptosis process. By this way these progenitor cells will keep proliferating and differentiating to produce erythrocyte [39].

2.2.4. Causes of anemia of chronic diseases (ACD)

Anemia remain as one of the serious and frequent problem of cancer mainly cancer of the gastrointestinal, liver, head and neck, ovarian and cervix. This is mainly caused by cytokines including interlukine-1, interlukine-6, interferon-γ and tumor necrosis factor-α produced by these cancer diseases. These cytokines caused impairment of erythropoietin (EPO) synthesis, reduce erythrocytes life span and prevent normal iron utilization. Other direct effect of tumor that cause anemia is bone marrow replacement which is associated with inhibition of the body ability for the production of RBC. This condition of bone marrow suppression is associated with specific types of cancers like breast, prostate, myeloma, lymphoma and acute leukemia. Also bone marrow suppression is mainly caused by chemotherapy and radiotherapy which are the main treatment for cancer. Mainly in cancer patients the major risk factors responsible for incidence and severity of anemia are the form of cancer as well as type and dose of chemotherapy administered to the cancer patients. [11, 33-36, 40, 41].

2.2.5. Diagnosis of anemia

Several parameters need to be checked for anemia diagnosis since each one is considered important and they are as follow: Family history, laboratory tests, X-ray, biopsy and bone examination [33, 35, 42].

2.2.6. Grades of anemia (levels)

The grades or severity of anemia will depend on several factors like hemoglobin level, velocity of onset of anemia, age, co-morbidities, extent of the underlining malignancy, intensity of treatment and the biological function of the patients organ. Anemia grades as follows:

Normal level (women Hb= 12.0 g/ dL-16.0 g/ dL, men Hb= 14.0 g/ dL- 18.0 g/ dL)

Mild Anemia Hb= 10g/ dL

Moderate Anemia Hb= 8.0 g/ dL- 10.0 g/ dL

Severe Anemia Hb= 6.5 g/ dL- 7.9 g/ dL

Life Threatening Anemia Hb= < 6.5 g/ dL [33, 36, 43].

2.2.7. Clinical signs and symptoms of anemia in cancer patients

The severity of signs and symptoms of anemia depend on several factors like Hb level, age, extent of the underlining malignant, comorbidity, rate of anemia onset, biological activity of patients vital organs and intensity of treatment used for anemia. Generally in elderly patients the clinical signs and symptoms appear with Hb level higher than that in younger patients. These symptoms usually appear gradually, starting with fatigue which is considered as one of the major signs happing in 60% to more than 90% of the anemic patients. Lethargy and lost of concentration will also take place as the Hb becomes lower than 12 g/ dL. When anemia becomes severe and chronic this will lead to decompensation of cadiorespiratory and impairment of several body organs and activities [36, 46].

2.2.8. Role of cancer patients ages

It has been found that the incidence of anemia and cancer increases as the age of the patient increases too. Anemia is much more related and significantly present as the age became higher than 60 years old and with steeper increases after age 80 years. Many studies showed that the hemoglobin levels remain stable between age 60 to 98 years old but there are several causes for the high incidence of anemia in the old age since there were high comorbidity, hematopoietic stress and reduce in function of many vital organs. For this reason there will be great association and increases in occurrence of anemia in elderly patients [44].

2.2.9. Cancer patients gender and anemia

As mention above anemia highly occur in patients older than 60 years old, but it has been found that among women, anemia happen at a younger age. The main difference between men and women are the presence of menstrual cycle i.e., blood loss and childbearing iron loss which make incidence and association of anemia higher in younger women as compared to men [44]. Besides that men and women who do not have menstruation, the amount of iron lost in one day is 1 mg. While, in women still with menstrual, the loss is about 0.6 to 2.5 times more than previous mentioned amount. The amount of iron lost during each menstruation cycle depends on the severity of bleeding. The standard iron lost per menstrual cycle for woman weighting about 60 kg is about 10 mg. So all of these evidences showed that anemia is associated with female as a gender more than male [45].

2.2.10. Cancer patients race

Race also play an important role in incidence of anemia since it is consider as one of the risk factor which play role in its occurrence. The prevalence of anemia in USA among white women is 7.1% and 25.1% among black women even after adjustment of iron level. Besides that black women are characterized by lower mean hemoglobin level compared to white women. Also black woman has a wide standard deviation in mean of hemoglobin than the white one has [45].

2.2.11. Mechanisms of anemia in cancer patients

2.2.11.1. Role of cancer disease

Occurrence and association of anemia with cancer depends on several factors including patients age, stage of cancer, presence or absence of infection and other comorbidities. Anemia prevalence is highly associated especially with lymphomas, genitourinary tumor, lung and multiply myeloma. The incidence of mild to moderate anemia with solid tumor is higher than incidence of severe anemia which occurs highly with hematological cancers than solid one [36, 46, 47]. The main mechanism whereby cancer causes anemia is by producing cytokines which are mainly tumor necrosis factor (TNF-α) and interleukin-1 and they have the ability to hamper EPO production and action, reduce the life span of RBC and preclude ordinary utilization of iron. Other mechanisms which will cause association of anemia with cancer will be separated from the cancer itself like Vit B_{12}, folic acid and iron deficiency. Renal, endocrinal disorders splenomegaly, clonogenic and cachexia occurrence with cancer also play a major role in occurrence of anemia [36].

2.2.11.2. Role of chemotherapy

Anemia is one of the common side effect of chemotherapy especially with the myelosuppressive type. Incidence and severity of anemia depend on several different factors which are the chemotherapy type, schedule and intensity as well as type of cancer. Chemotherapy cycles also play an important role in increasing the severity of anemia since multiply cycles will cumulatively inhibit or reduce erythropoiesis. It has been found by the European Cancer Anaemia Survey (ECAS) that the incidence of anemia after the first cycle is 19.5% and after second cycle is 34.3% while after the third the incidence was more than 40%. Also single or combination chemotherapy play a serious and major role in anemia incidence and severity since the use of combination chemotherapy regimen will leads to severe anemia more than the use of single chemotherapy drug [48-50]. Besides chemotherapy myelosuppression, anemia can take place as a result of direct destruction of the RBC (i.e., direct effect on the erythropoiesis in the bone marrow) or reduced erythropoietin production (i.e., impact on EPO production). When this chemotherapy drug or other drugs used repetitively this may lead to prolong production of anemia. Also the results that obtained from clinical trials showed that the probability of mild anemia incidence after the use of chemotherapy is 100%, while the probability of severe anemia incidence after chemotherapy is 80%. From these results and data it has been proven that chemotherapy is the major impact factor for anemia onset and severity in cancer patients [41, 48, 51-53].

2.2.12. Indications and options for anemia treatments

Anemia and its related symptoms have serious negative effects on patients quality of life (QOL) and anticancer treatment since it will leads to treatment delay. These effects may be tolerated in young patients even with very low hemoglobin levels. While in patients with multimorbidity would not be able to tolerate this and as a result of that many severe clinical signs and symptoms will developed even with minor reduction in the Hb levels [36, 54, 55]. The treatment strategies of anemia mainly based on the clinical situation, clinical signs and symptoms and on the underlining cause of anemia. These treatments will include red blood cell transfusion, corticosteroids, VitB12 and Epoetin alfa (recombinant human erythropoietin, rHuEPO). All these treatments were used to overcome anemia related signs, symptoms and to improve the anemic patients (QOL) [36].

2.3. Thrombocytopenia

Thrombocytopenia is a term used to denote abnormal decrease or drop in platelets numbers. The main function of these platelets is clot formation during bleeding in order to prevent blood lost. Thus a decrease in platelet number will leads to bleeding condition which ranges from mild bleeding from small blood vessels to severe bleeding from large blood vessels. Severe bleeding in the presence of severe thrombocytopenia or when is coupled with other clotting disorders can leads to serious morbidity or death. Thrombocytopenia is a common problem experience by cancer patients, which usually resulted from the use of conventional chemotherapy and at times is a dose limiting factor for chemotherapy administration. The incidence of thrombocytopenia among solid cancer patients is rather low i.e., ranging between 10%-25% among breast cancer, ovarian and germ cell cancer patients who were treated with intensive chemotherapy. However thrombocytopenia incidence is high among acute leukemia patients [56-63].

2.3.1. Platelets morphology and structure

Platelets or thrombocytes are irregular, disc shaped cells which are considered as the smallest cells in the blood (0.5 to 3.0 μm diameter). They are usually produce from the megakaryocytes which are large cells (80 to 150 μm diameter) found specifically in the spongy center of long bones by the stimulation of thrombopoietin (TPO) by process called endomitosis whereby each megakaryocyte cell produce about 2000 platelets. These platelets shared a characteristic of having a very short life span (five to nine days only) so the bone marrow of healthy individual continuously keep producing new platelets cells to replace the old dead ones. The thrombopoietin hormone is mainly synthesis and produce by the liver and plays a major role in stimulation of proliferation and maturation of platelets. The circulating platelets have no nucleus but they have alpha granules and dense granules [57, 64, 65]. Physiologically the platelets are removed from the blood circulation by two mechanisms. The first is being used at common sites of vascular injury like in the microcirculation, secondly to be phagocyte by macrophages cells predominantly in the spleen and liver [66].

2.3.2. Platelets function

Platelets have vital functions in immunity, wound repair and homeostasis. These functions mainly depend on platelets concentration in blood circulation. Platelets prevent bleeding by either sealing the hole in the blood vessel wall or by forming haemostatic plug or by liberating several chemicals that will activate more clotting formation by breaking down more of the platelets. The main steps for platelets action to form clot are the following:

1. Adhesion (Step 1): This reaction is mediated by release of granules and characterized by shape change of the platelets from disc shape to spiny spheres after their adhesion to collagen. The aggregation of the platelets in this face is reversible.

2. Aggregation (Step 2): In this step more of platelets adhere to each other and there will be an obvious shape change of these platelets. The main factors that stimulate this step are the chemical changes.

3. Release (Step 3): Here the aggregation caused by the dense granules released by the platelets themselves is irreversible. In addition vasoconstriction will take place as a result of thromboxane A_2 released by the platelets.

4. Stabilization of the clot (Step 4): This is the main reaction which is responsible for the thrombus formation, whereby the aggregate platelets will release factor V that will accelerate the aggregation of other platelets and this will lead to stabilized clot formation [64, 67].

From this it is clear that thrombocytopenia which is associated with decrease in platelets count in the blood of cancer patients such as leukemic patients is considered as a very serious problem. Thrombocytopenia prevalence in hematological patients is very high. While in case of solid tumor, thrombocytopenia happens because of chemotherapy uses and thus the incidence is rather low. However in some subgroups the incidence is higher than 20% and it still remain as a serious and dangerous problem [62].

2.3.3. Thrombopoietin hormone (TPO)

It is a single 353- amino acid protein, synthesized primarily in the liver. Its level will increase during thrombocytopenia and keep increasing in response to the decline in platelet mass. For this reason most of the studies found that when platelets is transfused to the thrombocytopenic patients the TPO level will decreased. TPO mainly act by increasing the numbers of megakaryocyte colony forming cells (Meg-CFC), increases their ploidy, size and growth to produce more of the platelets. Moreover, it will stimulate the hematopoietic stem cell of the bone marrow and it has been found that high doses of TPO will lead to reactivation of the mature platelets to some aggregation stimuli [61].

2.3.4. Main causes of thrombocytopenia

The main causes leading to occurrence of thrombocytopenia are:

1. Chemotherapy drugs.

2. Solid cancer.

3. Blood cancer (Leukemia).

4. Spleen cancer.

5. Anemia.

6. Hemorrhage which will lead to increases loss of platelets.

7. When the rate of platelets destruction is higher than the rate of bone marrow platelets production [57, 59, 65].

2.3.5. Role of age and gender

Repetto (2003) mentioned that anemia is highly prevalent and happened in the elderly cancer patients who receive chemotherapy. This is specifically because their senescent cells have low ability to repair DNA and their low mass of the hematopoietic stem cell causing slowing of their recovery ability. Repetto also mentioned in his study that the occurrence of grade 3 thrombocytopenia is highly associated with older female suffering from breast cancer and found that there is an association between age and gender with thrombocytopenia. While others retrospective studies of solid tumor patients found that there is no association between age and myelosuppression i.e., neutropenia, anemia and thrombocytopenia occurrence [68].

2.3.6. Chemotherapy and thrombocytopenia

Thrombocytopenia is a detrimental side effect of chemotherapy since it will lead to hemorrhage from vital organ particularly the brain specifically within solid cancer patients who were treated with chemotherapy. These chemotherapies caused thrombocytopenia by different mechanisms either by suppressing megakaryopoiesis leading to prevention of platelets production or by direct damaging of the platelets. Chemotherapies like antimetabolites and alkylating agents induced severe thrombocytopenia due to their ability in causing bone marrow suppression and specifically after the first cycle of chemotherapy [62, 69, 70, 71].

2.3.7. Mechanism of thrombocytopenia in solid cancer

The association between bleeding and thrombocytopenia in patient suffering from leukemia was first described in 1962. Later in 1878 and 1984 this was reported happening among patient suffering from solid cancer [72]. Thrombocytopenia as a serious side effect is usually associated with solid cancer as a result of its metastasis to bone marrow. Theoretically most of solid tumors can metastasis to bone marrow but the most frequent are breast, lung and prostate cancers. These cancers when metastasized to bone marrow will lead to bone marrow suppression resulting in neutropenia and thrombocytopenia with serious morbidity and mortality (Kilickap et al., 2007). Besides that Elting and his colleagues mentioned that solid cancer patients are characterized by several things which are poor performance status, low baseline for platelets count and bone marrow metastasis. Despite that the bleeding situation among solid cancer patients remain poor compare with hematological malignant unless all the above characteristic are all present [62].

2.3.8. Diagnosis of thrombocytopenia

Different parameters are taken into consideration in order to diagnose thrombocytopenia such as medical history and laboratory test. Platelets count which is considered as part of the complete blood count (CBC) is the main key for the diagnosis of thrombocytopenia. It measures the exact numbers of platelets in a measured volume of blood. If the test shows low number of platelets then a careful examination for spleen and bone marrow biopsy must be done since both have a direct association with thrombocytopenia occurrence. Usually in adults when the platelets count is less than 100,000 cell/ microliter it is considered low but sometimes this happen without any symptoms. Other important tests which are used to diagnose thrombocytopenia are the prothrombin time (PT), activated partial thromboplastin time (aPTT) and thrombin time (TT). The results of these tests play a critical role in the diagnosis and certification of the presence of thrombocytopenia. In addition to liver enzymes test, renal function test, erythrocyte sedimentation rate (ESR), Vit B_{12} and folic acid levels are also carried out [57, 59, 64, 65, 73, 74].

2.3.9. Grades of thrombocytopenia

The normal range of the platelets is between 150,000 and 450,000 cells per microliter of blood (i.e., 150-450×10^9/ L) while thrombocytopenia could be classified into three levels as follows:

1. Mild thrombocytopenia if platelets count < 150 and ≥ 100 × 10^9/ L.

2. Moderate thrombocytopenia if platelets count < 100 and ≥ 50 × 10^9/ L.

3. Severe thrombocytopenia if platelets count < 20 × 10^9/ L [75, 76].

2.3.10. Clinical signs and symptoms of thrombocytopenia

There are several signs and symptoms which occasionally happen with thrombocytopenia. These are bloody stool, dizziness, headache, hemorrhage, oral bleeding, nose bleeding, vaginal bleeding, black stool and petechiae (reddish purple spots in the skin) [57, 58, 74].

2.3.11. Options for thrombocytopenia treatments

There are different options for thrombocytopenia treatment but the selection will mainly depends on the etiology and severity of thrombocytopenia. Sometimes with asymptomatic thrombocytopenia treatment is not required like that in children with viral infection. But if thrombocytopenia incidence is because of spleen enlargement then splenectomy will be beneficial and effective in increasing the platelets counts. While for thrombotic thrombocytopenic purpura (TTP) treatment is needed since it can leads to renal failure. In case of idiopathic thrombocytopenic purpura (ITP) the treatment depends on severity of the case and the platelets counts. In the case of heparin induce thrombocytopenia and thrombosis (HITT) the treatment is by stopping heparin administration. If the cause of thrombocytopenia is due to patient's immune system causing destruction to the platelets then the use of corticosteroids is very effective so as to suppress immune response. While if the cause is due to chemotherapy then the decision to either continue the treatment with low chemotherapy doses or use of alternative drugs or use of platelets growth factors (i.e., thrombopoietic growth factor) (Oprelvekin, Neumega®) should be made. Recombinant human interleukin-11 (rhIL-11) will stimulate megakaryocyte maturation and proliferation and maintain platelets production. It has been proven by the Food and Drug Administration (FDA) that rhIL-11 is very effective in reducing and preventing of severe thrombocytopenia as well as it will decrease the need for platelet transfusions especially after myelosuppressive chemotherapy which could be continue with the same doses. In the case of severe thrombocytopenia (i.e., platelet level ≤ 20,000/ μL) which is due to intensive chemotherapeutics drugs treatment of hematological and solid cancer patients, in this case platelet transfusion is needed. At this point, patient will suffer from severe bleeding and the laboratory tests signify that platelets transfusion is very important and a required treatment. Platelets transfusion is one of the most important treatments for acute and severe thrombocytopenia, but there are some limitations to its use which are: the availability of the blood products since it must be freshly taken and used within 5 days, cost, refractoriness, transfusion reaction and diseases transmission [57-59, 63, 76, 77].

2.3.12. Thrombocytopenia and neutropenia

Acute thrombocytopenia has been described in patients given Hematopoietic Growth Factors. The main factor which play role in this incidence is neutropenia treatments which are either GM-CSF and/ or G-CSF. This rapid incidence for thrombocytopenia in association with these treatments is mainly because these treatments sometimes target the platelets or caused their destruction. But the main mechanism which is responsible for the incidence of neutropenia with thrombocytopenia together has not been defined yet [78].

2.4. Hypercalcemia

Hypercalcemia is a life threatening situation in which serum calcium level is elevated greater than 10.5 mg/ dl, while albumin concentration is lower than 4 g/ dl. It is a serious problem that occurs in about 10%-20% of all cancer patients especially lung, breast, head and neck cancer patients. While, in hematological cancer hypercalcemia also takes place specifically in the advanced phases of both myeloma and lymphoma. Besides that a very important point is that hypercalcemia is mainly caused by cancer without any effect or role from anticancer treatments. So many references consider hypercalcemia as a very serious and dangerous complication that caused a significant morbidity and mortality frequently in breast cancer patients. It can occur in patients with and without bone metastasis and the main cause of hypercalcemia is the pathological bone resorption. Bone resorption is caused by the secretion of cytokine like parathyroid hormone-related protein (PTHrP) leading to activation and differentiation of osteoclast cell. In normal condition normal breast cells also secreted PTHrP during lactation so as to stimulate bone resorption and skeletal calcium release which will be used in milk synthesis. In this situation hypercalcemia is asymptomatic since the elevation of calcium level is mild, but when serum calcium elevation became very high it will leads to significant morbidity and mortality. Hypercalcemia is highly associated with breast cancer more than other types of cancers [78-83].

2.4.1. Calcium homeostasis

Calcium in human body has multiply functions, it is one of the major components and mineral of the body skeleton and its concentration is maintained by influx and efflux to the extracellular fluid from kidney, bone and gut. This vital process is regulated by two hormones which are parathyroid hormone (PTH) and 1, 25 dihydroxyvitamin D. Serum calcium consist of calcium bounded to albumin 37%, bounded with globulin (10%), biologically active calcium (47%) i.e., ionized form and calcium complex with anion (10%) (like: phosphate, citrate, bicarbonate). The ionized serum calcium is the only form metabolically active and is regulated by homeostatic mechanisms [87, 90, 98]. Calcium also has other important role in regulation of the cellular metabolism function, since it is a co-factor for many of body enzymes reactions. Also, calcium is needed for cell adhesion, cell death, an important component of cellular electrical current and has a very important function in muscular contraction process [84, 85].

2.4.2. Kidney role in calcium homeostasis

Kidney plays a very important role in regulation of calcium concentration in the extracellular fluid and its capacity to clear the calcium is about 600 mg per day (15 mmol/ day). In adult approximately 98% of calcium is resorbed by kidney. This process of calcium absorption is mainly controlled by PTH and 65% of total reabsorbed calcium happens at the proximal tubules, 20-25% in the ascending loop of Henle, while only 10% in the distal convoluted tubules [86].

2.4.3. Gut role in calcium homeostasis

The daily amount of calcium absorbed ranges between 150-200 mg/ day and this is send to the extracellular fluid. This process of absorption is mainly regulated by 1, 25 dihydroxyvitamin D hormone and calcium concentration in the blood circulation. Besides that the amounts of calcium absorbed from the daily diet is affected by the amount of calcium in the diet and presence of other dietary components which may serve to increase (lactose, fatty acid) or decreases (oxalate, phosphate and phytate) calcium absorption. The absorption of calcium from the daily diet varies even in healthy adult from 20% to 70%. The main parts responsible for absorption are the ileum (65%) and jejunum (17%). This is because these parts are the longest parts and hence the longest time calcium will be absorbed [87].

2.4.4. Bone role in calcium homeostasis

Bone consider as the main storehouse of calcium which store 99% of the body calcium. The role of bone in calcium homeostasis is important in normal conditions since the process of bone formation is tightly coupled with processes of bone resorption i.e., the velocity of calcium influx and efflux between the extracellular fluid and bone. The extracellular calcium concentration will be disturbed when the rates of bone resorption increase more than the rate of bone formation. This is seen in cases of advanced cancer diseases which caused activation of the osteoclast cell of the bone marrow leading to increase in bone marrow destruction and increase in calcium efflux. This mainly happy when the cancer disease metastasis to bone marrow and is usually consider as a catastrophic situation. Metastasis to bone marrow happens in 30% of breast cancer patients and causing disturbances in the plasma calcium concentration. Thus it is clear that bone play a critical role in the maintenance of serum calcium level [86, 88].

2.4.5. Main hormones responsible for calcium control

The extra cellular calcium concentration is maintained in a narrow range of 8.5-10.2 mg/ dL (2.1-2.55 mmol/ L) by two main hormones which are:

1.   Parathyroid hormone (PTH)

2.   1,25-dihydroxy-vitamin D [1,25 (OH)$_2$ D]

Both act on the three main organs which are kidney, gut and skeleton but PTH is more important since it regulate calcium level from minute to minute (i.e., very rapid effect), PTH it is consists of 84 amino acid single chain polypeptides and is mainly secreted by the chief cells of the four parathyroid glands besides the thyroid gland in the neck. PTH secretion is regulated by the serum calcium level of the extracellular fluid. When calcium concentration increases, the PTH secretion will be suppressed and when the calcium concentration decreases, PTH secretion increases. PTH mainly regulates the calcium transportation between extracellular fluids and kidney, bone and gut. PTH has a direct effect on bone and plays a critical role in increasing the rate of bone formation and turnover. Its effect on bone came from its stimulation and activation for the osteoclast cells which will lead to increase in bone turnover and it also increases the rate for bone formation. This effect has been found to be dependent on the presence of other hormones like 1, 25-dihydroxyvitamin D. PTH effect on kidney will leads to an increase in distal tubules reabsorption of calcium. Here its effect is enhanced by 1, 25-dihydroxyvitamin D, but it has no direct effect on the gut [78, 85, 88]. 1, 25 dihydroxy-vitamin D is the major biological active metabolite of vitamin D. This steroid-like metabolite is derived either from skin during its exposure to ultraviolet light (i.e., sun light) or from plant ergosterol after its ingestion in the gut. It increases the absorption of calcium and phosphorus from the gut by active transport as well as it increases the bone resorption. 1, 25 dihydroxy-vitamin D is characterized by its slower action than PTH but it is more effective than PTH in long term control of the serum calcium level [83, 86, 89]. Besides these two hormones, calcitonin which is 32 amino acid peptide also is involved in calcium content. It is synthesis and secreted by parafollicular cells of the thyroid gland. Its main action is by inhibition of the osteoclast cell from resorption of the bone by causing their dissolution to mononuclear cells [85].

2.4.6. Causes of hypercalcemia

The main causes of hypercalcemia during solid or hematological malignancy are as follows:

1.   The direct effect of cancer diseases on the bone by causing bone destruction such as with breast cancer, lung cancer, multiply myeloma and leukemia. Hypercalcemia occurs in about 10%-20% of all cancer patients during specific stages of their malignant diseases. Lung and breast cancers are highly associated with hypercalcemia incidence beside head

and neck cancer. While myeloma and lymphoma are the most common hematological types of cancers associated with hypercalcemia.

2. Some cancers diseases lead to production of parathyroid hormone-related protein (PTHrP) which is mainly associated with solid cancer but not with malignant cancer.

3. Some cancer diseases decrease the ability of the kidneys to remove excess calcium also leading to decreases in the urination.

4. Dehydration due to nausea and vomiting which will lead to difficulties of the kidneys to remove excess calcium from the blood.

5. Decreases in the movement and activity of cancer patients which will lead to breakdown of the bone and hence increase in the release of the calcium into the blood [90-94].

2.4.7. Hypercalcemia diagnosis

Diagnosis of hypercalcemia is made based on serum calcium level and also on levels of phosphate, chloride, PTH and alkaline phosphates. Other tests for kidney function especially urea level, creatinine level and albumin level tests also performed because in hypercalcemia these are elevated. Bone scan, prospective computed tomography (CT) scan for neck, chest and magnetic resonance imaging (MRI) may help to determined whether the tumor has metastasized to the bone [95].

2.4.8. Hypercalcemia levels

Normal level of calcium in the blood ranges between 8.7 – 10.4 mg/ dl. Correct calcium level in the blood could be determined by using the following equation:

Corrected calcium (mg/ dl) = measured calcium + ([4- albumin (g/ dl)] × 0.8).

Serum calcium ranging between 10.5 – 12.0 mg/ dl indicates mild hypercalcemia.

Moderate hypercalcemia is being diagnosed when serum calcium is between 12.0 – ≤ 14.0 mg/ dl.

Severe hypercalcemia (hypercalcemia crisis) occurs when serum calcium is higher than 14.0 mg/ dl and is associated with acute signs and symptoms [87, 90-96].

2.4.9. Signs and symptoms of hypercalcemia

Since calcium has a wide range of physiological actions so it has a myriad of clinical effects on multi organs. On central nervous system (CNS), hypercalcemia will cause fatigue, depression, confusion, headache, difficulty in thinking and stupor. Cardiovascular system effects manifestation will range from abnormal electrocardiogram to arrhythmias. Gastrointestinal system signs will involve constipation, nausea and vomiting. Hypercalcemia will cause impaired kidney function and as a consequence will lead to decrease in the renal excretion of calcium and thus increase in the severity of hypercalcemia. Dehydration, bone pain and lost of appetite has also been observed. The hypercalcemia due to primary hyperparathyroidism is usually mild or moderate and the patient will be asymptomatic or only suffer from minor clinical signs mentioned above. While hypercalcemia occurs as a result of breast cancer is usually acute or subacute and the calcium level will be highly elevated and many of the clinical signs mentioned above will be manifested. While mild hypercalcemic patients will be asymptomatic and hypercalcemia will be detected fortuitously during routine laboratory screening [83, 97-99].

2.4.10. Hypercalcemia treatments and options

There are different types of treatments used for hypercalcemic patients whereby some are often use for daily cases and some others used for emergency cases of hypercalcemia:

1. Bisphosphonates (Etidronate, Clodronate and Pamidronate):

2. Plicamycin (Mithramycin)

3. Calcitonin (Calcimar®)

4. Zoledronic acid (Zometa®)

5. Glucocorticoids (Prednisone)

While for emergency cases with calcium level exceeding 13 mg/ dl the following treatments are preferred:

1. Normal saline 200-400 ml/ hour I.V.

2. Furosemide (Lasix®) 200-400 ml/ hour [83, 86, 87, 97-99].

2.4.11. Role of age and gender

Hypercalcemia is usually seen in aged female patients more than male where the main characteristic is the presence of hypercalcemia without any symptoms. The main cause is either malignant disease or hyperparathyroidism [83, 86].

2.4.12. Mechanisms of hypercalcemia occurrence with malignancy

Mechanism of hypercalcemia incidence in solid cancer patients can be divided into two groups. In the first group, hypercalcemia may or may not be associated with bone metastasis and the main factor is the solid cancer itself since it will produce systematic circulating humoral factors which will ultimately cause loss of calcium from the bone i.e., bone resorption. Moreover these factors will lead to increase in calcium reabsorption from renal tubules. So this group is named as humoral hypercalcemia of malignancy (HHM) which include lung, ovarian, head and neck, pancreas and kidney cancer but the most frequent are the lung and head and neck cancers. The main factors produced by the cancer cells responsible for this situation are PTH, PTH-like factors, transforming growth factors, colony stimulating factors and leukocyte cytokines. In the second group, hypercalcemia is mainly caused or produced by extensive bone metastasis (i.e., extensive localized bone destruction) which include breast cancer. Breast cancer is considered as the highest and the most frequent solid cancer associated with hypercalcemia caused by bone metastasis. This hypercalcemia is called local osteolytic hypercalcemia (LOH). The main difference is that in LOH, hypercalcemia is caused by localized bone destruction resulting from bone metastasis by the solid cancer, while in HHM the systematic humoral factor is the sole responsible factor and that hypercalcemia is unrelated to the extent of bone metastasis. In LOH, hypercalcemia is produced by direct effect of the solid cancer cells on the bone i.e., by acting like osteoclast cell producing acid protease (lysosomal enzymes) and collagens responsible for removing of mineral from bone and mainly lead to resorption of bone matrix and causing an increase in cAMP and inhibition of microtubule assembly by agents like colchicine. Resorption could also happened or take place independently of osteoclast cell activity. While for hematological cancers i.e., myeloma the main causes for hypercalcemia are increase bone resorption and glomerular filtration impairment. The main cause of hypercalcemia during lymphoma is bone resorption associated with increase in absorption of calcium from the gut [82, 86, 100].

2.4.13. Relation of hypercalcemia with nausea and vomiting

The main mechanism of hypercalcemia incidence in solid cancer is the metastasis of the cancer to the bone. Breast cancer which is the highest type of the LOH has shown to cause bone marrow destruction leading to hypercalcemia. Hypercalcemia will lead to many side effects mainly nausea and vomiting and there are studies indicating that hypercalcemia is one of the main risk factor for nausea and vomiting [16, 101].

2.5. Neurotoxicity

Neurotoxicity which induced by chemotherapy can occurs because of the direct or indirect effect and/ or damage that chemotherapy will cause to the central nervous system (CNS) or peripheral nervous system or any combination of these [102]. It is a critical matter to distinct between the two components of the nervous system. The CNS consists from the brain and the spinal cord. CNS mainly responsible for controlling neurological function of mental status, level of consciousness, motor power, sensory function, cerebral function and cranial nerve function. While for the peripheral nervous system it consists of peripheral nerves, this system mainly responsible for sensing pain, temperature and sensation [103].

This side effect i.e., neurological toxicity remain as one of the major critical side effect of chemotherapy treatment. Its clinical presentation varies significantly as a result of that it became very difficult to confirm the diagnosis [104].

2.5.1. General signs and symptoms of neurotoxicity

Symptoms associated with neurotoxicity may include cerebellar effects i.e., (tremor, loss of balance and fine motor movements), confusion, visual impairment, peripheral neuropathy, somnolence and auditory [102].

It has been found that neurotoxicity problems usually temporary i.e., resolving once treatment is completed, even so sometimes permanent neurological deficits may happened [102].

2.5.2. Blood-brain barrier and it's role in protecting CNS

Blood-brain barrier consider as a very efficient part of the nervous system that determine whether a chemotherapy agent is able to reach the nervous system or not. This barrier has the ability to block certain chemotherapy agents from entering nervous system at the cellular level [105]. Blood-brain barrier which surrounding the CNS varies from the one which surrounding the peripheral nervous system, as a result of this variation some chemotherapy agents such as vincristine significantly affect the peripheral nervous system but not the CNS. Chemotherapy agent will produce neurotoxic effects only if it has the ability to cross the blood-brain barrier [106].

2.5.3. Neurotoxicity and chemotherapy

Chemotherapy agents that significantly associated with neurotoxicity include the following: 1- Platinum compounds, 2- Taxanes, 3- Vinca alkaloid [104].

2.5.4. Factors associated with the incidence of neurotoxicity

There are many factors play role in the incidence of neurotoxicity but the most critical factors are the following::

1.   Chemotherapy doses.

2.   Route of chemotherapy administration [107].

2.5.5. Other factors

The incidence of neurotoxicity can be related to factors other than chemotherapy, these factors are:

1.   Primary or secondary tumor deposits, which may involve the nervous system.

2.   Metabolic or electrolyte imbalance which will leads to neurological disturbance.

3.   Neurological deficits [108].

2.5.6. Neurotoxicity evaluation and management

Treatment used for neurotoxicity that caused by chemotherapy agents is limited. The focus of care should be on early recognition of neurotoxicity and careful monitoring of patients at high risk of toxicity [109]. There are various agents that either block the development and/ or incidence of neurotoxicity that caused by chemotherapy agents. Even so the mechanisms of action for these agents still mysterious [110]. Example for agent used as antidote for encephalopathy cause by ifosfamide is the methylene blue [111], besides that amifostine and adrenocorticotropic hormone analogues have also been found to be an effective neuroprotective agents. But farther investigation still required to clarifying the role of these agents in overcoming and/ or preventing neurotoxicity problem which leads to either delay in chemotherapy schedule, reduction in chemotherapy doses or substitution with an alternative agent [104].

2.6. Cardiotoxicity

The major function of the heart is to pump the blood to the whole body to supply body organs with adequate oxygen and nutrition they need. This process will happened by contracting muscular walls of the left ventricle [112]. There are various factors which can leads to cardiac injury in the cancer patients. This may happened as a result of either infiltration of metastases to infections and/ or because of chemotherapy toxicity [112].

2.6.1. Major factors which cause cardiac damage in cancer patients

a-Cardiac tumors, b-Bacterial infections, c-Chemotherapy induce toxicity, e-Radiation induce toxicity, f-Fungal and/ or viral infection [113, 114].

Chemotherapy effects will be classified into two types: acute and chronic effects.

2.6.2. Acute toxic effect

Acute cardiotoxicity caused by doxorubicin came from combination of factors which are: mitochondrial changes, cellular degeneration and a loss of myocardial fibrils. The incidence of cardiotoxicity will be either during or after doxorubicin administration, this cardiotoxicity will leads to cardiac abnormalities which include: ST and T wave changes, sinus tachycardia, atrial and ventricular ectopics, complete heart block, supraventricular tachycardia and ventricular tachycardia [116, 117].

Although doxorubicin cause cardiotoxicity there is no specific treatment for this condition, but there is only a supportive treatments. Researchers and clinicians keep on using of cardioprotective agents that allow chemotherapy agents specifically anthracycline to be used at a higher dose without causing cardiotoxicity [114]. Example for these cardioprotective agents are dexrazoxane and amifostine [118].

2.6.3. Chronic toxicity

This type of toxicity is one of the most common toxicity caused by doxorubicin it is characterized by chronic dilated cardiomyopathy. This condition i.e., cardiomyopathy usually happened either at late of chemotherapy cycle or shortly after the end of it [119]. Cardiomyopathy is significantly attenuated by the chelation of iron. Moreover, cardiomyopathy has been diagnosed among the survivors of cancer patients who have been treated with doxorubicin during their childhood [120].

2.7. Pulmonary toxicity

It is one of the main side effects of chemotherapy, which become clinically obvious after weeks, months or even years of termination of chemotherapy. It usually associated with several clinical symptoms which are: dry cough, dyspnoea and progressive worsening of symptoms with a poor prognosis for recovery [121].

2.7.1. Chemotherapy and pulmonary toxicity

Chemotherapeutic agents will be divided into three groups, this will mainly based on their effects on pulmonary function:

1. Hypersensitive pulmonary reaction: Bleomycin, 6-mercaptopurine, methotrexate, mitomycin and procarbazine. This condition take place as a result of either desquamative interstitial pneumonitis or an eosinophilic pneumonitis [122, 123].

2. Non-cardiogenic pulmonary oedema: Cyclophosphamide, cytarabine and methotrexate. This condition will take place after few days of strating using of chemotherapy treatment.

3. Chronic pulmonary fibrosis: Bleomycin, busulfan, carmustine, cyclophosphamide, fludarabine, ifosfamide, methotrexate and mitomycin [122, 123]. This clinical condition will take place within months of using chemotherapy treatment.

Besides that it has been found that when mitomycin used in combination with vinca alkaloids and/ or gemcitabine with docetaxel or when the later two agents i.e., gemcitabine and docetaxel used alone they can cause pulmonary toxicity [124, 125, 126, 127].

2.7.2. Assessment of pulmonary function

It is very important to assess patients pulmonary function before start administration of chemotherapy, the assessment will include the following:1- Chest X-ray 2- Lung biopsy required to differentiate chronic fibrosis from lung metastasis [121].

2.7.3. Treatments used for pulmonary toxicity cases

Managements used for pulmonary problems i.e., toxicity will include the following: 1- Bronchodilator, 2- Corticosteroid 3- Expectorant 4- Oxygen 5- Antibiotics 6- Nebulised saline 7- Aminophylline and theophylline [128-129].

3. Conclusion

Cancer has become a major killer in the world which almost surpasses the cardiovascular diseases and will become the main lethal cause in this century. Although the global war against cancer leads to remarkable gain in understanding the main molecular mechanism for the cancer cell, this progress is still consider as slow and not enough especially in case of treatment of common solid tumor in adults. Besides that there are so many types of serious side effects caused by the tumor itself or because of its chemotherapy treatment.

Therefore it is an obligate for all the clinicians and physicians to focus on these main side effects that emerged as a result of cancer itself or its treatment and working to built and develop treatment guidelines to overcome or palliate these major side effects.

Acknowledgements

I would like to show and express my great appreciation and heartfelt thanks to my main supervisor Associate Prof. Dr. Zuraidah Mohd Yusoff, for her great support and guidance. Moreover, I'd like to express my great appreciation for my co-supervisors Associate Prof. Saad Bin Othman and Associate Prof. Dr Mohamed Azmi Hassali for their creative advice and guidance.

Also I'd like to express my grateful appreciation to Universiti Sains Malaysia and a special thanks to the School of Pharmaceutical Sciences. I'd like to thank those who represent the greatest support in my whole life, those who fill my life with all of colorful beauties of hope and nature, who always by their skillful advice made the correct scope for my life, my family specifically my great and marvelous father (Abdul Rasool), mother (Basma) and my daughter (Shams).

Author details

Bassam Abdul Rasool Hassan[1*], Zuraidah Binti Mohd Yusoff[1], Mohamed Azmi Hassali[2] and Saad Bin Othman[1]

*Address all correspondence to: bassamsunny@yahoo.com

1 Clinical Pharmacy Discipline, School of Pharmaceutical Sciences, Universiti Sains Malaysia, Minden, Penang, Malaysia

2 Discipline of Social and Administrative Pharmacy, School of Pharmaceutical Sciences, Universiti Sains Malaysia, Minden Penang, Malaysia

References

[1] Carson-DeWitt RCancer. In: Longe JL. (ed.) The Gale Encyclopedia of Medicine Farmington Hills. Gale Group; (2002). , 631-638.

[2] Markman, M. Principles of cancer screening. In: Aziz K., & Wu GY. (ed.) Cancer screening A Practical Guide for Physicians. New Jersey: Humana Press; (2002). , 170-189.

[3] Dolan, S. Thrombocytopenia. In: Brighton D., Wood M. (ed.) The Royal Marsden Hospital Handbook of Cancer Chemotherapy. London: Churchill Livingstone; (2005). , 231-247.

[4] Henry, L. Malnutrition. In: Brighton D., Wood M. (ed.) The Royal Marsden Hospital Handbook of Cancer Chemotherapy. Churchill Livingstone: Elsevier; (2005). , 177-184.

[5] Sitamvaram, R. Gastrointestinal effects In: Brighton D., Wood M. (ed.) The Royal Marsden Hospital Handbook of Cancer Chemotherapy. Churchill Livingstone: Elsevier; (2005). , 161-164.

[6] Stephens, M. Nausea and Vomiting. In: Brighton D., Wood M. (ed.) The Royal Marsden Hospital Handbook of Cancer Chemotherapy. Churchill Livingstone: Elsevier; (2005). , 155-160.

[7] Weir-hughes, D. Foreword. In: Brighton D., Wood M. (ed.) The Royal Marsden Hospital Handbook of Cancer Chemotherapy. London: Elsevier / Churchill Livingstone; (2005). p ix.

[8] Rizzo, T, & Cloos, R. Chemotherapy. In: Thackery E. (ed.) The Gale Encyclopedia of Cancer. Detroit: Gale Group; (2002). , 225-233.

[9] Abrams, A. C. Drugs Used in Oncologic Disorders. In: Repchinsky C. (ed.) Clinical Drug Therapy. 36 ed. Ontario: Canadian Pharmacists Association; (2001). , 17-29.

[10] Koda-Kimble LYYWayne A., Kradjan BJG., Brain KA., Robin LC. Applied Therapeutics the Clinical Use of Drugs. In: Troy D. (ed.) Hand Hook of Applied Therapeutics. Philadelphia: Lippincott Williams & Wilkins; (2002). , 212-234.

[11] Haggerty, M. Nausea and Vomiting. In: Donna O., Christine J., Karen B. (ed.) The Gale Encyclopedia of Medicine. Farmington Hills: Gale Research; An International Thomson company; (1999). , 21-34.

[12] Oberleitner, M. G. Nausea and Vomiting In: Ellen T. (ed.) The Gale Encyclopedia of Cancer. Detroit: Gale group; (2002). , 37-52.

[13] Coates, A, Abraham, S, & Kaye, S. B. On The Receiving End-Patient Perception of The Side-Effects of Cancer Chemotherapy. European Journal of Cancer & Clinical Oncology (1983). , 19, 203-208.

[14] Lebourgeois, J. P, Mckenna, C. J, & Coster, B. Efficacy of an Ondansetron Orally Disintegrating Tablet: A Novel Oral Formulation of This 5-HT3 Receptor Antagonist in The Treatment of Fractionated Radiotherapy-Induced Nausea and Emesis. Clinical Oncology (1999). , 11, 340-347.

[15] Morrow, G. R, Hickok, J. T, Roscore, J. A, & Matteson, S. A Biobehavioral Perspective of Nausea and Emesis In: Hesketh PJ. (ed.) Management of Nausea and Vomiting in Cancer and Cancer Treatment. Mississauga: Jones and Barlett; (2005). , 119-146.

[16] Hesketh, P. J. Management of Nausea and Vomiting in Cancer Treatment: Introduction, Scope of The Problem. In: Hesketh PJ. (ed.) Management of Nausea and Vomiting in Cancer and Cancer Treatment. Mississauge: Jones and Bartlett; (2005). , 1-14.

[17] Rudd, J. A. Andrews PLR. Mechanisms of Acute, Delayed and Anticipatory Emesis Induced by Anticancer Therapies In: Hesketh PJ. (ed.) Management of Nausea and Vomiting in Cancer and Cancer Treatment. Mississauge: Jones and Bartlett; (2005). , 1-14.

[18] Oberleitner, M. G. Nausea and Vomiting In: Ellen T. (ed.) The Gale Encyclopedia of Cancer. Detroit: Gale group; (2002). , 71-89.

[19] Mitchell, E. P, & Schein, P. S. Gastrointestinal Toxicity of Therapeutics Agents. In: Perry MC., Yarbro JW. (ed.) Toxicity of Chemotherapy. Orlando: Grune & Stratton; (1984). , 55-65.

[20] Bartlett, N, & Koczwara, B. Review: Control of Nausea and Vomiting After Chemotherapy: What is The Evidence?. Internal Medicine Journal (2002). , 32, 401-407.

[21] Molassiotis, A, & Börjeson, S. Nausea and Vomiting In: Kearney N., Richardson A., editor. Nursing Patients With Cancer/ Principles and Practice. Philadelphia: Churchill Livingstone; (2006). , 415-437.

[22] Navari, R. M. Overview of The Updated Antiemetic Guidelines for Chemotherapy-Induced Nausea and Vomiting. Community Oncology (2007). , 4(4), 3-11.

[23] Hesketh, P. J. Potential Role of The NK1 Receptor Antagonists in Chemotherapy-Induced Nausea and Vomiting. Supportive Care in Cancer. (2001). , 9, 350-354.

[24] Osoba, D, Zee, B, Warr, D, Latreille, J, Kaizer, L, & Pater, J. Effect of Postchemotherapy Nausea and Vomiting on Health-Related Quality of Life. Support Care Cancer (1997). , 5, 307-313.

[25] Rubenstein, E. The Role of Prognostic Factors in Chemotherapy Induced Nausea and Vomiting In: Hesketh PJ. (ed.) Management of Nausea and Vomiting in Cancer and Cancer Treatment. Mississauga: Jones and Bartlett; (2005). , 87-97.

[26] Ballatori, E, & Roila, F. Methodological Issues in The Assessment of Nausea and Vomiting. In: Hesketh PJ. (ed.) Management of Nausea and Vomiting in Cancer and Cancer Treatment Mississauga: Jones and Bartlett; (2005). , 67-85.

[27] Hesketh, P. J. Comparative Review of 5-HT3 Receptor Antagonists in The Treatment of Acute Chemotherapy-Induced Nausea and Vomiting. Cancer Invest (2000). , 18, 163-73.

[28] Kris, M. G, Gralla, R. J, & Clark, R. A. Incidence, Course and Severity of Delayed Nausea and Vomiting Following the Administration of High-Dose Cisplatin. Journal of clinical oncology (1985). , 3, 1379-84.

[29] Jordan, K, Kasper, C, & Schomll, H-J. Chemotherapy-Induced Nausea and Vomiting: Current and New Standards in The Antiemetic Prophylaxis and Treatment. European Journal of Cancer (2005). , 41, 199-205.

[30] Grunberg, S. M, & Dugan, M. Integrated Therapy of Nausea and Vomiting. In: Hesketh PJ. (ed.) Management of Nausea and Vomiting in Cancer and Cancer Treatment. Mississauga: Jones and Bartlett; (2005). , 147-160.

[31] Gross, S. A, Bridge, S, & Shenfield, G. M. Pharmacokinetic of Tolbutamide in Ethnic Chinese. Journal of Clinical Pharmacology (1999). , 47, 151-6.

[32] Ruzilawati, A. B. Mohd Suhaimi AW, Gan SH. Genetic Polymorphisms of CYP3A4: CYP3A4*18 Allele is Found in Five Healthy Malaysian subjects. Clinica Chimica Acta (2007). , 383, 158-162.

[33] Haut, A. Anemia. In: Weil J, Blumel D, Tylor R, Geller E. (ed.) Encyclopedia of Science and Technology. New York McGraw-Hill; (2007). , 12-31.

[34] Blaser, L. Anemia. In: Mcgrath KA, Lachford SB. (ed.) The Gale Encyclopedia of Science. Farmington Hills: Gale group; (2001). , 201-211.

[35] Brown, T, & Olde, T. G. Anemia. In: Longe JL. (ed.) The Gale Encyclopedia of Cancer2. Detroit Gale group; (2005). , 341-352.

[36] Pohl, G, & Ludwig, H. Positive Effects of Correction of Anemia in Malignant Diseases. In: Weiss G., Gordeuk VR., Hershko C. (ed.) Anemia of Chronic Disease. New York: Taylor & Francis; (2005). , 489-557.

[37] Gordeuk, V. R. Iron Therapy and the Anemia of Chronic Disease In: Weiss GG VR., Hershko C. (ed.) Anemia of Chronic Disease New York Taylor & Francis Group; (2005). , 381-395.

[38] Marx JJMErythrophagocytosis and Decreased Erythrocyte Survival In: Weiss G., Gordeuk VR., Hershko C. (ed.) Anemia of Chronic Disease New York: Taylor & Francis group; (2005). , 201-227.

[39] Metzen, E, & Jelkmann, W. Erythropoietin and Erythropoiesis In: Weiss GG., Gordeuk VR., Hershko C. (ed.) Anemia of Chronic Disease New York: Taylor & Francis Group; (2005). , 61-85.

[40] Gordon, M. S. Managing Anemia in The Cancer Patient: Old Problems, Future Solutions. Oncologist. (2002). , 7, 331-41.

[41] Beguin, Y. Endogenous Eryhthropoietin in The Anemia of Chronic Disorders In: Weiss G., Gordeuk VR., Hershko C. (ed.) Anemia of Chronic Disease. New York: Taylor & Francis group; (2005). , 145-200.

[42] Punnonen, K, & Rajamaki, A. Usefulness of Old and New Diagnostic Test in ACD. In: Weiss GG., Gordeuk VR., Hershko C. (ed.) Anemia of Chronic Disease New York: Taylor & Francis Group; (2005). , 349-364.

[43] Pronzato, P. Cancer-Related Anaemia Management in The 21st Century. Cancer Treatment Reviews. (2006). , 32, 1-3.

[44] Balducci, L. Anemia, cancer, and aging. Cancer Control. (2003). , 10(6), 478-86.

[45] Killip, S, Bennett, J. M, & Chambers, M. D. Iron deficiency anemia. American Family Physician. (2007). , 75, 671-678.

[46] Reed, W. R, Hussey, D. H, & Degowin, R. L. Implications of The Anemia of Chronic Disorders in Patients Anticipating Radiotherapy. The American Journal of Medical Sciences. (1994). , 308, 9-15.

[47] Ludwig, H, & Fritz, E. Anemia in Cancer Patients. Semin Oncol. (1998). , 25, 2-6.

[48] Groopman, J. E, & Itri, L. M. Chemotherapy-Induced Anemia in Adults: Incidence and Treatment. Journal of the National Cancer Institute (1999). , 91(19), 1616-34.

[49] Barrett-lee, P. J, Ludwig, H, Birgegård, G, Bokemeyer, C, Gascón, P, Kosmidis, P. A, & Krzakowski, M. Nortier JWR, Kongable G, Schneider M, Schrijvers D, Van Belle SJ. Independent Risk Factors for Anemia in Cancer Patients Receiving Chemotherapy: Results From the European Cancer Anaemia Survey. Oncology (2006). , 70, 34-48.

[50] Ruggiero, A, Attinà, G, Haber, M, Coccia, P, Lazzareschi, I, & Riccardi, R. Assessment of Chemotherapy-Induced Anemia in Children with Cancer. Central European Journal of Medicine (2008). , 3(3), 341-345.

[51] Glaspy, J, Jadeja, J. S, & Justice, G. A dose-Finding and Safety Study of Novel Erythropoiesis Stimulating Protein (NESP) For The Treatment of Anaemia in Patients Receiving Multicycle Chemotherapy. British Journal of Cancer (2001). , 84(1), 17-23.

[52] Cazzola, M. Mechanisms of Anaemia in Patients With Malignancy: Implications For The Clinical Use of Recombinant Human Erythropoietin. Medical Oncology (2000). , 17(1), 11-16.

[53] Danova, M, Aglietta, M, & Pierelli, L. The Use of Erythropoietin Alpha in Programs of High Dose Chemotherapy. Recenti Prog Med (2000). , 91, 681-9.

[54] Manegold, C. The Causes and Prognostic Significance of Low Hemoglobin Levels in Tumor Patients. Strahlenther Onkol (1998). , 174(4), 17-19.

[55] Sabbatini, P. The Relationship Between Anemia and Quality of Life in Cancer Patients. Oncologist (2000). , 5(2), 19-23.

[56] Dolan, S. Thrombocytopenia. In: Brighton D., Wood M. (ed.) The Royal Marsden Hospital Handbook of Cancer Chemotherapy. London: Churchill Livingstone; (2005). , 15-28.

[57] De Bellis, D. Thrombocytopenia. In: Olendorf D., Jeryan C., Boyaden K. (ed.) The Gale Encyclopedia of Medicine. Farmington Hills: Gale Research, An international Thomson company; (1999). , 75-88.

[58] Miller, B, & De Bellis, D. Thrombocytopenia. In: Longe JL. (ed.) The Gale Encyclopedia of Cancer 2. Detroit: Gale group; (2005). , 115-123.

[59] Dolan, S. Haemorrhagic problems. In: Grundy M. (ed.) Nursing in Haematological Oncology. London: Bailliere Tindall; (2000). , 11-19.

[60] Terranova, L, Gerli, G, & Cattaneo, M. Platelet Disorders in The Elderly. In: Bladucci L., Ershler W., de Gaetano G. (ed.) Blood Disorders in The Elderly. Cambridge: University Press; (2007). , 420-431.

[61] Kuter, D. J. Thrombopoietin: Biology and Potential Clinical Applications In: McCrae KR. (ed.) Thrombocytopenia New York: Taylor & Francis Group; (2006). , 17-51.

[62] Elting, L. S, Rubenstein, E. B, Martin, C. G, Kurtin, D, Rodriguez, S, Laiho, E, Kanesan, K, Cantor, S. B, & Benjamin, R. S. Incidence, Cost, and Outcomes of Bleeding and Chemotherapy Dose Modification Among Solid Tumor Patients With Chemotherapy-Induced Thrombocytopenia. Journal of Clinical Oncology (2001). , 19(4), 1137-1146.

[63] Cantor, S. B, Elting, L. S, Hudson, D. V, & Rubenstein, E. B. Pharmacoeconomic Analysis of Oprelvekin (Recombinant Human Interleukin-11) For Secondary Prophylaxis of Thrombocytopenia in Solid Tumor Patients Receiving Chemotherapy. American Cancer Society (2003). , 97(12), 3099-3106.

[64] Castellone, D. Overview of Hemostasis and Platelet Physiology. In: Ciesla B. (ed.) Hematology in practice. Philadelphia: F. A. Davis Company; (2007). , 229-244.

[65] Miller, B, & De Bellis, D. Thrombocytopenia. In: Longe JL. (ed.) The Gale Encyclopedia of Cancer 2. Detroit: Gale group; (2005). , 315-322.

[66] Mckenzie, S, & Reilly, M. Platelet Clearance In: McCrae KR. (ed.) Thrombocytopenia New York: Taylor & Francis group; (2006). , 101-114.

[67] Groeger, J. S. Critical Care of The Cancer Patient. St Louis: Mosby Year Book; (1991).

[68] Repetto, L. Greater Risks of Chemotherapy Toxicity in Elderly Patients With Cancer. The Journal of Supportive Oncology (2003). , 1(2), 18-24.

[69] Zeuner, A, Signore, M, Martinetti, D, Bartucci, M, Peschle, C, & De Maria, R. Chemotherapy-Induced Thrombocytopenia Derives From the Selective Death of Megakaryocyte Progenitors and can be Rescued by Stem Cell factor. Cancer Research (2007). , 67(10), 4767-4773.

[70] Margaglione, M. Congenital Platelet Disorders. In: Hoffbrand AV., Catovsky D., & Tuddenham EGD. (ed.) Postgraduate Haematology. Massachusetts: Blackwell Publishing Ltd; (2005). , 925-936.

[71] Avvisati, G, Tirindelli, M. C, & Annibali, O. Thrombocytopenia and Hemorrhagic Risk in Cancer Patients. Critical Reviews in Oncology/ Hematology (2003). , 48, 13-16.

[72] Elting, L. S, Cantor, S. B, Martin, C. G, Hamblin, L, Kurtin, D, Rivera, E, Vadhan-raj, S, & Benjamin, R. S. Cost of Chemotherapy-Induced Thrombocytopenia Among Pa-

tients with Lymphoma or Solid Tumors. American Cancer Society (2003). , 97(6), 1541-1550.

[73] Betrosian, A. P, Theodossiades, G, & Lambroulis, G. Heparin-Induced Thrombocytopenia with Pulmonary Embolism and Disseminated Intravascular Coagulation Associated with Low-Molecular-Weight. American Journal of Medicine Sciences (2003). , 325, 45-7.

[74] WikipediaThrombocytopenia Wikipedia the Free Encyclopedia: WKIPEDIA. http:// en.wikipedia.org/wiki/updated (2008). cited] (accessed 17th August 2008).

[75] Lea, B, Anna, P, Shakuntala, N, & Rajeev, M. Thrombocytopenia Related Neonatal Outcome in Preterms. Indian Journal of Pediatrics (2007). , 74, 269-74.

[76] Mcclure, M. W, Berkowitz, S. D, Sparapani, R, Tuttle, R, Kleiman, N. S, Berdan, L. G, Lincoff, A. M, Deckers, J, Diaz, R, Karsch, K. R, Gretler, D, Kitt, M, Simoons, M, Topol, E. J, Califf, R. M, & Harrington, R. A. Clinical Significance of Thrombocytopenia During a non-ST-Elevation Acute Coronary Syndrome The Platelet Glycoprotein IIb/ IIIa in Unstable Angina: Receptor Suppression Using Integrilin Therapy (PURSUIT) Trial Experience. Journal of the American Heart Association (1999). , 99, 2892-2900.

[77] Milman, E, Berdon, W. E, Garvin, J. H, Cairo, M. S, Bessmertny, O, & Ruzal-shapiro, C. Periostitis Secondary to Interleukin-11 (Oprelvekin, Neumega) Treatment for Thrombocytopenia in Pediatric Patients. Pediatr Radiol (2003). , 33, 450-452.

[78] Mcfarlane-parrott, S. Oprelvekin. In: Thsckery E. (ed.) The Gale Encyclopedia of Cancer: Farmington Hills; (2002). , 33-47.

[79] Aster, R. H, & George, J. N. Drug-Induced Thrombocytopenia. In: McCrae KR. (ed.) Thrombocytopenia New York: Taylor & Francis Group; (2006). , 145-177.

[80] Helft, P. R, & Rudin, C. M. Metabolic and Electrolyte Complications of Malignancy In: Vokes EE., Golomb HM. (ed.) Oncologic Therapies Chicago: Springer-Verlag Berlin Heidelberg (1999). , 244-257.

[81] Dolan, S. Electrolyte abnormalities In: Brighton D., Wood M. (ed.) The Royal Marsden Hospital Handbook of Cancer Chemotherapy Churchill Livingstone Elsevier (2005). , 205-208.

[82] Swartout-corbeil, D. Hypercalcemia In: Thackery E. (ed.) Gale Encyclopedia of Cancer Detroit: Gale group; (2002). , 516-518.

[83] Swartout-corbeil, D. Hypercalcemia In: Longe JL. (ed.) Gale Encyclopedia of Cancer 2. Detroit: Gale group; (2005). , 579-581.

[84] Ericson, K. Hypercalcemia. In: Olendorf D., Jeryan C., Boyaden K. (ed.) Gale Encyclopedia of Medicine. Farmington Hills: Gale Research, An International Thomson company; (1999). , 1500-1503.

[85] Broadus, A. E. Mineral balance and homeostasis. In: Favus MJ. (ed.) Primer on The Metabolic Bone Diseases and Disorders of Mineral Metabolism. Washington: Asbmr; (2003). , 702-744.

[86] Juppner, H. W, Gardella, T. J, Brown, E. M, Kronenberg, H. M, & Potts, J. T. Parathyroid Hormone and Parathyroid Hormone Related Peptide in The Regulation of Calcium Homeostasis and Bone Development. In: Degroot LJ., Jameson JL. (ed.) Endocrinology. Philadelphia: WB Saunders; (2001). , 557-569.

[87] Mundy, G. R. Calcuim Homeostasis: Hypercalcemia and Hypocalcemia/ General Concepts of Calcuim Homeostasis.. Dunitz M. (ed.) Cambridge: The University Press; (1990). , 75-89.

[88] Mundy, G. R. Calcuim Homeostasis-Role of The Gut, Kidney and Bone. Dunitz M. (ed.) Cambridge: The University Press; (1990). , 103-121.

[89] Mundy, G. R. Mechanisms of Bone Metastasis/ Skeletal Complications of Malignancy. Cancer supplement (1997). , 80(8), 1546-1556.

[90] De Mauro, S, & Wysolmerski, J. Hypercalcemia in Breast Cancer: An Echo of Bone Mobilization During Lactation? Journal of Mammary Gland Biology and Neoplasia (2005). , 10, 157-67.

[91] Edelson, G. W, & Kleerekoper, M. Hypercalcemic Crisis. Medical Clinical of North America (1995). , 79, 79-92.

[92] Walls, J, Ratcliffe, W. A, Howell, A, & Bundred, N. J. Parathyroid hormone and parathyroid hormone-related protein in the investigation of hypercalcaemia in two hospital populations. Clinical Endocrinology (Oxford) (1994). , 41, 407-413.

[93] Gurbuz, A. T, & Peetz, M. E. Giant Mediastinal Parathyroid Cyst: An Unusual Cause of Hypercalcemic Crisis-Case Report and Review of The Literature. Surgery (1996). , 120, 795-800.

[94] Potts, J. J. Hyperparathyroidism and Other Hypercalcemic Disorders. Advance in Internal Medicine (1996). , 41, 165-212.

[95] Hiraki, A, Ueoka, H, Takata, I, Gemba, K, Bessho, A, Segawa, Y, Kiura, K, Eguchi, K, Yoneda, T, Tanimoto, M, & Harada, M. Hypercalcemia-leukocytosis syndrome associated with lung cancer. Lung Cancer (2004). , 43, 301-307.

[96] Bilezikian, J. P. Clinical review 51: Management of Hypercalcemia. Journal of Clinical Endocrinology Metabolism (1993). , 77, 1445-1449.

[97] Bushinsky, D. A, & Monk, R. D. Calcium. Lancet (1998). , 352, 306-311.

[98] Ariyan, C. E, & Sosa, J. A. Assessment and Management of Patients with Abnormal Calcium. Critical Care Medicine (2004). , 32, 146-154.

[99]   Leboff, M. S, & Mikulec, K. H. Hypercalcemia: Clinical Manifestations, Pathogenesis, Diagnosis and Management. In: Favus MJ. (ed.) Primer on The Metabolic Bone Diseases and Disorders of Mineral Metabolism. Washington ASBMR (2003). , 631-651.

[100] Swartout-corbeil, D. Hypercalcemia In: Longe JL. (ed.) Gale Encyclopedia of Cancer 2. Detroit: Gale group; (2005). , 579-581.

[101] Wysolmerski, J. J, & Broadus, A. E. Hypercalcemia of Malignancy: The Central Role of Parathyroid Hormone-Related Protein. Annual Review of Medicine (1994). , 45, 189-200.

[102] Molassiotis, A, & Börjeson, S. Nausea and Vomiting In: Kearney N., Richardson A. (ed.) Nursing Patients With Cancer/ Principles and Practice Philadelphia Churchill Livingstone (2006). , 415-437.

[103] Groenwald, S. Hansen Frogge M., Goodman M. Cancer Nursing: Principles and Practice. 4th edn. Boston: Jones and Bartlett; (1997).

[104] Armstrong, T, Rust, D, & Kohtz, J. Neurologic, Pulmonary and Cutaneous Toxocities of High Dose Chemotherapy. Oncology Nursing Forum (1997). , 24(1), 23-33.

[105] Merien-bennett, R. Chemotherapy-Induced Neurological Toxicities. In: Brighton D. (ed.) The Royal Marsden Hospital Handbook of Cancer Chemotherapy. New York: Churchill Livingstone; (2005). , 213-215.

[106] Cline, M. J, & Haskel, C. M. Cancer Chemotherapy. Philadelphia: WB Saunders; (1980).

[107] Holmes, S. Cancer Chemotherapy. A Guide For Practice. Surrey: Asset Books; (1997).

[108] Kaplan, R, & Wiernik, P. Neurotoxicity of Antineoplastic Drugs. Seminars in Oncology (1982). , 16-103.

[109] Wilson, J, & Marsarryk, T. Neurological Emergencies in The Cancer Patient. Seminars in Oncology Journal (1989). , 16, 490-503.

[110] Cameron, J. Ifosfamide Neurotoxicity: A Challenge For Nurse, A Potential Nightmare For Patients. Cancer Nursing Journal (1993). , 16(1), 40-46.

[111] Gilbert, M. Neurologic Complications. In: Abeloff M, Armatige J., Lichter A. (ed.) Clinical Oncology. 2nd Edition. Edinburgh: Churchill Livingstone; (2000). , 1000-1020.

[112] Kupfer, A, Aeschlimann, C, & Cerny, T. Methylene Blue and The Neurotoxic Mechanisms of Ifosfamide Encephalopathy. European Journal of Clinical Pharmacology (1996). , 50(4), 249-259.

[113] Dolan, S. Cardiac Effects. In: Brighton D. (ed.) The Royal Marsden Hospital Handbook of Cancer Chemotherapy. New York: Churchill Livingstone; (2005). , 217-219.

[114] Zennhausern, R, Tobler, A, & Leoncini, L. Fatal Cardiac Arrhythmia After Infusion of Dimethyl Sulfoxide-Cryopreserved Hematopoietic Stem Cells in a Patient With Se-

vere Primary Cardiac Amyloidosis and End-Stage Renal Failure. Annals of Hematology (2000). , 79(9), 523-526.

[115] Whedon, M. B, & Wujcik, D. Blood and Marrow Stem Cell Transplantation. Boston: Jones and Bartlett (1997).

[116] Groeger, J. S. Critical Care of The Cancer Patient. St Louis: Mosby Year Book; (1991).

[117] Von Herbay, A, Drorken, B, & Mall, G. Cardiac Damage in Autologous Bone Marrow Transplant Patients: An Autopsy Study. Klinische Wochenschrift (1988). , 66, 1175-1181.

[118] Nelson, M. A, Frishman, W. H, & Seiter, K. Cardiovascular Considerations With Anthracycline Use in Patients With Cancer. Heart Disease Journal (2001). , 3(3), 157-168.

[119] Lefrak, E. A, Pitha, J, & Rosenheim, S. A Clinicopathologic Analysis of Adriamycin Cardiotoxicity. Cancer (1973).

[120] Ferrans, V. J, Clark, J. R, & Zhang, J. Pathogenesis and Prevention of Doxorubicin Cardiomyopathy. Tsitologiia (1997). , 39(10), 928-937.

[121] Stephens, M. Pulmonary Effects. In: Brighton D. (ed.) The Royal Marsden Hospital Handbook of Cancer Chemotherapy. New York: Churchill Livingstone; (2005). , 221-223.

[122] Rosenow, E. C, & Limper, A. H. Drug-Induced Pulmonary Disease. Semin Respir Infect Journal (1995). , 10, 86-95.

[123] Helman Dl Jr, Byrd JC, Ales NC. Fludarabine-Related Pulmonary Toxicity: A Distinct Clinical Entity in Chronic Lymphoproliferative Syndromes. Chest (2002). , 122(3), 785-790.

[124] Dunsford, M. L, Mead, G. M, & Bateman, A. C. Severe Pulmonary Toxicity in Patients Treated With Combination of Docetaxel and Gemcitabine for Metastatic Transitional Cell Carcinoma. Annals of Oncology (1999). , 10(8), 943-947.

[125] Rivera, M. P, Kris, M. G, & Gralla, R. J. Syndrome of Acute Dyspnea Related to Combined Mitomycin Plus Vinca Alkaloid Chemotherapy. American Journal of Clinical Oncology (1995). , 18(3), 245-250.

[126] Lanzowsky, P. Manual of Pediatric Hematology and Oncology. 3rd edition. San Diego: Academic Press; (2000).

[127] Stover, D. E. Pulmonary Toxicity. In: DeVita VT, Hellman SH, Rosenberg SA. Cancer; Principles and Practice of Oncology. 4th edition. Philadelphia: Lippincott; (1993). , 1993, 2362-2370.

[128] Bruera, E, Macmillan, K, & Pither, J. Effects of Morphine on The Dyspnea of Terminal Cancer Patients. Journal of Pain and Symptoms Management (1990). , 5, 341-344.

[129] Filshi, J, Penn, K, & Ashley, S. Acupuncture For The Relief of Cancer-Related Breath-
       lessness. Palliative Medicine (1996). , 10, 145-150.

Perspectives in Cancer Biology and Modeling

Chapter 6

Sialyl Salivary–Type Amylase Associated with Ovarian Cancer

Takanori Moriyama

Additional information is available at the end of the chapter

1. Introduction

1.1. Review of related literature

Studies of tumor-producing amylase originated with Weiss et al.'s 1951 report illustrating a case of bronchogenic carcinoma associated with elevated serum amylase levels [1]. Since then, many reports have focused on lung cancer-producing amylase [2-11], and there have been similar reports in pancreatic [12], stomach [13], uterine [14], and ovarian cancers [15, 16]. Moreover, there have been reports of non-epithelial amylase-producing osteosarcoma [17] and multiple myeloma [18-20]. In these cases, the amylase had the salivary phenotype. However, pancreatic-type amylase has been reported in one case of uterine cancer [21] and two cases of breast cancer [22, 23]. Among those reported cases, determine of the total amylase activity in the sera and amylase isoenzyme electrophoretic analysis have been contributed much to the diagnosis and treatment.

In contrast, Sudo and Kanno [24] reported so-called sialic-acid-containing amylase in the sera of patients with lung and pancreatic cancer. It was similarly detected in the sera of patients with IgA-type [25] and IgD-type multiple myeloma [26], and identified to be sialyl salivary-type amylase by electrophoretic study with neuraminidase treatment and immunological characterization [26]. In 2004, Shigemura et al. [27] demonstrated, using cell culture and immunohistochemical techniques, that sialyl salivary-type amylase, together with normal salivary amylase (defined by electrophoretic characteristics), was produced by myeloma cells. In 2006, Yokouchi et al. [28] also detected the same type of amylase in culture medium from the amylase-producing lung adenocarcinoma cell line IMEC-2. In 2008, the author reported that the characterization of sialyl salivary-type amylase associated with ovarian cancer using conserved sera that were obtained from a retrospective study of amylase zymograms [29]. That by this paper, universally seen sialyl salivary-type amylase has been revealed in the patients' sera with those malignancies.

1.2. Ovarian cancer–producing amylase

When you focus on ovarian cancer-producing amylase, many studies have been published so far [30-46]. In these reports, the important thing is the following three points.

1. Amylase is directly produced from tumor cell and it can be thought of as of one of the important tumor marker.

2. Serum levels of amylase is decreased after removal the tumor and/or treatments.

3. The phenotype has been deflected to the salivary-type.

In those reports [30-46], in 1988, Henriksen and Brock had been already reported about "fast-migrated amylase isoenzymes" in the patient's serum, cyst fluid, and tumor tissue. They reported that electrophoretic separation of the amylase revealed fast-migration forms in serum 10 of 47 (21.3%) patients with malignant ovarian neoplasms. Unfortunately, they did not characterize the fast-migrating amylase isoenzyme forms [45], however, it is considered in the perspective of today think and as "sialyl salivary-type amylase" similar to our reports [25, 28, 29]. In the following, describe the research results that led to the identification of the amylase found in the sera with ovarian cancer.

2. Materials and methods

2.1. Subjects

Three patients' sera were chosen from strictly retrospective observation of routine amylase isoenzyme electrophoresis data, 2,850 specimens, which were analyzed from April 1988 to March 1999 in the Clinical Laboratory, Asahikawa Medical College Hospital, Hokkaido, Japan. The criteria were: a S3 to S2 ratio of over 1.0 and/or acidic fast-migrated sub-bands from S4 to S6. The sera were stored at -80ºC until required.

A sample with a normal amylase isoenzyme electrophoretic pattern was used as control in the analyses of neuraminidase treatment, reaction with anti-salivary monoclonal antibody, and size-exclusion HPLC.

2.2. Measurement of total amylase activity

Total serum amylase activity was measured on a Hitachi 7170 automated analyzer with G4-CNP as substrate (Toyobo, Osaka, Japan) at 37ºC. The reference interval of total serum amylase activity was from 40 to 160 U/L.

2.3. Amylase isoenzyme electrophoresis

The electrophoresis was performed for 60 min at 300 V using a cellulose acetate membrane (Titan III lipo, Helena Labs, Beaumont, TX, USA) with discontinuous buffer system [47]. Amylase activity was detected by blue starch staining, according to the technique described by Leclerc and Forest [48]. This electrophoretic technique is the most convenient way to have a high resolution.

2.4. Treatment with neuraminidase

Neuraminidase from *Arthrobacter ureafaciens* (specificities: α-2→3, α-2→6 and α-2→8) and *Clostridium perfringens* (specificities: α-2→3 and α-2→6) were purchased from Nakalai Tesque (Kyoto, Japan) and Sigma (St. Louis, MO, USA), respectively. Neuraminidase treatment was performed at 37ºC for 1 h and the treated sample was analyzed by amylase isoenzyme electrophoresis. It was confirmed, using samples from previous reports that the results of both treatments did not differ between whole serum and a purified amylase fraction sample obtained by size-exclusion chromatography [25, 26]. Whole sera were used for this treatment and the next reaction with monoclonal antibody, because the sample volumes were very low.

2.5. Reaction with anti-human salivary monoclonal antibody

Inhibitory monoclonal antibody against human salivary amylase was obtained from an amylase isoenzyme PNP kit (Roche Diagnostics, Tokyo, Japan) based on the method of Gerber et al. [49]. The monoclonal antibody solution was concentrated 5-fold with Minicon B15 clinical sample concentrators (Millipore, Billerica, MA, USA). The monoclonal antibody binds specifically to salivary amylase and inhibits *ca.* 90% of total activity. The whole serum was mixed with this antibody, and incubated at 37°C for 1 h then at 4°C for 18 h. After the reaction, amylase isoenzyme electrophoresis of the mixture was performed.

2.6. High performance liquid chromatography (HPLC)

Size-exclusion HPLC analysis was carried out on a Pharmacia (Uppsala, Sweden) fast-protein liquid chromatography (FPLC) apparatus with a Superose 12 HR column (30 cm 1.0 cm) [50]. The serum (100 μL) was eluted with a phosphate buffer (50 mmol/L, pH 7.2) containing NaCl (150 mmol/L). The volume of each fraction was 0.8 mL. Protein was monitored by absorbance at 280 nm, and amylase activity (absorbance at 600 nm) was monitored with an amylase test kit purchased from Iatoron Labs, Tokyo, Japan.

3. Results

3.1. Ages, serum total amylase activities, amylase isoenzyme electrophoretic analyses, and clinical diagnoses of selected sera

Three specimens came from female patients, and afterward it was found out that they had been diagnosed with ovarian cancer based on medical histories. The patients' ages, total serum amylase activities, and amylase isoenzyme electrophoretic data at the time of amylase electrophoretic analysis are summarized in Table 1. Their total amylase activities were 300, 772, and 798 U/L and the ratios of activity to the upper reference interval were 1.88, 4.20, and 4.99, respectively. Amylase isoenzymes with abnormal anodic migration were detected in all three patients' sera and are shown in Fig. 1A (lane 3), B (lane 3), and C (lane 3). Table 1 gives the ratios of total fast-migrated isoenzymes to S1 and S2 isoenzymes ((S3+S4+S5+S6)/(S1+S2)) and of S3 to S2 (S3/S2). These ratios approximately indicate the proportion of sialyl salivary-type amylase in the total salivary amylase fraction. In cases 2 and 3, the S3 sub-bands were slightly more dominant than the S2 sub-bands, but the ratio of S3 to S2 was below 1.00 only in case 1. The ratio of abnormal anodic bands (from S3 to S6) to normal salivary sub-bands (S1 and S2) was highest for case 3. Unfortunately, these cases were not recognized as having an abnormal amylase pattern in the routine electrophoretic analyses. It was considered that the S3 sub-bands were obviously dominant over the S2 sub-band in previous cases of multiple myeloma [25, 26]; this was less pronounced in the cases here.

3.2. Neuraminidase treatment

The serum samples of the three cases were treated with neuraminidase and submitted to electrophoretic analyses. The results using neuraminidase from *Arthrobacter ureafaciens* are shown in Fig. 1A (lane 2), 1B (lane 2), and 1C (lane 2). The abnormal anodic bands (from S3 to S6) showed a reduction of electrophoretic mobility compared with those in untreated sera, and shifted to the cathodic side corresponding to normal salivary isoenzymes in all cases. Both S1 and S2 bands were resultantly stained more strongly, respectively. These densitometric data are shown in Table 1 together with original amylase isoenzyme data. Neuraminidase from *Clostridium perfringens* had similar effects (data not shown). Therefore, it was considered that the binding pattern of the sialic acid residue was α-2$\rightarrow$3 or α-2$\rightarrow$6 in those cases. It has been previously confirmed that normal serum shows no change in electrophoresis under the same neuraminidase treatment conditions [25].

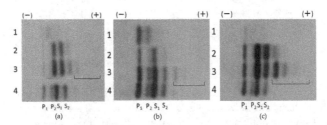

A, Case 1; B, Case 2; C, Case 3. 1, After reaction with anti-salivary amylase monoclonal antibody; 2, after neuraminidase treatment; 3, patient's original serum; 4, normal serum. The fast-migrated amylase isoenzymes were indicated by the bracket.

Figure 1. Amylase isoenzyme electrophoretic analysis of three patients' sera treated with anti-salivary monoclonal antibody and neuraminidase.

3.3 Reaction with an anti-salivary amylase monoclonal antibody

The fast-migrating bands found in the three cases disappeared from the electrophoretic patterns, together with residual normal salivary bands, on reaction with the anti-salivary amylase monoclonal antibody, and a faint broad band of amylase activity was observed on the original patterns. Formation of the faint broad band is evidence that the fast-migrating amylase reacted completely with the monoclonal antibody [25]. These results are shown in Fig. 1A (lane 1) 1B (lane 1), and 1C (lane 1), respectively. It was confirmed previously that the salivary amylase bands in normal serum disappeared from the electrophoretic pattern following similar treatment [25].

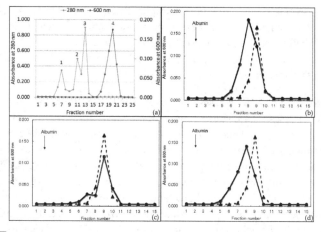

A, Elution profile of normal serum amylase. Protein concentration and amylase activity were monitored at 280 nm (blue line) and 600 nm (red line), respectively. Peak 1, IgM; peak 2, IgG; peak 3, alubumin; peak 4, normal amylase. B, Elution profile of amylase in the serum of case 1; C, that of case 2; D, that of case 3. Amylase activity was monitored at 600 nm. Amylase activities of normal and patient were indicated by the broken line and solid line, respectively. In case 1 and 3, amylase activity was eluted in a broad peak. In case 2, amylase activity was eluted in two peaks. Fraction numbers 7 and 9 correspond to the peak of sialyl salivary-type amylase and the normal serum amylase, respectively.

Figure 2. Elution profiles of amylase from normal serum and three patients' sera by HPLC on a Superose 12 HR column.

3.4. HPLC analysis

Normal serum and the patients' sera were subjected to HPLC using a Superose 12 column, and the elution patterns are shown in Fig. 2. Typically, normal serum amylase is eluted as a single peak far from sharp in the low-molecular-weight albumin, indicated in Fig. 2A. From Fig. 2B to 2D, elution patterns of the three cases are shown in comparison with normal amylase peak. Normal serum amylase eluted in fraction number 9, illustrated with a broken line. In contrast, two amylase activity peaks were noted in case 2, in fractions 7 and 9 (Fig. 2C). In cases 1 and 3, the amylase activity eluted in a large peak, fraction number 8 (Fig. 2B and D). It has been confirmed using isoamylase electrophoretic characterization that fraction 9 corresponds to normal salivary and pancreatic amylase, fraction 8 corresponds to a mixture of fast-migrating abnormal amylases with normal amylases, and fraction 7 corresponds to the fast-migrating abnormal amylase [25].

4. Discussion

The fast-migrating amylase isoenzyme bands found in the three cases of ovarian cancer were determined to be a sialyl salivary-type amylase from the following results:

1. The isoenzyme bands showed reduced electrophoretic mobility to the cathodic side following neuraminidase treatment.

2. The isoenzyme bands disappeared from the amylase zymograms, and faint broad bands were formed, on reaction with anti-human salivary amylase monoclonal antibody.

3. The isoenzyme bands could be separated by Superose 12 HR size-exclusion HPLC. Thus, an apparent extra high-molecular-mass peak was observed on the chromatogram.

These characteristics of sialyl salivary-type amylase were also demonstrated in the author's first report of myeloma [25]. The three characteristics above were considered simultaneously as strict criteria to detect sialyl salivary-type amylase. The author would like to recommend that, in the future, at least neuraminidase treatment and size-exclusion HPLC analysis should be used for identification.

Many investigators have reported amylase-producing ovarian cancer and reported that serum amylase is an important tumor marker [15, 30-44]. In particular, amylase isoenzyme electrophoresis has been helpful [6, 32] in making an early diagnosis and distinguishing from pancreatitis; the amylase phenotype was generally salivary. In contrast, there have been a few unique reports [30, 40, 44, 45] describing acidic amylase and/or fast-migrating amylase found in the sera or ascites associated with ovarian cancer. Unfortunately, neuramidase treatment and characterization of other properties were not performed in these studies. The author considers those amylases, from the findings of this and previous reports [25-28], to be most likely sialyl salivary-type. It seems likely that sialylated salivary-type amylase is directly produced together with normal salivary amylase by ovarian cancer cells, as in multiple mylelona cells [27] and lung cancer cells [28].

In contrast, acidic amylase from ovarian cystic fluids [51, 52] can be distinguished clearly from sialyl salivary-type amylase because the cystic amylases are unaffected by treatment with neuraminidase. These amylases are thought to result from aging transformation of cystic amylase, as reported by Warshaw and Lee [53], and Weaver et al.[54]. Therefore, neuraminidase treatment is expected to provide a very important and useful means of distinguishing between aging salivary amylase and sialyl salivary-type amylase. For contrast, we previously published the electrophoretic pattern of aging sialyl salivary-type amylase in pleural effusion with IgD-type multiple myeloma [26].

Size-exclusion HPLC characteristic is another important means of distinguishing sialyl salivary-type amylase from normal salivary amylase. The molecular mass of sialyl salivary-type amylase from myeloma was determined by immunoblotting to be approximately 60,000 Da, the same as normal salivary amylase [25]. Unfortunately, the equivalent experiment could not be repeated in this study, owing to the small serum sample sizes, but as the elution profiles in this report were the same as in previous reports [25-28], the molecular mass is assumed to be the same. However, the sialyl salivary-type amylases were well separated by Superose 12 HPLC analyses. Moreover, the peak of the amylases did not change following neuraminidase treatment; such elution behavior can probably be explained by the unusual protein conformation of this abnormal salivary-type amylase [25].

Recently, Shigemura et al.[55] reported that sialyl salivary-type amylase was detected in serum from 7 out of 11 (63.6%) subjects with multiple myeloma. It was emphasized that sialyl salivary-type amylase is a useful marker of disease activity in multiple myeloma, and that sialylation of the amylase molecule might be concerned with oncogenic transformation or chromosomal abnormalities. Moreover, it was disclosed that sialyl salivary-type amylases could be detected in the serum of patients with a normal serum amylase level and apparently normal electrophoretic patterns. In our cases, although even cases 2 and 3 were not recognized at the time of the samples were taken, the electrophoretic pattern of case 1 was close to normal. However, there certainly were some (small) abnormal fast-migrating sub-bands; those observations were extremely significant. Accordingly, if amylase isoenzyme electrophoresis is more widely and carefully applied to hyperamylasemia with ovarian cancer, it seems likely that more cases will be detected. Serum sialyl salivary-type amylase will no doubt prove a useful marker of ovarian cancer, as for multiple myeloma [55].

In this study, a case of salivary amylase genetic variant [56] might be experienced by unexpectedly. In amylase zymogram of case 1, S2 sub-band was equal or dominant to S1 sub-band. However, further studies could not be performed in this study and there are no evidences. Isoamylase analysis of saliva and/or tumor extract should been carried out to characterize the variant [57].

Sialyl salivary-type amylase has been found in the sera of patients with lung cancer [24, 28], pancreatic cancer [24], multiple myeloma [25], and ovarian cancer [29]. Therefore, it is expected that the sialyl salivary-type amylase will be found generally in patients with amylase-producing tumors. The author especially recommends that amylase isoenzyme electrophoresis should be applied to hyperamylasemia with malignancies, in place of immunological amylase isoenzyme analysis [49] or that a rapid immunological technique for sialyl salivary-type amylase should be developed in future.

Zakrzewska and Pietrynczak [58] had already elucidated that the total serum and urinary amylase activity and salivary isoenzyme were significantly decreased after surgical removal of the tumor with different types of ovarian cancer. Moreover, they demonstrated that those activities in the serum of the patients with ovarian carcinoma with various types were significantly decreased after radiotherapy [59]. Although the frequency of salivary amylase and/or sialyl salivary-type amylase in ovarian cancer has not been revealed those amylase could be definitely considered as a nonspecific tumor maker [60]. Therefore, the author would like to propose that this old and new amylase should be added with standard tumor marker CA125 [61, 62] in the routine treatment and surgery in ovarian cancer

5. Conclusion

Sialyl salivary-type amylase was detected in the sera of the patients with ovarian cancer. The amylase was considered to have been directly produced together with salivary-type amylase from tumor cells. These studies have contributed to the research into amylase-producing tumors, particularly into amylase-producing ovarian cancer.

Acknowledgements

The author extremely grateful to the deceased Professor Tatsuo Tozawa, Department of Laboratory Medicine, Hyogo College of Medicine, Nishinomiya, Hyogo, Japan, for encouragement and helpful discussions.

Author details

Takanori Moriyama

Address all correspondence to: moriyama@hs.hokudai.ac.jp

Medical Laboratory Science, Faculty of Health Sciences, Hokkaido University, Kitaku, Sapporo, Japan

References

[1] Weiss MJ, Edmondson HA, Wertman M. Elevated serum amylase associated with bronchogenic carcinoma; report of case. Am J Clin Pathol. 1951 Nov;21(11):1057-61.

[2] Ammann RW, Berk JE, Fridhandler L, Ueda M, Wegmann W. Hyperamylasemia with carcinoma of the lung. Ann Intern Med. 1973 Apr;78(4):521-6.

[3] Gomi K, Kameya T, Tsumuraya M, Shimosato Y, Zeze F, Abe K, et al. Ultrastructural, histochemical, and biochemical studies of two cases with amylase, ACTH, and beta-MSH producing tumor. Cancer. 1976 Oct;38(4):1645-54.

[4] Yokoyama M, Natsuizaka T, Ishii Y, Ohshima S, Kasagi A, Tateno S. Amylase-producing lung cancer: ultrastructural and biochemical studies. Cancer. 1977 Aug;40(2): 766-72.

[5] Morohoshi T, Nakamura N, Hayashi K, Kanda M. Amylase producing lung cancer. Electronmicroscopical and biochemical studies. Virchows Arch A Pathol Anat Histol. 1980;387(2):125-32.

[6] Maeda M, Otsuki M, Yuu H, Saeki S, Yamasaki T, Baba S. Salivary-type hyperamyla-
     semia in primary lung cancer: observation of a possible precursor of the salivary-
     type isoamylase. Eur J Cancer Clin Oncol. 1982 Feb;18(2):123-8.

[7] Yoshida Y, Mori M, Sonoda T, Sakauchi F, Sugawara H, Suzuki A. Ultrastructural,
     immunohistochemical and biochemical studies on amylase and ACTH producing
     lung cancer. Virchows Arch A Pathol Anat Histopathol. 1985;408(2-3):163-72.

[8] Tomita N, Matsuura N, Horii A, Emi M, Nishide T, Ogawa M, et al. Expression of
     alpha-amylase in human lung cancers. Cancer Res. 1988 Jun 1;48(11):3292-6.

[9] Tsukawaki M, Izawa M, Yoshida M, Araki N, Hashiba Y, Nakagawa H, et al. A case
     of amylase-producing lung cancer. Intern Med. 1992 Jan;31(1):60-3.

[10] Grove A. Amylase in lung carcinomas. An ultrastructural and immunohistochemical
     study of two adenocarcinomas, and a review of the literature. APMIS. 1994 Feb;
     102(2):135-44.

[11] Lenler-Petersen P, Grove A, Brock A, Jelnes R. alpha-Amylase in resectable lung can-
     cer. Eur Respir J. 1994 May;7(5):941-5.

[12] Shimamura J, Fridhandler L, Berk JE. Nonpancreatic-type hyperamylasemia associat-
     ed with pancreatic cancer. Am J Dig Dis. 1976 Apr;21(4):340-5.

[13] Nomura H, Tokumitsu SI, Takeuchi T. Ultrastructural, cytochemical, and biochemi-
     cal characterization of alpha-amylase produced by human gastric cancer cells in vi-
     tro. J Natl Cancer Inst. 1980 May;64(5):1015-24.

[14] Ueda G, Yamasaki M, Inoue M, Tanaka Y, Inoue Y, Nishino T, et al. Immunohisto-
     chemical demonstration of amylase in endometrial carcinomas. Int J Gynecol Pathol.
     1986;5(1):47-51.

[15] Corlette MB, Dratch M, Sorger K. Amylase elevation attributable to an ovarian neo-
     plasm. Gastroenterology. 1978 May;74(5 Pt 1):907-9.

[16] Nakayama T HY, Kitamura M, editor. Onco-developemental gene expression. New
     York: Academic Press; 1976: 455-62.

[17] Masiar PJ. Serum amylase and isoamylases in malignant bone tumors. Neoplasma.
     1984;31(3):351-9.

[18] Hata H, Matsuzaki H, Tanaka K, Nomura H, Kagimoto T, Takeya M, et al. Ectopic
     production of salivary-type amylase by a IgA-lambda-type multiple myeloma. Can-
     cer. 1988 Oct 15;62(8):1511-5.

[19] Fujii H, Yashige H, Kanoh T, Urata Y. Amylase-producing multiple myeloma. Arch
     Pathol Lab Med. 1991 Sep;115(9):952-6.

[20] Delannoy A, Hamels J, Mecucci C, Fally P, Wallef G, de Fooz C, et al. Amylase-pro-
     ducing IgD-type multiple myeloma. J Intern Med. 1992 Nov;232(5):457-60.

[21] Matsuyama M, Inoue T, Ariyoshi Y, Doi M, Suchi T, Sato T, et al. Argyrophil cell carcinoma of the uterine cervix with ectopic production of ACTH, beta-MSH, serotonin, histamine, and amylase. Cancer. 1979 Nov;44(5):1813-23.

[22] Weitzel JN, Pooler PA, Mohammed R, Levitt MD, Eckfeldt JH. A unique case of breast carcinoma producing pancreatic-type isoamylase. Gastroenterology. 1988 Feb; 94(2):519-20.

[23] Inaji H, Koyama H, Higashiyama M, Noguchi S, Yamamoto H, Ishikawa O, et al. Immunohistochemical, ultrastructural and biochemical studies of an amylase-producing breast carcinoma. Virchows Arch A Pathol Anat Histopathol. 1991;419(1):29-33.

[24] Sudo K, Kanno T. Sialic acid containing abnormal amylases in human sera. Clin Chim Acta. 1975 Nov 3;64(3):303-6.

[25] Moriyama T, Tozawa T, Yamashita H, Onodera S, Nobuoka M, Makino M. Separation and characterization of sialic acid-containing salivary-type amylase from patients' sera with immunoglobulin A-type myeloma. J Chromatogr. 1991 Nov 15;571(1-2):61-72.

[26] Moriyama T, Tozawa T, Nobuoka M, Ikeda H. Sialyl salivary-type amylasemia associated with immunoglobulin D-type multiple myeloma. Clin Chim Acta. 1995 Jan 16;233(1-2):127-34.

[27] Shigemura M, Moriyama T, Endo T, Shibuya H, Suzuki H, Nishimura M, et al. Myeloma cells produce sialyl salivary-type amylase. Clin Chem Lab Med. 2004;42(6): 677-80.

[28] Yokouchi H, Yamazaki K, Asahina H, Shigemura M, Moriyama T, Takaoka K, et al. Establishment and characterization of amylase-producing lung adenocarcinoma cell line, IMEC-2. Anticancer Res. 2006 Jul-Aug;26(4B):2821-7.

[29] Moriyama T. Sialyl salivary-type amylase associated with ovarian cancer. Clin Chim Acta. 2008 May;391(1-2):106-11.

[30] Sandiford JA, Chiknas SG. Hyperamylasemia and ovarian carcinoma. Clin Chem. 1979 Jun;25(6):948-50.

[31] Cramer SF, Bruns DE. Amylase-producing ovarian neoplasm with pseudo-Meigs' syndrome and elevated pleural fluid amylase: case report and ultrastructure. Cancer. 1979 Nov;44(5):1715-21.

[32] Norwood SH, Torma MJ, Fontenelle LJ. Hyperamylasemia due to poorly differentiated adenosquamous carcinoma of the ovary. Arch Surg. 1981 Feb;116(2):225-6.

[33] Takeuchi T, Fujiki H, Kameya T. Characterization of amylases produced by tumors. Clin Chem. 1981 Apr;27(4):556-9.

[34] Shapiro R, Dropkin R, Finkelstein J, Aledort D, Greenstein AJ. Ovarian carcinomatosis presenting with hyperamylasemia and pleural effusion. Am J Gastroenterol. 1981 Oct;76(4):365-8.

[35] Hodes ME, Sisk CJ, Karn RC, Ehrlich CE, Lehrner LM, Roth LM, et al. An amylase-producing serous cystadenocarcinoma of the ovary. Oncology. 1985;42(4):242-7.

[36] Hayakawa T, Kameya A, Mizuno R, Noda A, Kondo T, Hirabayashi N. Hyperamylasemia with papillary serous cystadenocarcinoma of the ovary. Cancer. 1984 Oct 15;54(8):1662-5.

[37] Yagi C, Miyata J, Hanai J, Ogawa M, Ueda G. Hyperamylasemia associated with endometrioid carcinoma of the ovary: case report and immunohistochemical study. Gynecol Oncol. 1986 Oct;25(2):250-5.

[38] Teshima H, Kitamura H, Mizoguchi Y, Hino S, Mizutani K, Mori H, et al. Immunohistochemical and immunoelectron microscopic study of an amylase-producing, CA19-9 positive ovarian mucinous cystadenocarcinoma. Gynecol Oncol. 1988 Jul; 30(3):372-80.

[39] Schlikker I, Nakad A, Gerbaux A, Azzouzi K, Kadou J, Lezaire P, et al. Hyperamylasemia with papillary serous cystadenocarcinoma of the ovary. Acta Clin Belg. 1989;44(4):255-8.

[40] Brophy CM, Morris J, Sussman J, Modlin IM. "Pseudoascites" secondary to an amylase-producing serous ovarian cystadenoma. A case study. J Clin Gastroenterol. 1989 Dec;11(6):703-6.

[41] Tohya T, Shimajiri S, Onoda C, Yoshimura T. Complete remission of ovarian endometrioid adenocarcinoma associated with hyperamylasemia and liver metastasis treated by paclitaxel and carboplatin chemotherapy: a case report. Int J Gynecol Cancer. 2004 Mar-Apr;14(2):378-80.

[42] Srivastava R, Fraser C, Gentleman D, Jamieson LA, Murphy MJ. Hyperamylasaemia: not the usual suspects. BMJ. 2005 Oct 15;331(7521):890-1.

[43] Kavitha S, Balasubramanian R. Elderly lady with ascites. J Assoc Physicians India. 2006 Apr;54:325-6.

[44] Kosches DS, Sosnowik D, Lendvai S, Bank S. Unusual anodic migrating isoamylase differentiates selected malignant from nonmalignant ascites. J Clin Gastroenterol. 1989 Feb;11(1):43-6.

[45] Henriksen R, Brock A. Amylase activity and fast-migrating amylase isoenzymes in serum and cyst fluid from patients with ovarian neoplasms. Acta Obstet Gynecol Scand. 1988;67(1):65-70.

[46] Bruns DE, Mills SE, Savory J. Amylase in fallopian tube and serous ovarian neoplasms: immunohistochemical localization. Arch Pathol Lab Med. 1982 Jan;106(1): 17-20.

[47] Kohn J. Separation of haemoglobins on cellulose acetate. J Clin Pathol. 1969 Jan;22(1): 109-11.

[48] Leclerc P, Forest JC. Electrophoretic determination of isoamylases in serum with commercially available reagents. Clin Chem. 1982 Jan;28(1):37-40.

[49] Gerber M, Naujoks K, Lenz H, Gerhardt W, Wulff K. Specific immunoassay of alpha-amylase isoenzymes in human serum. Clin Chem. 1985 Aug;31(8):1331-4.

[50] Moriyama T YK, Takebe T, Makino I, Nobuoka M, Makino M. Purification of the pancreatic stone protein by high-performance liquid chromatography. J Chromatogr. 1989;493:164-9.

[51] Zakowski JJ, Bruns DE. Improved DEAE-Sephadex column chromatography in measuring amylase in serous ovarian neoplasms, and results for 13 cases. Clin Chem. 1982 Oct;28(10):2095-8.

[52] Zakowski JJ, Gregory MR, Bruns DE. Amylase from human serous ovarian tumors: purification and characterization. Clin Chem. 1984 Jan;30(1):62-8.

[53] Warshaw AL, Lee KH. Aging changes of pancreatic isoamylases and the appearance of "old amylase" in the serum of patients with pancreatic pseudocysts. Gastroenterology. 1980 Dec;79(6):1246-51.

[54] Weaver DW, Bouwman DL, Walt AJ, Clink D, Sessions S, Stephany J. Aged amylase: a valuable test for detecting and tracking pancreatic pseudocysts. Arch Surg. 1982 May;117(5):707-11.

[55] Shigemura M, Moriyama T, Shibuya H, Obara M, Endo T, Hashino S, et al. Multiple myeloma associated with sialyl salivary-type amylase. Clin Chim Acta. 2007 Feb; 376(1-2):121-5.

[56] Ward JC, Merritt AD, Bixler D. Human salivary amylase: genetics of electrophoretic variants. Am J Hum Genet. 1971 Jul;23(4):403-9.

[57] Moriyama T NM, Ikeda H. Properties of dominant amylase-2 found in routine electrophoreric analysis. Jpn J Electroph. 1995;39:195-200.

[58] Zakrzewska I, Pietrynczak M. [Changes in activity of alpha amylase and its salivary isoenzyme in serum and urine after surgical treatment of ovarian neoplasms]. Ginekol Pol. 1996 Oct;67(10):504-9.

[59] Zakrzewska I, Pietrynczak M. The alterations in the activity of amylase and its salivary isoenzyme in the serum of patients with ovarian carcinoma, submitted to radiotherapy. Rocz Akad Med Bialymst. 1997;42(1):229-35.

[60] Seyama K, Nukiwa T, Takahashi K, Takahashi H, Kira S. Amylase mRNA transcripts in normal tissues and neoplasms: the implication of different expressions of amylase isogenes. J Cancer Res Clin Oncol. 1994;120(4):213-20.

[61] Bast RC, Jr., Xu FJ, Yu YH, Barnhill S, Zhang Z, Mills GB. CA 125: the past and the future. Int J Biol Markers. 1998 Oct-Dec;13(4):179-87.

[62] Bast RC, Jr., Badgwell D, Lu Z, Marquez R, Rosen D, Liu J, et al. New tumor markers: CA125 and beyond. Int J Gynecol Cancer. 2005 Nov-Dec;15 Suppl 3:274-81.

Chapter 7

Life-Cycling of Cancer: New Concept

Marina Shaduri and Marc Bouchoucha

Additional information is available at the end of the chapter

1. Introduction

The best way to deal with a tricky and unpredictable disease is to understand its essence, causes and triggers.

- Why and how become some normal cells "rebellious" and aggressive? Are there any common processes and rules that govern the transformation of normal cells into malignant neoplasm?

- What is the main cause of cancer diversity and individualism?

- Why do some cancers give metastasis and some do not?

- There are overlaps between benign and malignant lesions. Can we define cancer accurately? Is there a clear margin or a criterion that differentiates benign and slowly progressing malignant neoplasm?

The basic questions about cancer must be answered to demystify this scary disease and solve the "Oncogenic Paradox" described by the Nobel Prize laureate Albert Szent-Gyorgyi [1]: "The malignant transformation of tissues … is a very specific process which must involve very specific changes in a very specific chemical machinery. Accordingly, one would expect that such transformation can be brought about only by a very specific process, as locks can be opened only by their own keys. Contrary to this, a malignant transformation can be brought about by an infinite number of unspecific influences, such as pieces of asbestos, high-energy radiation, irritation, chemicals, viruses, etc. It is getting more and more difficult to find something that is not carcinogenic".

A new promising way of understanding malignant neoplasia and its paradoxes rests upon integrating biomedical and physical knowledge. Several years ago the US National Cancer Institute funded a major research program to bring insights into the cancer problem from the standpoint of physical science; the hope was that physicists could introduce some radical new ideas to the table. In the manuscript we focus mainly on the physical aspects of cancer origin pushing aside biochemical, immunological and gene-associated findings that do not presently add much to the conceptual framework for cancer theory. Our model of carcinogenesis incorporates certain recently discovered physical phenomena [2-4] that elucidate many peculiarities of malignant processes.

New concept of cancer origin is a particular example of the more general model of system-genesis published last year [5]. According to this hypothesis, a malignant neoplasm originates within a small isolated area of a larger organism as a new functional unit with its individual mechanisms of self-control and self-regulation; the cells that are deprived of nutrients and oxygen do pass through several stages of dramatic transformations that lead to the formation of toti- or pluripotent cells with altered genetic makeup. The future fate of this "potential neoplasm" depends on a combination of some physical factors and on the proper timing of successive events that include the unification of enclosed cells and their preparation for aggressive expansion through the physical effect of "Random Lasing" [2]. Hence, contrary to a widely spread opinion of cancer being a chaotic and poorly controlled pull of rebellious cells that are "driven mad" by some mutations, we consider malignant neoplasm to be a strictly controlled and adaptive system of cooperatively acting primitive cells. Some researchers share this point of view regarding cancer as a self-organizing adaptive system or a parasite-like organism [6, 7].

Our model of carcinogenesis is the result of 12-year-long experimental and clinical work in the emerging scientific field of Biological Holography. All illustrations presented in the manuscript are obtained with the computer-assessed device (CID-system) developed specially for cancer detection and visualization [5]. This hardware-software system is the ever first cancer-detecting and monitoring tool convenient for mass-screening purposes; it is capable of detecting and monitoring of any malignant process disregarding its type and location in the body. The non-invasive and automatable method of any cancer detection through a single and short-term procedure is already implemented in diagnostic practice: the patients with and without malignancies are distinguished by spectral information emitted from their body surfaces.

2. Cancer origin theories: State-of-the-art

Malignant neoplasia of normal cells remains a source of misunderstanding and controversy. There is a vast literature on cancer theories. In this section we briefly describe only some of the most acknowledged and interesting ideas. Although none of the debatable hypothesis of carcinogenesis elucidates the general scenario applicable to all cases of cancer, they are nevertheless helpful in generalization of the state-of-the-art knowledge.

A central feature of today's view of cancer is that it does not develop all at once but evolves as a result of complex succession of events over time. According to Hanahan and Weinberg [8] there are several essential alterations in cell physiology typical for malignant cell growth. These hallmarks of cancers include: 1) Self sufficiency in growth signals, 2) Insensitivity to anti-growth signals, 3) Evading apoptosis, 4) Limitless replicative potential 5) Sustained angiogenesis, 6) Tissue invasion and metastasis, and 7) Genome instability. It is also widely accepted that cancers express aerobic glycolysis regardless of their tissue or cellular origin [9]. Abnormal segregation of chromosomes during mitosis (aneuploidy) and genome instability are found almost in all cancers [10], though the reason(s) of these abnormalities are not clarified.

The somatic mutation theory of carcinogenesis has been dominant since the beginning of the 20th century. It is known that cancer cell genomes carry somatic mutations in DNA that may include base substitutions, small insertions and deletions, rearrangements, and copy number alterations. As the tumor progresses, mutations accumulate and the cell eventually becomes cancerous. Apart of successive alterations in genetic material (somatic events), some germ-line mutations can also predispose a person to heritable or familial cancer. Certain defects in DNA are known to be responsible for a variety of hereditary cancer predisposition syndromes including non-polyposis colorectal carcinoma, Bloom syndrome, ataxia-telangiectasia, Fanconi anaemia, etc. [11,12]. Molecular genetics has identified some oncogenes that, along with tumor suppressor genes, can reproduce many aspects of cancer progression. In fact, each tumor is unique in its genetic makeup [13] and, correspondingly, has a unique phenotype akin to an individual organism. Many researchers consider the above theory unsatisfactory because no strict correlation exists between gene mutations and malignancy; besides, it is unclear which factors trigger the gen-associated events that lead to neoplasia. Evidently, the genomic instability per se is not sufficient to initiate a malignant tumor. The somatic mutation theory can explain neither genetic variability within individual tumors, nor many other observable phenomena in cancer biology.

The **cancer-stem-cell (CSC) concept** is becoming increasingly popular, since non-differentiated, relatively primitive and pluri- or totipotent cells have the ability to self-renew and to give rise to distinct types of malignant cells. It is now generally accepted that the CSC sub-population of cancer cells plays significant role in initiation, progression and recurrence of cancer. The CSC concept was first demonstrated in the study of leukemia, which was found to be associated with the "stem-cells" having specific surface antigen profiles [14, 15]. Italian researchers who spotted CSCs in human primary bone sarcomas highlighted CD133 as a pivotal marker for their identification [16]. In recent years similar cells were found in human cancers of brain, breast, colon, pancreas and other tissues [17]. Kornelia Polyak from Dana-Farber Cancer Institute (Boston, US) demonstrated that the frequency of tumor cells positive for stem cell–like and more differentiated cell markers varies according to tumor subtype and histological stage [18]; the question whether malignancy arises from normal stem cells due to maturation arrest or due to transformation of mature cells into CSC is still open.

The Viral/Microbial Theory of Cancer that regards viruses/microbes as potential triggers of a neoplastic process has long history. First finding concerned the avian leucosis virus as a cause of leukemia in chickens [19]; Two years later after this discovery P. Rous presented his theory about ultramicroscopic organisms capable to induce cancer in humans and animals [20]. Since then many viral infections have been linked to malignant processes. Recent studies have provided cogent evidence that some "oncoviruses", e.g., human papillomavirus, hepatitis B and hepatitis C virus, Epstein-Barr virus, etc. are indeed associated with increased incidence of human cancers [21, 22]. Over the years, scientists have proposed a number of mechanisms to explain this link. However, numerous cases of cancer can originate and develop independently of any viruses, fungi or bacteria.

A major cohort of scientists supports the **embryonal theory of cancer.** A type of similarity between embryogenesis and carcinogenesis was first mentioned by John Beard, who put forward The Unitarian Trophoblastic Theory of cancer [23]. The main idea behind his theory is that certain fetal cells or atavistic genes give rise to a neoplasm. Prominent physicist Paul Davis argues that ancient genetic toolkit active in the earliest stages of embryogenesis gets switched back on, re-activating the Proterozoic developmental plan for building cell colonies [7]. Rippert [24] suggested that cells expressing embryonic potential arise due to the process of dedifferentiation. According to the proponents of the embryonal theory, some immature cells such as the remnants of fetal tissues, become eventually malignant due to altered blood supply, e.g., after tissue traumas or mechanical isolation of a small area from nutrients and oxygen. Remarkably, the development of the zygote up to the blastula stage is more or less the same in all mammals, so one can assume that the early phases of cancer "prenatal life" would be of the same nature. Whether we should blame the atavistic genes or there are some other factors that eventually "fertilize" the host-cells producing neoplasm remains an open question.

The embryonal theory is closely related to the hypothesis dubbed **the "speciation theory"** that regards cancers as new species. Duesberg and his UC Berkeley colleagues, who studied aneuploid nature of a cell karyotype across numerous cell cultures, came to a conclusion that some cell-destructive events cause chromosomal mutations and result in cells with totally new phenotypes [25]. The authors argue that carcinogenesis is initiated by a disruption of chromosomes that alters the balance of tens of thousands of genes. The result of these processes is a cell with new traits – that is, a new phenotype or a new organism. According to these researchers, "cancer is comparable to a bacterial level of complexity, but still autonomous; ... it doesn't follow orders like other cells in the body, and it can grow where, when and how it likes" [ibid]. M. Vincent [26] also considers cancer as a programmed and evolutionarily conserved formation rather than just a random series of disease-causing mutations.

Malignant neoplasm develops within host tissues, so the state of entire body and traits of **the micro-environment** of a "cancer-nursery" must be taken in account while searching cancer initiation factors. Gene mutations are only part of the process that leads to cancer, which involves an interaction between neoplasm and surrounding tissue. The importance of changes in the micro-environment during tumor progression has been recognized thanks to pertinent enthusiastic scientists, who were moving against the mainstream science to prove their hypothesis [27-29]. The existence of histologically abnormal tissue beyond a neoplastic area that predisposes to tumor formation is a characteristic feature of many cancers. Interesting data were published by a team of American researchers who established that in the course of tumor development the normal cells in tumor stroma may lose more regions of DNA than do the cancer cells [30]. Another team of American scientists demonstrated that stromal cells actively participate in carcinogenesis [31]. Sonnenschein and Soto from Tufts University in Boston [32] put forward the tissue organization field theory arguing that dynamic breakdown of cellular communication and signal transduction prompts disoriented cells to mistakenly revert to pro-growth patterns of behavior.

The theoretical considerations listed above are substantiated by empiric evidence, but they deal with particular events and manifestations of carcinogenesis. These hypotheses are essentially complementary to each other rather than contradictory; they describe various contributing factors and peculiarities of a neoplasm but no data are available concerning the general scenario and common physical processes that take place at early stages of any cancer genesis. No doubt that there is an urgent need for such a theory capable to reconcile existing hypotheses and empiric findings by establishing the reasons and physical laws that drive normal cells towards malignant neoplasia.

3. Malignant neoplasm as a new organism

Our model of cancer origin has much in common with the embryonal and speciation hypotheses mentioned above; however, it brings new insights into physical mechanisms of cancer emergence and elucidates some details of its "prenatal" life. In this section we will discuss the general peculiarities of complex adaptive systems and show that malignant neoplasm being a system of cooperatively acting cells, behaves as an autonomous organism with its own mechanisms of self-control and self-regulation. Evidently, the whole spectrum of distinct cells, tissues and organs in human body comes out from a bunch of initially identical cells produced by a single zygote - the same processes would be expected in cancers. Lloyd J. Old has found common genetic programs at work in tumor cells and gametes that led him to describe cancer as a "somatic cell pregnancy" [33]. In sections 6 and 7 of the manuscript we will search an answer to the question: how a normal and well-differentiated (somatic) cell becomes "pregnant" in the absence of fertilizing agents?

One can suggest that a cluster of young cancer-cells would not survive in the heavily populated competitive environment unless their development is driven by powerful autonomous mechanisms of self-regulation and adaptation. Such self-organizing entities belong to the class of complex adaptive systems (CAS) which are capable to learn from their experience while functioning in variable ambience. Adaptive evolution (evolvability) and the emergence phenomenon are their yet unexplained characteristics. Emergence implies appearance of certain unpredictable and qualitatively new functions that pop up out of the multiplicity of relatively simple interactions.

It is widely accepted, that all CASs share the following common characteristics: 1) robustness – the ability to maintain a basic level of dynamic equilibrium; 2) resilience – all CASs are capable to restore the quasi-equilibrium state after various perturbations; 3) multi-level organization in terms of complex structural and functional hierarchy; 4) self-organization that implies creation of more complex internal structures without external resources or information and, of course, 5) adaptability in the sense that any CAS can vary its strategy and tactics according to a new or previously experienced situation. The listed hallmarks of autonomously functioning systems are unimaginable without synergy, which implies an orchestrated, synchronized and interdependent behavior of all system-components.

We argue that cancer has all the traits typical for any CAS: cancer cells are hard to destroy even by chemical toxins and radiation, since they coordinate their action in order to survive as an entity. Only united and self-organizing system of cooperating cells would be able to start the vital struggle against the powerful host-organism. The cancer-system shares the phase-space with the host-CAS which is its rival and breadwinner at the same time. New organism should either defeat its host, or, alternatively, obey its rules and commands adapting to the variable ambience.

3.1. Adaptive behavior and diversity of cancers

There are about 200 types of cancers each type comprising multiple "families" and sub-types of cells. The scientists from the Wellcome Trust Sanger Institute in Hinxton, England, recently announced 73 different combinations of disease-causing mutations in the breast tumors each involving up to six different genes from a set of 40 driver genes [34]. Canadian researchers have shown that the cells taken from patients with acute lymphoblastic leukemia are actually composed of multiple families of genetically distinct leukemia cells [35]. No doubt, that the treatment of such a diverse pathology would not be efficient without understanding of the most general regulatory mechanisms common for all cancers.

What is the reason of cancer diversity? Are its cells the clones of distinct "cancer-stems" that originate simultaneously, or they emerge as new cells due to clashes with surrounding cells that produce odds and ends of damaged cellular components?

We assume that an interaction of poorly differentiated cells with the bystander elements of stroma can yield various karyo- and phenotypes through the same mechanisms that take place in the first "nursery" of emerging cancer. The tumor micro-environment is a complex system of many cell types, including endothelial cells and their precursors, smooth-muscle cells, fibroblasts, granulocytes, lymphocytes, macrophages, etc. Taking into consideration the features of CAS, one can suggest that adaptation of young, meta-stable and extremely motile cancer cells to variable and heterogeneous micro-environment plays crucial role in the process of cell diversification; however, there is another possibility to provide diverse "stems" and their clones. This "fresh" idea about recurrent (iterative) cycles of carcinogenesis that imply successive production of less complex generations of malignant cells is described in section 7.

Many cancers adapt to chemo- and radiation therapy: according to some researchers, the clonal selection leads to the resistance of recurrent tumors [36]. If "cancer-embryos" are nurtured in various conditions before they proceed to active life-cycling, they might give birth to distinct "clones". This process cannot be considered as selection, but as the emergence of new organisms by the same scenario as in the first act of carcinogenesis.

It should be noted that the adaptation itself is not a well understood phenomenon. Elusive non-molecular processes of information exchange between the cells/tissues are difficult to study. As a result, we often ignore an obvious fact that no process of learning (gaining experience) is possible without data storage. No doubt that some mechanisms of data memorizing should exist in all, even in simplest entities capable to adapt and develop: ambient information has to be perceived, processed and stored in a readily accessible (usable) form. We argue that a kind of associative memory must be an embedded feature of all adaptive systems, among them, of cancers, since autonomous functioning, adaptation and development are unimaginable without the available information on previously experienced states [5]. The physical basis of a system memory is closely related to real-time holographic mechanisms that are basic for any CAS. These poorly understood mechanisms that imply the wave-wave and wave-matter interactions ensure the unification and integration of many separate elements into an autonomously functioning system of interdependent agents (see below).

3.2. Collective behavior of malignant cells

Cells and other elements of complex biological systems are functionally interdependent – they exhibit evident signs of collective behavior being organized as a hierarchy [37-39]. If cancers are integral and adaptive organisms, the action of malignant cells should be strictly coordinated. Indeed, nontrivial spatial correlations between malignant cells have been found by various researchers. The cooperative behavior, namely, collective migration of malignant cells during their invasion into healthy tissues seems to follow essentially the same pathways as healthy cells that participate in embryological development and damaged tissue reparation [40]. Cells performing collective migration share many biological characteristics with independently migrating cells but, by affecting one another mechanically and via signaling, these cell groups are subject to additional regulation and constraints [41, 42].

Experimental and clinical observations support the suggestion that cancer cells form a complex and integrated system. G. Lambert studied the collective response of breast cancer tissues to drug-induced stress and found a similarity between the rapid evolution of drug resistance in cancers and the behavior of bacterial colonies under starvation conditions [43]. Professor P. Davies, principal investigator of a major research program funded by the National Cancer Institute, argues that cancer is not a random bunch of selfish rogue cells behaving badly, but a highly-efficient pre-programmed response to stress, honed by a long period of evolution. [7, 44].

Hence, one can regard cancer as a life-tenacious organism created by and incorporated into relatively mature tissues of the host-body. This complex adaptive system, which is doomed to conduct a life-long battle with its superior ancestor - parental body, has its own powerful self-regulation mechanisms, a flexible primitive structure and enough power to hunt the preys – host cells.

4. New approach to the cancer non-invasive study

Cancer remains an elusive, unpredictable and scary disease mostly because the malignant processes are difficult to detect and monitor. The most efficient methods of cancer conventional diagnostics are either harmful or too costly to be used in vivo as often as necessary. Oncologists lack a non-invasive, reliable, user-friendly, automatable and non-expensive test for tracking the malignant processes on the organism-level. We were lucky to find the solution to this problem thanks to an unexpected discovery of a previously unknown physical effect - "the holographic diffraction" which turned out to be characteristic of all biological objects [4-5, 45]. Detailed description of the innovative technology developed and tested by the authors was published earlier [46, 47]; in this manuscript we present concise information about this principally new approach to the detection and monitoring of malignant processes for a better understanding of our empiric data.

The computer-assessed diagnostic system "CID" provides reliable and comprehensive spectral information valuable for non-invasive detection and monitoring of malignant processes of any location and type [5]. The CID-system belongs to the class of the imaging technology dubbed BHT (Bio-holographic tomography) which is both – a diagnostic and research tool. The device is not cumbersome or difficult to operate: examinations can be conducted right at a patient's bed and the interface is so simple that even novice users can collect data in the form of BHT-grams. The whole procedure of the BHT-examination lasts several minutes: distal body-parts (usually 10 fingertips) are exposed to the pulsed electric fields that are strong enough to initiate the discharge of air; the relaxation of excited atoms and molecules in ionized gas produces optical radiation, which is captured for further processing and analysis; cancer-specific optical signatures are determined by analyzing effects of electric impulses on the body distal "terminals". A computer operates the device and performs analyses of recordings (fig. 1).

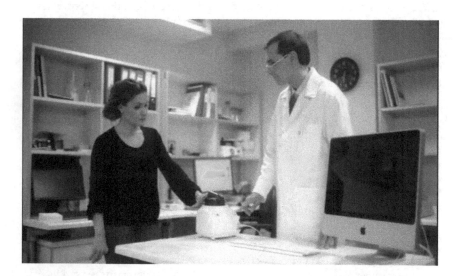

Figure 1. BHT-examination implies the recording of ten fingertips' emission that takes only 2-3 minutes.

In observational research, results can be changed or biased by the act of measurement itself. The distal areas of human body are used as a source of information because they provide less distorted spectral information about entire body-state avoiding "an observer/measurement effect". A set of images-tomograms of 10 fingertips (each showing a 2D momentary "slice" of the 3D system) is recorded for the detection and monitoring of malignant processes in human body. The fingertips are exposed to electric impulses of distinct frequencies, so that one gets comparable information on the character of resonant responses to electric impulses of particular frequencies in 10 distant areas of human body (necessary for mapping of pathological process). The harmless and short-term procedure of a person examination can be conducted as often as necessary.

In clinical practice various modalities are used for imaging of body parts, including radiography, computed tomography, magnetic resonance imaging (MRI), and positron emission tomography-computed tomography (PET-CT). All these modalities focus on particular areas of human body in order to get the images of organs/tissues that physicians need to examine. In BHT there is no necessity to screen entire body part by part, since the holography-based mechanisms spread the scaled information about the deviations from normal functioning of cells and tissues throughout the whole body acting akin to a wireless system of bio-communication. Experimental and clinical study of various patients (with and without diseases) enabled us to reveal some cancer-specific spectral signatures in fingertip BHT-grams [5, 48] that prompted subsequent research in oncology. The CID is a portable, easy-to-use and non-costly tool of the whole body examination; it allows the determination of the spatiotemporal distribution of malignant processes throughout an intact organism. The CID-system is already implemented in routine diagnostic practice.

Pre-existing devices of the same class [49, 50] failed to provide reliable and reproducible information on cancer-specific emission and on the dynamics of systems. In order to stabilize the air discharge plasma and obtain the informative optical data it became indispensable to modify the device and alter the examination procedure. We have filtered out the most variable and non-informative spectral components thus getting reproducible and comparable recordings of fingertip emission. Stabilization of the discharge plasma and improvement of data quality have been achieved through the limitation of the gas transit-time across the discharge zone, the restriction of particle upward scattering/dissipation, etc.

It became necessary to conduct a plethora of probes on hundreds of patients with distinct types and stages of cancer before we understood the principles of the holographic imaging and developed the system of data interpretation. Close collaboration with clinicians made it possible to define the matrix of correlations between clinical diagnoses and spectral information obtained in various conditions of data acquisition. Experimental and clinical work conducted during several years led us to the conclusion that interference patterns emitted from body surfaces in response to high frequency electric impulses carry encoded information on the shapes, densities, complexity and dynamic features of the most problematic areas/processes disregarding their type, size and location in human body (fig. 2).

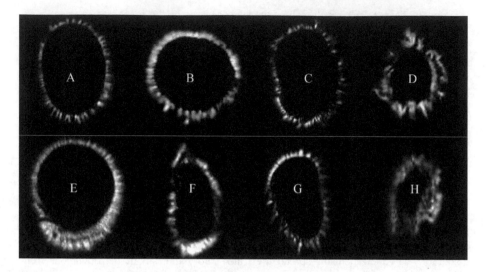

Figure 2. The geometry and texture of fingertip BHT-grams is altered according to certain characteristics of the most affected tissues and organs: A - a healthy person's uniform emission; B – a case of prostate cancer (a chestnut–like flattened shape); C – cancer of the left kidney (the shape of a bean); D – the lactation state; E – gastrointestinal cancer; F – the shoulder malfunctioning (complex elongated shape); G – lung cancer, advanced stage; H – colorectal cancer (terminal stage).

A system in a quasi-balanced state radiates evenly thanks to intrinsic processes of the destructive interference (similar waves propagating in opposite directions cancel one other and do not affect neighboring waves), whereas any perturbation caused by pathological processes results in constructive interference and phase-shifts that upsets the whole system of interdependent waves. Actually, all non-uniformities on fingertip BHT-grams represent the interference patterns, namely the replicas-holograms of the most malfunctioning tissues and cells – the source of wave-imbalance.

This extraordinary capability of system-waves to scale the information on any abnormal process and to deliver it to all body-elements enables the BHT-analysts to observe many structural nuances of pathological areas like in a microscope (fig.3).

The discovery of the astonishing peculiarity of biological systems that act like "bio-microscopes" became a great stimulus for subsequent theoretical and experimental research. This natural phenomenon enabled us to get and analyze the interference patterns/holograms of real anatomic structures using human fingertips as a source of the otherwise invisible and non-measurable information. New approach to the evaluation of the body problematic areas can be referred to as the "Holographic Imaging". Owing to non-locality of holographic information and because of spectral differences between immature cancer-cells and differentiated host-cells, it has become possible to detect malignant pathology with high accuracy [45]. It should be noted that contrary to the spectral analysis of BHT-grams, the visual interpretation of the holographic replicas is not an automatable task.

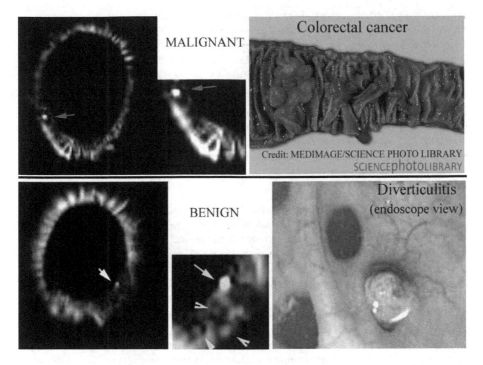

Figure 3. Holograms of the small body-structures are displayed on BHT-grams like in a microscope (see section 5 for explanations of the scaling effects). Two fingertip "coronas" and their enlarged parts are shown next to photographs of similar pathologies. Red arrows (upper images) point to a very bright inclusion embedded into a dark zone. Such a contrast between bright "spot" and dark background is typical for invasive cancer: the degrading host-cells around invasive tumors emit weakly. In the case of benign diverticula (bottom image, white arrows) no signs of degradation are present next to rounded inclusions and the center of relatively intensive emission.

5. Spectral information is distinct in benign and malignant cases of pathology

Waves play enormous role in integration and self-organization of complex adaptive systems, though their contribution to the functioning of human body is still grossly underestimated. Some oscillatory and cyclic bio-activities are studied in the process of functional diagnostics in conventional medicine (e.g., ECG, EEG, etc.); however, organization of nonlinear waves within intact body (especially on micro- and nano-scales) was never explored experimentally.

All physical objects radiate in response to incident electromagnetic waves that are always present in the environment. The spectrum emitted by simple objects such as particles, atoms, molecules and chemical substances, can be recorded and studied much easier than that of complex dynamical systems where internal waves interact with each other. Natural radiation of human body is extremely variable and weak; besides, any perturbation of observable waves causes their instant change, so direct measurements cannot provide reliable spectral information. Only resonant enhancement of body emission and its distant probing can bring the relevant data on the dynamics and character of intrinsic processes. In our model of carcinogenesis we focus mainly on dynamic processes and interactions rather than on various participants (the solid components) in biological processes.

The hardware-software system "CID" records a resonant response of a body to applied electric impulses of high frequencies. This spectral information is valuable for investigation and understanding of yet unknown functional mechanisms in human organism. An elusive and extremely fragile system of organized and interdependent physical waves of various types ensures not only the self-control and self-regulation of the system, but also its interaction with ambient waves and fields [5].

Waves are carriers of energy and information, so their internal "life" and exchange with environment is worth to study. One can ask whether various non-molecular signals, waves and their interference patterns emitted by nontransparent and dynamic organisms carry non-distorted (and interpretable) information on the state of various tissues, cells, intercellular communications and other peculiarities of internal processes. Experimental findings of many researchers prove that the answer to the posed question is positive: G. Hyland has shown that some biological objects emit highly focused coherent electromagnetic waves of ultra-low intensity. The author assumes that such an emission is an outward sign of an orderly functioning metabolism [51]. Japanese researchers caught sound waves generated by bacteria and showed that bacterial cells can enhance the proliferation of neighboring cells through acoustic waves. It is suggested that sounds can function as growth-regulatory signals for entire colony of cells [52]. The alteration of bacterial growth and the synchronization of light emission of adjacent cultures were observed by M. Trushin [53]. An ability of placental mammalian cells to generate pulsating light signals in response to near-ultraviolet light irradiation was discovered by G. Albrecht-Buehler [54]. Such a reversible enhancement of autofluorescence can be used by cells for the "quorum sensing" and coordinated action. And finally, our own experimental and clinical data provide arguments on behalf of the well organized system of interacting waves whose rules and mechanisms are already disclosed (at least partially). The coordinated vibrations and waves of a system medium turned out to be crucial for system integrity and self-regulation via real-time holographic mechanisms (see below).

Although the study of weak radiation of complex biological objects is still in its infancy, spectral analysis of cells, tissues and entire organisms offers great potential being a source of readily automatable biomedical information. The development of spectral methods for Biomedicine was prompted by recent advances in computer sciences, since enormous amount of spectral data requires specific tools and appropriate concepts for data interpretation. There are many approaches to spectroscopic studies of biological samples. Here are some examples that demonstrate the usefulness of spectra for medical studies:

• American researchers developed a novel microscopy technique, called nonlinear interferometric vibrational imaging (NIVI) intended for quantitative analysis of tissue specimens [55]. The NIVI can differentiate cancer versus normal tissue sections with greater than 99% confidence interval in a preclinical rat breast cancer model and define cancer boundaries in fresh unstained tissues.

• Extremely detailed study of cells in their natural state without the need of fixatives has been performed through Raman spectroscopic analysis [56].

• Surface-enhanced Raman spectroscopy in conjunction with imaging was found to be informative in the studies of the chemical composition of the live cells [57].

• Fluorescence emission spectrum of blood components was found to be efficient in distinguishing normal from early-stage and advanced-stage breast cancer. The sensitivity and specificity of the method are 80.4% and 100%, respectively, in distinguishing subjects with breast cancer from normal controls [58].

• Fourier Transform Infrared (FTIR) spectroscopic studies and Fluorescence Emission Spectroscopy (FES) have been effectively employed in the qualitative and quantitative analyses of rat tissues. The study showed that the spectral profiles are different when the tissue of a particular organ is affected with tumor [59].

• Near-infrared light (NIR) is used to differentiate oxygenated vs. deoxygenated forms of hemoglobin and myoglobin. Illumination of intact tissue with NIR allows qualitative assessment of changes in the tissue concentration of these molecules [60].

• Over the last few years infrared microspectroscopy has been used to study cells and tissues. Research work is now aimed at characterizing spectral biomarkers for cancer diagnosis [61]. Dynamic IR imaging with image-processing-guided frequency analysis is a promising modality for breast cancer detection and may not have the tissue-dependent limitations of mammography. The IR imaging process recognizes the cancer area independently of tissue density, cancer size, and cancer appearance on mammography [62].

• Photoacoustic tomography (PAT) is an automatable emerging technique for spectroscopic analysis and imaging live tissue at depths up to 10 cm for detecting tumors and cancer research. The method enables in vivo study of melanomas with both exquisite sensitivity and high specificity [63, 64]. Besides, it can provide anatomical, functional, metabolic, molecular, and genetic contrasts of vasculature, hemodynamics, oxygen metabolism, biomarkers, and gene expression.

• Angle-resolved low coherence interferometry (a/LCI) during endoscopic examination has been found to be convenient for esophageal cancer diagnosis [65]. Physicians shine short bursts of light at locations of suspected disease and sensors capture and analyze the light as it is reflected back.

It is evident that spectral characteristics of actively developing immature cells differ from the emission of normal cells due to increased metabolic rate and proliferative activity of cancer-cells. Much more difficult is to explain how a small cluster of malignant cells alters the emission of distant body-parts, e.g., human fingertips.

The "Holographic Imaging" of abnormally functioning internal structures through non-transparent body is, in fact, a mind-boggling effect. Nobody could ever imagine that it was possible to observe the structural and functional nuances of internal cells, tissues and microscopic areas via assessment of fingertip emission; neither could it be suspected that our organism is able to scale the holograms of real anatomic structures and to expose on a huge scale only those cells and tissues that do not obey the general rules of entire system. This "holographic imaging" is a physical phenomenon and it has been explained as a manifestation of background activity of the system nonlinear medium (phase-space) that acts akin to an organizing holographic grating of a body [5].

In complex adaptive systems (CAS), where all components are well-controlled and there exists a strong subordination between the levels of a system hierarchy, a permanent interaction of "each" and "all" (non-locality) is of utmost importance. In order to achieve interdependence of all agents of a CAS, the periodic grating and synchronicity of vibrations within whole medium must be set from the very first moments of a new system emergence. In the next section we will discuss the role of focused coherent waves in the processes of a system-unification that makes it possible to create an integral system of cooperatively acting agents out of separate elements.

Can the waves generated within human body affect the motion of small neutral particles, molecules and cells? Physicists know that certain waves (e.g., light) can serve to bind neutral matter in new organized forms. It has been established that high frequency oscillations of intense fields interact with micron-size dielectric objects trapping and bounding small particles. The artificial holographic/diffractive setups allow the simultaneous production of very high numbers of such traps generated by superimposing coherent beams either through the wave-interference or through the interaction of several beams previously fanned-out by diffractive optical elements [66]. Hence, a kind of feedback interactions really exists between the waves and solid particles of a CAS. If the suggestion about interdependent action of all system-waves and solid "particles" is correct, the medium waves of a biological system would mirror the state of corresponding solid elements (atoms, molecules, cells, etc.) as all these "agents" are enclosed in the partially bounded space. Any alteration in one of these two complementary realms would affect another - either directly or via some intermediate mechanisms; so, one can evaluate the system-wave behavior/patterns (interference) in order to get information on both - the features of background waves and the state of their complementary (solid) structures.

The permanent wave-wave and wave-matter interactions within a bounded space can explain the effect of the "holographic imaging" discovered by our team 12 years ago; it was an exciting day when we were all huddled round the computer puzzled by the similarity between some BHT-grams and real anatomic structures (see section 8).

As mentioned earlier, an integral system of interfering waves is too sensitive to be studied directly: the wave functions collapse as soon as an observer tries to probe this fragile "structure". That is why we take only the most distant minor areas of human body for BHT-examination – the minor "terminals" of a system provide us with less perturbed system-information.

The background order within the medium/space of a system can explain many peculiarities of CASs. This unifying and organizing realm of a system must be preserved during the whole life-cycle; obviously, the ordered motion of a system-medium and the wave interactions set at initial stage of the system-genesis become more and more complex in parallel with its growth and development. The invisible activity of waves in the phase-space occupied by a CAS can be considered as a "wireless" system of communication between all system-components.

Information propagates in the form of a signal or a message that cannot alter behavior of the solid matter directly but can instead be sent simultaneously to all system-waves. Obviously, diverse "recipients" of information would not react to one and the same message in a similar way; however, weak interactions ensure delivering of a message to a large "audience", actually to the whole system, so that the instructions and commands would not miss their targets.

The question arises whether there are any specific mechanisms that a biological system utilizes for the reinforcement/amplification of the most urgent and/or essential information; it is also very important to understand how a system controls its "misbehaving agents" and which mechanisms are able to transform weak signals into an effective force? We have reasoned that the system-mechanisms of self-control and self-organization require the interaction between weak (information-associated) and strong (energy-associated) waves; powerful or focused waves can play the role of mediators between the information-associated processes and the processes that affect distinct particles, molecules and cells. The reinforcement of information without actual participation of the solid matter in the process of signal amplification is possible via the holography-based mechanisms.

The holographic principle and real-time holography are the only concepts that can explain the imaging of scaled internal structures on the surfaces of autonomous systems. A characteristic feature of any static and dynamic hologram is that any part of a holographic record can be used for the reconstruction of the whole recorded scene. In physics the principle of holography implies that information about a 3D space-volume is encoded in 2D form on its boundary [67-69]. We argue that permanent encoding and decoding of information is a natural phenomenon specific for all autonomously functioning systems; it should not be confused with the conventional process of technical holography.

The real-time holography enables a rapid successive recording and read-out of the information (interference patterns); in the case of a CAS the amount of the processed information can be very high (terabits/s), since the operation is performed in parallel within the entire volume. When creating a hologram, the ordered reference waves (aka the ordered medium-waves of the body) interfere with disordered waves generated by perturbed waves/particles. This information can be reconstructed if the reference waves are subtracted, e.g., by conjugated waves that propagate in the opposite direction. The original object's field/image is reconstructed when the waves deflect in the hologram structure. The refresh rate (update) of information correlates with the periods of phase-conjugated waves, so the reaction of the entire system to any disorder in a high frequency range would be much more "acute" than in the case of a mismatch in slower processes.

We argue that the holographic mechanisms play crucial role in the self-organization of any CAS. These mechanisms imply existence of a hidden order in the background medium where all waves comprise a harmonious structure of vibrations and standing waves; the same mechanisms are critical for the adaptation (decentralized memory) and the resilience of biological systems. Any perturbation, disregarding its actual cause and culprit, would result in constructive interference and phase-shifts of corresponding waves thus altering the entire (scale-invariant) system of background harmonics. Besides, the principle of holography makes it possible to observe the most disordered tissues and organs via assessment of their holographic replicas on distant surfaces of a system (e.g., fingertip BHT-grams), since the "whole" and its "part" can equally reconstruct the entire "holo-image".

The scaling of information in a system of natural origin depends greatly on the frequency/ wavelengths of the most perturbed intrinsic waves. Thanks to the fractal nature of body wave-structure, its self-similarity and scale-invariance, the high frequency signals from excited cells (short waves correspond to small structures) can reach the body surface only after their scaling through the waves of lower frequency (longer waves correspond to larger structures of a system): the fingertips BHT-grams display the interference patterns with the resolution that is proportional to the frequency of constructively interfering waves.

On the way towards the body surface, the upward propagating waves of high frequency (complementary to cells and other microscopic structures) are scaled through the doubling of their amplitudes and periods at each successive level of the hierarchy; that is why the interference patterns/holograms of cells and their constellations are emitted with higher resolution compared to holograms of larger parts of the body. This peculiarity of the multilevel and self-similar structure of interacting waves enables us to observe and analyze the most active processes and also malignant cells/tissues via assessment of fingertip BHT-grams (see section 8 for examples of the cell-holograms).

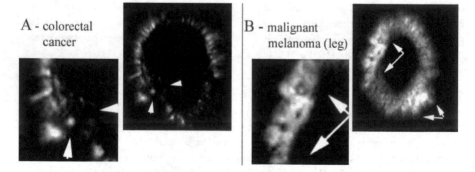

Figure 4. Examples of cancer-signatures on fingertip BHT-grams. In the case of colorectal cancer (A) a part of growing neoplasm paves its way through degrading surrounding tissues (dark zone around to bright inclusion). In the case of malignant melanoma (B) the rapidly proliferating cancer-cells produce an effect of diffuse illumination. The multidirectional radiation that illuminates major parts of BHT-grams is a hallmark of the high frequency coherent emission generated by large conglomerates of poorly differentiated cells (see section 6 for more explanations).

In the cases of cancer, two autonomously functioning entities occupy a shared phase-space and compete for available resources. The conflicting organisms that are "trapped" within a shared body are not able to synchronize their individual rhythms and achieve a state of a quasi-balance. Hence, the BHT-grams of the patients with cancer would display the replicas (interference patterns) of aggressive neoplasm with huge resolution. In certain cases of malignant pathology the fingertip "coronas" demonstrate dark areas around brighter inclusions that present the "remnants" of cells destroyed by cancer-cells (fig.3 and fig. 4,a); The effect of illumination by diffuse light is a BHT-characteristic of actively proliferating non-differentiated cells (fig. 4,b).

6. Emergence of cancer via random lasing

Waves – the carriers of energy and information - are the sole candidates to perform the task of information reinforcement in living systems. In a bounded system of interdependent mechanical and electromagnetic waves of various intensities, wavelengths and frequencies, any perturbation propagates throughout the entire system. The higher coherence and intensity of waves the greater their influence on the solid matter. The interaction of the information- and energy-associated events ensures synergy and coordination of all system-components.

The recently discovered physical effect of "Random Lasing" [2, 3] which implies the focusing and amplification of light in a non-uniform and disordered medium, e.g., in biological tissues, casts new light on the interaction between information and energy-related biological mechanisms. The reinforcement of information through the real-time holographic mechanisms differs from the principles that focus and amplify waves in random lasing; the random lasing implies a complex process of wave-trapping and releasing by disordered excitable material. Emitted waves become much more focused and coherent than those that have been initially "arrested", which explains the term "lasing" (light amplification by lasers).

Conventional lasers that amplify light through the stimulation of photonic emission, require an excitable medium (gain medium) and some feedback mechanisms that temporarily trap the light before emitting a narrower spectrum beams. Usually the gain medium in lasers is excited by pumped energy supplied as an electrical current, or as light of different wavelength, while the photons are confined between mirrors in optical resonator.

Back in 2000, several teams of researchers announced the creation of microlasers exploiting a disordered dielectric material as gain medium [70, 71]. A disordered material that comprises the scattering elements in random positions was found capable to exhibit a laser-like behavior [72]. Electromagnetic waves bounce from one scattering center/cavity to another and such a recurrent scattering on a microscopic length scale temporarily traps light. Hence, the random lasers do not possess large cavity or mirrors typical for conventional lasers; they contain only multiple non-uniformities that scatter light (or other waves). Small irregularities in the material act just like artificial mirrors in laser resonators preventing the light from escaping too quickly. These non-uniformities can be presented by particles, bubbles, droplets of dye, density fluctuations in fluids, surface roughness, cells in organisms, textile fibers in clothing, etc. In polymer films and biological tissues the lasing effects take place because of naturally formed cavities and non-uniformities that temporarily trap energy of waves through internal resonances.

Coherent amplified emission and dramatic spectral narrowing take place only if excitable medium gains energy above the threshold of its excitation [73, 74]. The random micro-laser characteristics can be tuned by varying the geometry of the scatterers' clusters, since each cluster operates at its own specific wavelength, depending on its shape and size.

In some cases constructive interference of backscattered waves brings transport of light to a complete halt (Anderson localization). Philip Anderson was awarded the Nobel Prize in physics for the theory of light localization in disordered medium [75]. In principle, not only electrons and photons, but actually any wave can be localized in a similar way: successful experiments aimed at the sound-wave localization in the strongly disordered 3D samples (composed of aluminum beads) have been described in 2008 [76].

The effects of light amplification and lasing have been found in various vegetable and animal tissues as well as in human tissues from various organs [77]. Even individual cells are capable to produce narrowband laser emission remaining alive after prolonged lasing action: these data were published by researchers from Harvard Medical School, who created biological cell "lasers" based on green fluorescent protein [78]. The team engineered human embryonic kidney cells to produce this protein; when they placed such a cell in the optical micro-resonator and exposed it to pulsed blue light, the cell started to emit a directional laser beam visible with the naked eye.

We have described the random lasing effect and wave interactions in detail because these findings elucidate the energy-mediated mechanism by which information in the form of weak waves affects inert material and creates an "order out of chaos" within the whole system (essential for the system-resilience); besides, the random lasing can account for the appearance of anaplastic cells – the process referred to as the "dedifferentiation" [79]. The spectra narrowing and light amplification are equally important for the understanding of cancer aggressive behavior as the focused light can readily destroy surrounding tissues and facilitate the neoplasm progression.

Indeed, intensity and character of lasing in malignant neoplasm were found to be distinct from benign tissues of the same origin. The Utah University researchers have demonstrated that the malignant colon tissues, when soaked in the laser dye Rhodamine 6G and excited by laser light, emit many more coherent lines than benign tissues in the same colon [2]. The disorder in cancerous tissue was much more chaotic than that in a benign tissue due to a mixture of distinct cells and processes of degradation; however, the increased intensity of coherent radiation in cancerous tissues is indicative of the aggressive behavior and active signaling between elements of neoplasm. The Utah University scientists have experimented with various healthy and cancerous colon tissues taken from different patients, as well as from other parts of the human body such as kidney, with very similar results.

It is acknowledged that the radiation pressure from the focused laser beams is able to trap and physically move small dielectric particles acting like a kind of tweezers. S. Kawata and T.

Sugiura were the first to demonstrate that the field can be coupled to the particles in proximity on the order of 100 nanometers [80]. Optical interaction forces are able to organize microscopic objects with sub wavelength accuracy; they can be very long range and oscillate in sign at the optical wavelength [66, 81]. Continuous evanescent field that originates in conditions of multiple internal reflections within a small bounded area can guide a large number of particles into a preferred direction.

The field-wave-matter interactions discussed above can be considered the key mechanisms of the self-organization in live cells, since a complex system of organized waves is able to direct and unify diverse elements into an indivisible "whole".

Random lasing creates a perfect order out of extreme disorder. This effect takes place in a chaotic excited medium and it might facilitate creation of a new ordered system out of "ashes" of the host-body degrading cells. Such "Phoenix Paradigm" was proposed by researchers of the Pittsburgh Cancer Institute: their experiments with the Kaposi Sarcoma-associated Herpesvirus resulted in the conclusion that excessive cell death, rather than its absence, may be a defining force that drives the cancer emergence [82]. In a stressful situation, e.g., when deprived of energy and oxygen, living cells can act as a gain medium for wave reinforcement. The increase in internal pool of energy that results in excitement of cellular matrix can be caused by many "cancer-promoting" factors: the degradation of intracellular substances, intrusion of some toxic substances or viruses/microbes into cells, increased temperature during inflammatory reactions, etc. can contribute to random lasing within a small bounded area; however, all these factors should be evaluated from the standpoint of their energy-associated effects upon an emerging system.

Coherent radiation of any cellular constellation can reach the body surface if cellular emission is strong and distinct from less intensive radiation of surrounding tissues. The signatures of random lasing are especially prominent on BHT-grams of the patients with aggressive malignant processes (fig. 5).

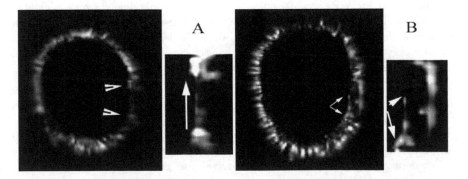

Figure 5. Examples of coherent beams produced by cancer cells. Enlarged and slightly contrasted parts of fingertip coronas are shown next to the raw BHT-grams. A – gastrointestinal cancer, ongoing radiation therapy; B – non-treated renal cancer with spreading metastasis. White arrows point to the scaled holograms of straight tiny lines (focused light).

7. New concept of cancer origin: Dramatic events within a "cancer-nursery"

Cancer, as a new system with altered karyo- and phenotype, originates within a larger and more mature host-system only if a cluster of genetically altered cells builds up its real-time holographic mechanisms of control and regulation. The physical processes within a bounded area of the host-organism play critical role in the cancer-emergence.

We argue that the early carcinogenesis is a multistep process and it starts in a small "nursery", isolated from the matter, energy and information. Such a segregated "nursery" is deprived of oxygen and nutrients having no access to blood supply for this or that reason (a trauma, fibrosis, etc.). A number of starving ischemic cells undergo a chain of metabolic and structural alterations that include the shift of metabolism from aerobic to anaerobic glycolysis, significant increase of Hypoxia-Inducible Factors [83], activation of cell-death programs, disruption of cellular membranes, release of energy from complex substances through their degradation, and other dramatic events typical for metabolic and hypoxic stress in "cut out tissues".

A growing body of evidence supports the view that hypoxia can contribute to the development of cancer. Some researchers established that hypoxia drives cancer progression by promoting genomic instability and that inactivation of apoptosis is essential for tumor-cell survival during this process [84, 85]. Chinese researchers demonstrated that hypoxia inhibits serum withdrawal-induced apoptosis in endothelial progenitor cells [86], while Australian scientists determined that certain monocyte/macrophage populations survive better under conditions of low oxygen [87].

Low oxygen levels characterize the micro-environment of both stem cells and rapidly growing tumors. Moreover, hypoxia is associated with the maintenance of stem-cell–like phenotypes and increased invasion, angiogenesis and metastasis in cancer patients [88]. Recent observations demonstrate the parallelism existing in hypoxia responses of embryonic, adult and cancer stem cells: the mechanisms involved in hypoxia-dependent processes related to stem cell features and tumor progression include the maintenance of the undifferentiated state, cell proliferation, tumor neovascularization, extra-cellular matrix degradation and motility factor up-regulation [89]. Hypoxia often leads to increased aggressiveness and tumor resistance to chemotherapy and radiation [90]. All the findings about the effects of hypoxia and starvation on the state of bounded cellular constellations were taken into account while working on the new concept of cancer emergence.

According to our hypothesis, not only hypoxia, but also isolation from other environmental processes should be considered as the key factors that initiate carcinogenesis. The degradation of starving cells should be tightly regulated in order to rescue at least some of confined cells. It is well known that autophagy is a highly conserved self-digestion process to promote cell survival in response to nutrient starvation and other metabolic stresses [91-92]; however, the role of autophagy that may lead either to cell survival or to cell death is poorly understood in the context of early carcinogenesis.

The autophagy is the chief machinery for bulk elimination and reutilization of aberrant cell components - constituents of cytoplasm and organelles. In the cases of cancer this "self-digesting" mechanism plays an essential role at all stages of the disease, since it helps to prevent tumor cell necrosis by mitigating metabolic stress while acting in concert with apoptosis [93]; the autophagy provides an alternate energy source by degrading damaged proteins and organelles that allow some tumor cells to survive during extended periods of starvation [94]. In the absence of phagocytes, apoptosis would be less efficient as the debris cannot be eliminated from the isolated "nursery" (the disposal of debris is necessary in apoptosis). So, the autophagy seems to dominate over apoptosis in early carcinogenesis though cooperation or alternated action of both mechanisms is not excluded especially just after cessation of the blood supply. Increasing evidence points to the selectivity of autophagy: it helps to "sort" vacuolar enzymes, to remove the aggregate-prone proteins and to destruct only excessive organelles [95].

There is a kind of similarity between neoplasm and budding primitive organisms (see fig.11 in section 8 – holograms of proliferating cells). A key role of recycling of cellular organelles via autophagy and *de novo* purine biosynthesis was found while studying caloric restriction effects on the longevity of budding yeast (Saccharomyces cerevisiae). This yeast is an effective model for the analysis of genes and cellular pathways. Researchers have shown that additional genes appear to contribute to the restriction of either amino acids or sugar, and that defects in autophagy prevent lifespan extension induced by limitation of nutrients in the growth media [96]. An international team of researchers found that the autophagy helps some starving cells to recover, whereas the cells with a disrupted mitochondrial transmembrane potential inexorably die even under optimal culture conditions [97].

Taking all the above findings into account, one can speculate that a complex action of death-programs maintains viability of some cells at the expense of others and that debris of sacrificed cells serve as the sources of energy and nutrients for a cluster of rescued cells. The most viable cells with primitive organization, increased pool of free energy, altered genetic material and the capability to proliferate without additional resources, start to colonize the "nursery" and prepare themselves for the cooperative functioning.

New genetic makeup of surviving cells might have many reasons, such as partial degradation of cellular DNA, abnormal mitosis due to metabolic stress [98], fusion of cells or their "remnants", functional impairment of DNA repair pathways, the shattering and rebuilding of chromosomes named chromothripsis [99, 100], etc. In chromothripsis the chromosomes exhibit a Humpty Dumpty-like behavior: multiple fragments of chromosomes stuck back together after almost complete "pulverization". Such a massive genomic rearrangement acquired in a single catastrophic event can lead stressed cells towards neoplasia [ibid]; however, the effect of coherent waves on the genetic material of cells should not be ignored, since extreme disorder in overexcited biological tissues would initiate the random lasing processes and the laser-like coherent beams would be able to cut/weld distinct macromolecules and other cellular structures.

Thus, dramatic events within a bounded area are accompanied by the release of free energy that excites the trapped mass of degrading cells. Random lasing takes place in the extremely disordered overexcited medium full of debris where the clusters of nanoparticles, macromolecules and the remnants of cells have their own unique sets of lasing frequencies

[73,74]. Intensive motion of the enclosed mass becomes ordered thanks to the organizing effects of powerful waves in the medium [66, 80, 81].

The wave interactions and the motion of solid matter within an isolated area inevitably reach a state when all dynamic processes become synchronous and coordinated. Increasing laser-like radiation of excited cells can help them to break through the isolation and invade host-tissues. "Cancer embryos" do not and cannot manage their logistic problems at the stages of division, compaction and unification that take place in isolation (prenatal phase); such a neoplasm needs to gain power and become "armed" with laser-weapons before it proceeds to the stages of expansion and growth. At the stage of unification via ordered vibrations and organized motion, the entire cluster of new cells acquires its individual rhythm of functioning and becomes a self-organizing entity ready to grow and struggle for resources.

Duration and timing of all "prenatal" stages are the factors of great importance in any system-genesis. For example, one can deduce that if a "cancer-embryo" is ready for independent functioning but the barrier around its nursery cannot be breached yet, the cells would continue to "chop" internal structures and eventually die. Without supply of nutrients, oxygen and some "building blocks" from surroundings, the trapped energy would be spent on the self-destructive work yielding a cyst filled with fluids/semi-solid material; if, on the contrary, the passage of nutrients through the isolating barrier is open earlier than enclosed cells become integrated and "armed", the neoplasm would grow and develop like a benign tumor.

In the manuscript we do not discuss the "postnatal" behavior of the neoplasm in detail; however, once adaptive malignant organism left its nursery and started the life-long battle with its host-rival, it would repeat the same (formerly experienced) scenario whenever possible by blocking blood supply to minor areas and creating the nurseries for new "generations" within the host or its own tissues (the latter is a source of metastasis). Cancer easily adapts to variable situation thanks to the holographic mechanisms of data storage [5] and its first "experience" determines the behavior of its clones. This proclivity of the neoplasm to execute the learned schema of action multiple times in the same or in a slightly changed form can explain the exponential progression, diversity, resistance to the stress posed by "aggressive treatment" and other yet unsolved peculiarities of cancer. The arrangement of new nurseries in various host tissues can be regarded as a kind of adaptive de-evolution: malignant cells produce new generations of "stems" whose structure becomes more and more primitive in each successive cycle.

The schema presented on figure 6 describes the main stages of such an iterative carcinogenesis.

It is established that non-differentiated stem-cell-like sub-populations of cancer (CSCs) are resistant to chemo- and radiation therapy [101]. Since a "cancer-stem" that yields CSCs originates from the remnants of partially degraded progenitor cells, a kind of genetic kinship exists between the host and malignant tissues. The same can be said about a relatively mature neoplasm and its metastasis: the features of metastasis though distinct from primary cancer cells are usually distinguishable from the metastasis of other types of cancer.

The Stages of Carcinogenesis

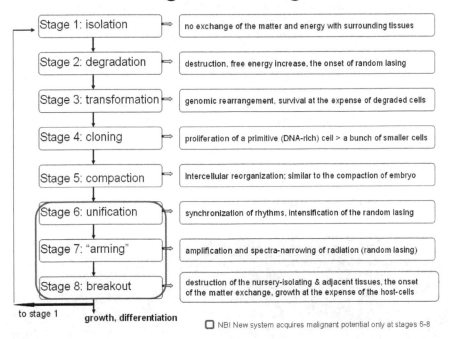

Stage	Description
Stage 1: isolation	no exchange of the matter and energy with surrounding tissues
Stage 2: degradation	destruction, free energy increase, the onset of random lasing
Stage 3: transformation	genomic rearrangement, survival at the expense of degraded cells
Stage 4: cloning	proliferation of a primitive (DNA-rich) cell > a bunch of smaller cells
Stage 5: compaction	Intercellular reorganization; similar to the compaction of embryo
Stage 6: unification	synchronization of rhythms, intensification of the random lasing
Stage 7: "arming"	amplification and spectra-narrowing of radiation (random lasing)
Stage 8: breakout	destruction of the nursery-isolating & adjacent tissues, the onset of the matter exchange, growth at the expense of the host-cells

to stage 1   **growth, differentiation**

☐ NBI New system acquires malignant potential only at stages 6-8

Figure 6. The host-cells should pass through "prenatal" stages before the malignant system leaves its "nursery". Note, that some malignant tissues can start the whole process anew. Each successive cycle would generate less differentiated cells.

To summarize, we argue that malignant neoplasia presents an iterative process of the recurrent system-genesis: one and the same scenario is repeated multiple times within various tissues, in various conditions and with accelerated "prenatal" periods. Such course of the disease can explain the capability of many types of neoplasm to give metastasis through successive rejuvenation of its "daughter-spores". Multiple execution of described tactics of the self-reproduction and the creation of new (younger and less differentiated) generations enables the primary clone of malignant neoplasm to progress exponentially, conquer more and more space at the expense of diverse tissues, resist new stresses and ultimately destroy its breadwinner host. From this point of view, certain stresses posed by standard chemo- and radiation therapy should be considered as the factors that in some cases facilitate the genesis of extremely aggressive and resistant clones of new primitive "organisms".

An unpredictable nature of cancer and dubious efficiency of the methods of its treatment often raise the question whether intervention into the disease course is better than the watchful waiting. For instance, the breast ductal carcinoma in situ, which is a low grade (well differentiated) malignant tumor, can become invasive after more than 30 years since its first manifestation [102]; many patients with low-risk prostate cancer lead a normal life for about 10 years without any treatment: "some prostate cancers might never have developed into serious disease… surgery or radiation therapy may not outweigh the substantial side effects of these treatments" [103].

No doubt, it is urgent and critical to understand the most common rules and principles of malignant neoplasia. We hope that an interdisciplinary approach to the problem and fresh ideas would help everyone involved in healthcare and medical decision-making to plot a clear course through the cancer-paradoxes.

8. Holo-imaging: Some examples

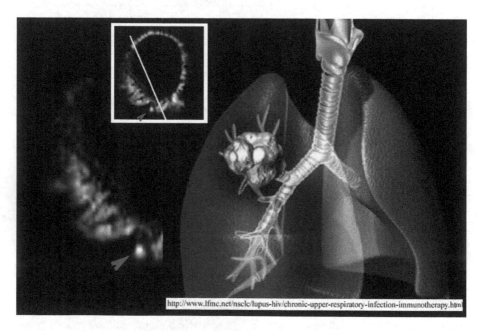

http://www.lfmc.net/nsclc/lupus-hiv/chronic-upper-respiratory-infection-immunotherapy.html

Figure 7. BHT-gram of the patient with treated lung carcinoma. Prominent functional and/or structural disorder in large areas of the body alters major parts of coronas displaying characteristic features of affected tissues in a slightly distorted form. The holographic replica of the most affected lobe of the lung occupies 2/3 of the index finger BHT-gram. Red arrow points to the replica of a growing metastasis.

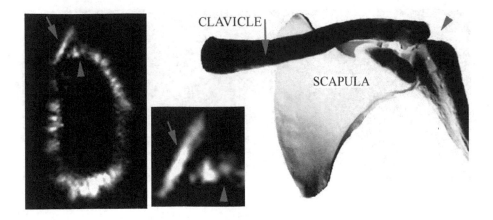

Figure 8. Shapes of presented corona's parts are distorted resembling a shoulder joint (blue arrows); a replica of the most affected bone – clavicle - is displayed with higher quality (red arrows). This is a case of the shoulder malfunctioning (former trauma).

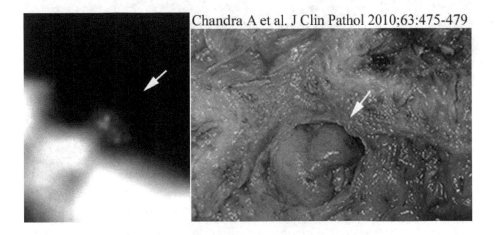

Chandra A et al. J Clin Pathol 2010;63:475-479

Figure 9. Small areas provide their holographic replicas with higher resolution than the large ones. A case of malignant polyp in the urinary bladder (left) is shown next to the photograph of the bladder cancer.

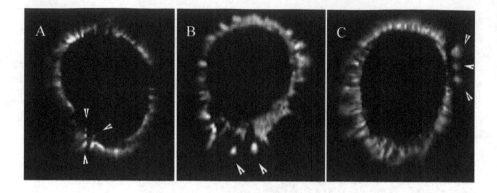

Figure 10. Spreading metastases are displayed on BHT-grams as bright balls on a dark background (indicated): A –
Colorectal carcinoma with liver metastasis; B – Colorectal carcinoma with regional metastasis; C – Renal carcinoma
with metastasis in regional lymph-nodes.

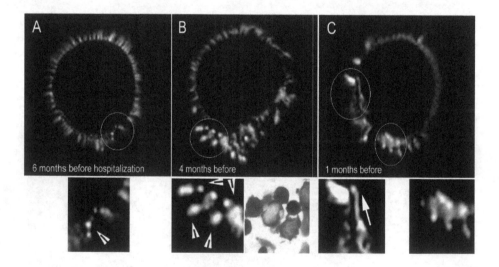

Figure 11. A case of refractory dysmyelopoietic anemia transformed to acute leukemia and liver metastasis. BHT-signs
of the disease aggravation have been revealed 4 months before the clinical manifestation of acute leukemia (B). Lab-
analyses were not informative a month prior to urgent hospitalization of the patient (C). Abnormally proliferating cells
are displayed with huge resolution (B, enlarged part). Compare these holograms of "budding" cancer-cells to the
bone marrow smear of a patient with acute leukemia (color-image from http://www.washington.edu/news/
2011/09/06/gene-defect-that-predisposes-people-to-leukemia-discovered/).

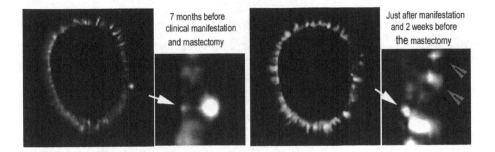

Figure 12. The case of the breast cancer (relapse). BHT revealed the tumor 7 months prior to its detection by conventional imaging methods. Pay attention to powerful diffuse light that consists of multidirectional coherent beams. Such a "fireball" is typical for the neoplasm that just came out of its "nursery" (dark surroundings). Several months later the neoplasm became less uniform and poorly outlined; it grows, multiplies and creates the nurseries for new generations (red arrowheads).

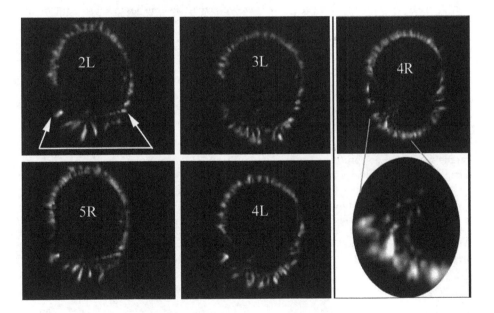

Figure 13. A case of the breast cancer (treated). Almost all BHT-grams display similar replicas of unusually shaped structures. Such a similarity of disordered coronas is typical for an aggravating (sub-acute, transitory) state. A chain of enlarged lymph-nodes in the upper thorax-neck was found to be responsible for the similarity of interference patterns.

9. Conclusion

Presented work was inspired by the discovery of previously unknown physical effects specific to complex adaptive systems of natural origin [5]. The model of carcinogenesis discussed above is a particular example of the more general scenario of system-genesis [5]. According to our data, the "prenatal" life of malignant cells starts in isolation from normally functioning host-tissues. This segregated "nursery" of cancer cells can be compared to a closed box with the famous "Schrödinger's cat" whose fate is totally unpredictable: no direct observation is possible unless the box is transparent to the observer's eye. Conventional biomedical approaches to *in vivo* diagnostics and monitoring are not efficient in such cases. However, we managed to look into the "cancer-nursery" with the help of the waves that in autonomously functioning systems of natural origin act as "wireless" means of the communication between all system-components; back in 2000 we found that cancer provides specific spectral signatures and that aggressive behavior of its cells can be detected via non-invasive analysis of the body-surface radiation. Thanks to complex nonlinear mechanisms of information scaling and transfer across the system, it became possible to conduct a non-perturbing observation of some physical processes that take place in early carcinogenesis. Presented hypothesis focuses on very early stages of cancer emergence; however, we suggest that the described scenario of the system-genesis within more mature organism is equally responsible for the generation of distinct clones and metastasis.

The general model of iterative carcinogenesis reconciles many existing hypotheses and also significantly reduces the number of possible causes and triggers of malignant neoplasia; besides, it opens wide horizons for new experiments and theoretical considerations that can result in the development of more targeted methods of cancer treatment. Apart of the widely known facts about biochemical and genetic features of cancer cells, our model takes into account some physical aspects of malignant neoplasia.

Fragile non-molecular processes within biological systems were largely ignored by official science due to their elusive and non-measurable nature. The findings of the physicists who demonstrated the ability of live cells to manipulate and focus intra- and intercellular waves (e.g., light) should be acknowledged as a giant leap forward, towards the official recognition of the critical role that background nonlinear processes play in the system life-cycling.

We hope that empiric generalization of the biomedical and physical information together with the new possibility to study the "secret" life of the neoplasm would cast light on many puzzles and paradoxes of malignant processes and also help to build foundation for more efficient diagnostic and cancer-treatment strategies.

Acknowledgements

This research would not have been possible without the support of many enthusiastic and open-minded people. Medical professionals, engineers, software developers, biologists, physicists and friends contributed to this work. We would like to extend our sincere thanks to all of them. We express our gratitude to Dr. Raymond Samak – the oncologist from Nice, France and to Dr. Marina Abuladze from the Institute of Physics (Tbilisi, Georgia), who kindly assisted us in the course of the manuscript preparation. We are also much indebted to Professor Andrea Peracino and Dr. Emanuela Folco from the Lorenzini Foundation (Milan, Italy) for their help, valuable advices and encouragement. Deepest gratitude is due to the staff of many collaborating hospitals, clinics and private medical cabinets in France and Italy; without their assistance our work would not have been successful.

Author details

Marina Shaduri[1,2] and Marc Bouchoucha[1]

1 Center of Bioholography, Tbilisi, Georgia

2 Advanced BioResearch & Technology, Luxemburg

References

[1] Szent-Gyorgyi A. The Living State and Cancer. Proc. Natl. Acad. Sci. Biophysics 1977; 74(7) 2844-2847.

[2] Polson R, Vardeny Z. Random lasing in human tissues. Appl. Phys. Lett 2004; 85: 1289-1292

[3] Martorell J, Lawandy N. Observation of inhibited spontaneous emission in a periodic dielectric structure. Phys. Rev. Lett 1990; 65, 1877–1880.

[4] Shaduri M. The Holographic Principle and Emergence Phenomenon. In: Rosen J. (ed.) Holography, Research and Technologies. Rijeka: InTech; 2012. p27-54. Available from: http://www.intechopen.com/books/holography-research-and-technologies/the-holographic-principle-and-emergence-phenomenon

[5] Shaduri M. Secondary holodiffractional radiation of biological systems. Kybernetes – The International Journal of Systems & Cybernetics 2005; 34 (5) 666-680.

[6] Deisboeck T, Berens M, Kansal A. et al. Pattern of Self-Organization in Tumour Systems: Complex Growth Dynamics in a Novel Brain Tumour Spheroid Model, Cell Prolif 2001; 34 115-134

[7] Davies P, Lineweaver C. Cancer Tumors as Metazoa 1.0: Tapping Genes of Ancient Ancestors, Phys. Biol 2011; 8 015001, p. 7

[8] Hanahan D, Weinberg R. The Hallmarks of Cancer. Cell 2000; 100 57-70

[9] Seyfried T, Shelton L. Cancer as a Metabolic Disease (review). Nutrition & Metabolism 2010; 7: 7. Available from http://healthycuriousity.blogspot.com/2012/01/cancer-as-metabolic-disease.html

[10] Nikholson J, Duesberg P. On the Karyotypic Origin and Evolution of Cancer Cells. Cancer Genet Cytogenet 2009;194(2):96-110.

[11] Croce C. Oncogenes and Cancer, N Engl J Med 2008; 358: 502-511

[12] Charames G, Bapat B. Genomic Instability and Cancer, Curr Mol Med 2003; 7: 589-596.

[13] Hameroff S. A New Theory of the Origin of Cancer: Quantum Coherent Entanglement, Centrioles, Mitosis, and Differentiation. BioSystems 2004;77:119–136

[14] Lapidot T. A Cell Initiating Human Acute Myeloid Leukaemia After Transplantation into SCID Mice. Nature 1994; 367: 645–648

[15] Dick J, Lapidot T. Biology of Normal and Acute Myeloid Leukemia Stem Cells. Int J Hematol 2005: 82(5) 389-396

[16] Tirino V, Desiderio, Paino F, et al. Human Primary Bone Sarcomas Contain CD133+ Cancer Stem Cells Displaying High Tumorigenicity In Vivo. FASEB J 2011 Jun;25(6): 2022-30

[17] Avall Lundqvist E, Sjövall K, Eneroth P. Initial Experiences with Serum Alkaline DNase Activity in Monitoring the Effects of Therapy for Carcinoma of the Uterine Cervix. Eur J Cancer 1991;27(10): 1313-1315.

[18] Polyak K. Heterogeneity for Stem Cell–Related Markers According to Tumor Subtype and Histologic Stage in Breast Cancer. Clin Cancer Res 2010; 16(3): 876–887

[19] Ellerman V, Bang O. Experimentelle Leukaemia bei Hühnern, Zentralbl. Bakt 1908; 46:595:7

[20] Rous P. A Sarcoma of the Fowl Transmissible by an Agent Separable from the Tumor Cells (1911) Downloaded from jem.rupress.org on August 3, 2012.

[21] Thompson M, Kurzrock R. Epstein-Barr Virus and Cancer. Clin Cancer Res 2004;10:.803OF

[22] Yu Y, Clippinger A, Alwin J. Viral Metabolism: Changes in Glucose and Glutamine Utilization During Human Cytomegalovirus Infection. Trends in Microbiology 2011; 19(7): 360-367

[23] Beard J. The Enzyme Treatment of Cancer and its Scientific Basis, 1911; Available from http://vitamincfoundation.org/beard/ (accessed 06 August 2012).

[24] Rippert H. Das Carcinom des Menschen. Geschwulstlehre. 2011; Cohen(ed), Bonn.

[25] Duesberg P, Mandrioli D, McCormack A, Nicholson JM. Is Carcinogenesis a Form of Speciation? Cell Cycle 2011; 10(13):2 100-114.

[26] Vincent M. Cancer: A De-repression of a Default Survival Program Common to All Cells? BioEssays 2012; 34(1): 72–82

[27] Hu M, Yao J, Carroll D. et al. Regulation of in situ to Invasive Breast Carcinoma Transition. Cancer Cell 2008; 13(5): 394-406.

[28] Rønnov-Jessen L, Bissell M. Breast Cancer by Proxy: Can the Microenvironment be Both the Cause and Consequence? Trends Mol Med 2009; 5: 5–13

[29] Kenny P, Lee G, Bissell M. Targeting the Tumor Microenvironment. Frontiers in Bioscience.2007; 12: 3468-3474.

[30] Fukino K, Shen L, Matsumoto S. et al. Combined Total Genome Loss-of-heterozygosity Scan of Breast Cancer Stroma and Epithelium Reveals Multiplicity of Stromal Targets, Cancer Res 2004; 64: 7231-7236.

[31] Tlsty T, Coussens L. Tumor Stroma and Regulation of Cancer Development. Annual Review of Pathology 2005; 1: 119-150.

[32] Sonnenschein C, Soto A. Theories of Carcinogenesis: An Emerging Perspective. Semin Cancer Biol 2008; 18(5): 372–377.

[33] Old LJ. Cancer is a Somatic Cell Pregnancy. Cancer Immun 2007; 7: 19-21

[34] Stratton M, Campbell P, Futreal P. The Cancer Genome. Nature 2009; 458: 719-724.

[35] Wang J, Dick J. Cancer Stem Cells: lessons from leukemia. Trends in Cell Biology 2005; 15(9) 494-501.

[36] Radosevich J, Elseth K, Vesper B. et al. Long-Term Adaptation of Lung Tumor Cell Lines with Increasing Concentrations of Nitric Oxide Donor. The Open Lung Cancer Journal 2009; 2: 35-44

[37] Deisboeck T, Berens M, Kansal A. et al. Pattern of Self-Organization in Tumour Systems: Complex Growth Dynamics in a Novel Brain Tumour Spheroid Model. Cell Prolif 2001; 34(2): 115–134.

[38] Kenny P, Nelson C, Bissell, M. The Ecology of Tumors. The Scientist 2006; 20(4): 31–35.

[39] Bonnet D, Dick J. Human Acute Myeloid Leukemia is Organized as a Hierarchy that Originates from a Primitive Hematopoietic Cell. Nature Medicine 1997; 3: 730 – 737.

[40] Friedl P, Hegerfeldt Y, Tusch M. Collective cell migration in morphogenesis and cancer. Int. J. Dev. Biol 2004; 48: 441-449.

[41] Rørth P. Collective Cell Migration. Annual Review of Cell and Developmental Biology 2009;25: 407-429.

[42] Subra Suresh S. Biomechanics and Biophysics of Cancer Cells. Acta Biomater 2007; 3(4): 413–438.

[43] Lambert G. Emergent Collective Behavior of Microorganisms. PhD thesis. Princeton University; 2011.

[44] Davies P, Demetrius L, Tuszynski J. Cancer as a Dynamical Phase Transition, Theoretical Biology and Medical Modelling 2011; 8:3. doi:10.1186/1742-4682-8-30.

[45] Shaduri M, Benford M, Bouchoucha M, Sukhin D, Lebedev V. Holo-imaging - the principle of holography and its practical application: proceedings of the Int. conf. Actual problems of modern physics, 15 June 2008, Krasnodar, Russia. Kuban State University; 2009.

[46] Shaduri M, Tshitshinadze G, Davitashvili T. Investigation of biological systems' holographic properties. Bulletin of the Georgian Academy of Sciences 2002; 2: 264-267.

[47] Shaduri M. A Device to Detect Malignant Processes in Living Organisms - patent. International Application No.: PCT/GE2008/000003.

[48] Shaduri M. Principle of holography in complex adaptive systems. Kybernetes – The International Journal of Systems & Cybernetics 2008; 37(6): 732-738.

[49] Korotkov K. Human Energy Field: study with GDV Bioelectrography. NewYork, USA: Backbone Publishing Co; 2002.

[50] Canetos J, Herbepin P, Reynes J. Method and Installation for Determining the Physical Properties of an Object. US Patent Application, Publication No AU2001031853, May 22, 2003.

[51] Hyland G. Physics and biology of mobile telephony. The Lancet 2000; 356 (9244) 1833 – 1836.

[52] Matsuhashi M, Shindo A, Ohshima H, et al. Cellular Signals Regulating Antibiotic Sensitivities of Bacteria. Microb Drug Resist 1996; 2(1):91-3.

[53] Trushin M. Studies on Distant Regulation of Bacterial Growth and Light Emission. Microbiology 2003; 149: 363–368

[54] Albrecht-Buehler G. Reversible Excitation Light-Induced Enhancement of Fuorescence of Live Mammalian Mitochondria. FASEBJ. 2000; 14: 1864-1866.

[55] Chowdary P, Jiang Z, Chaney E, et al. Molecular Histopathology by Spectrally Reconstructed Nonlinear Interferometric Vibrational Imaging. Cancer Res 2010; 70(23): 9562-9.

[56] Salzer R, Steiner G, Mantsch H. et al. Infrared and Raman Imaging of Biological and Biomimetic Samples. Fresenius' J Anal Chem 2000; 366:712-716.

[57] Kneipp K, Haka AS, Kneipp H, et al. Surface-enhanced Raman Spectroscopy in Single Living Cells Using Gold Nanoparticles. Appl Spec 2002; 56:150–154.

[58] Kalaivani R, Masilamani V, Sivaji K, et al. Fluorescence Spectra of Blood Components for Breast Cancer Diagnosis. Photomed Laser Surg. 2008; Jun;26(3):251-6.

[59] Sankari G, Aishwarya T, Gunasekaran S. Fourier Transform Infrared Spectroscopy and Fluorescence Emission Spectroscopic Investigations on Rat Tissue. Recent Research in Science and Technology 2010; 2(11): 20-31.

[60] Gussakovsky E, Jilkina O, Yang Y. et al. Non-invasive Measurements of Hemoglobin + Myoglobin, their Oxygenation and NIR Light Pathlength in Heart in vivo by Diffuse Reflectance Spectroscopy. Proc. of SPIE 2009; 7161 71612L. doi: 10.1117/12.807715.

[61] Sulé-Suso J, Cinque G. Infrared Microspectroscopy in Cancer Diagnosis. Do We Need Synchrotron Light? Microscopy and Analysis 2010; 140: 25-28.

[62] Lääperi J, Järvenpää D, Kuukasjärvi R. et al. A Dynamic Infrared Imaging-Based Diagnostic Process for Breast Cancer. Acta Radiol. 2009; 50(8):860-9.

[63] Chulhong Kim, Eun Chul Cho, Jingyi Chen et al. In Vivo Molecular Photoacoustic Tomography of Melanomas Targeted by Bioconjugated Cold Nanocages. ACS Nano 2010; 4(8) 4559–4564.

[64] Geng Ku, Bruno D, Fornage M. Et al. Thermoacoustic and Photoacoustic Tomography of Thick Biological Tissues Toward Breast Imaging. Technology in Cancer Research & Treatment 2005; 4(5): 559-565.

[65] Terry N, Zhu Z, Rinehart M. et al. Detection of Dysplasia in Barrett's Esophagus With In Vivo Depth-Resolved Nuclear Morphology MeasurementsGastroenterology 2011; 140(1): 42-50.

[66] Fournier J, Burns M, Golovchenko J. Writing Diffractive Structures by Optical Trapping. Proc. SPIE 1995; 2406: 101-111.

[67] Bousso R. The holographic principle. Reviews of Modern Physics 2002; 74: 825-870.

[68] Bekenstein, J. Universal Upper Bound on the Entropy-to-Energy Ratio for Bounded Systems. Physical Review D 1981; 23(2) 287-298.

[69] Shaduri M, Davitashvili T. Holo-diffraction in Biological Systems. Bulletin of the Georgian Academy of Sciences 2004; 3: 477-481.

[70] Van Soest G, Poelwijk F, Sprik R, Lagendijk A. Dynamics of a Random Laser above Threshold. Phys. Rev. Lett 2001; 86: 1522–1525.

[71] Polson R, Chipouline A, Vardeny Z. Random Lasing in π-Conjugated Films and Infiltrated Opals. Advanced Materials 2001; 13(10): 760–764.

[72] Lawandy Nabil M. Disordered Media: Coherent Random Lasing. Nature Physics 2010. 6: 246 – 248.

[73] Apalkov V., Raikh M and Shapiro B. Random Resonators and Prelocalized Modes in Disordered Dielectric Films. Phys. Rev. Lett. 2002; 89(1), 016802: 4

[74] Cao H. Waves in Random Media. Institute of Physics Publishing; 2003;13 R1PII: S0959-7174(03)39997-5.

[75] Folli V, Conti C. Anderson Localization in Nonlocal Nonlinear Media. Optics Letters 2012; 37(3) 332-334.

[76] Hefei H, Strybulevych A, Page J. et al. Localization of Ultrasound in a Three-Dimensional Elastic Network. Nature Physics 2008; 4: 945 – 948.

[77] Song Qinghai, Xiao, Shumin, Xu, Zhengbin et al. Random Lasing in Bone Tissue. Optics Letters 2010; 35(9) 1425-1427.

[78] Malte C, Gather M, Seok Hyun Yun. Single-Cell Biological Lasers. Nature Photonics 2011; 5: 406–410.

[79] Jopling C, Boue S, Belmonte J. Dedifferentiation, Transdifferentiation and Reprogramming: Three Routes to Regeneration. Nature Reviews Molecular Cell Biology 2011; 12: 79-89.

[80] Kawata S, Sugiura T. Movement of Micrometer-Sized Particles in the Evanescent Field of a Laser Beam". Optics letters 1992; 17 (11): 772.

[81] Mohanty S, Andrews J, Gupta P. Optical Binding Between Dielectric Particles. Optics Express 2004; 12(12) 2746-2753.

[82] Zhao J, Punj V, Matta H, Mazzacurati L, Schamus S, et al. K13 Blocks KSHV Lytic Replication and Deregulates vIL6 and hIL6 Expression: A Model of Lytic Replication Induced Clonal Selection in Viral Oncogenesis. PLoS ONE 2007: 2(10): e1067.

[83] Ke Q, Costa M. Hypoxia-Inducible Factor-1 (HIF-1). Mol Pharmacol 2006;70:1469–80.

[84] Nelson D., Tan T, Rabson B, et al. Hypoxia and Defective Apoptosis Drive Genomic Instability and Tumorigenesis, Genes Dev. 2004; 18: 2095–2107.

[85] Harris A. Hypoxia — a key regulatory factor in tumour growth. Nature Rev. Cancer 2001; 2: 38–47.

[86] Dai T, Zheng H, Fu GS. Hypoxia Confers Protection Against Apoptosis via the PI3K/Akt Pathway in Endothelial Progenitor Cells. Acta Pharmacol Sin 2008; 29: 1425–1431.

[87] Roiniotis J, Hang Dinh, Masendycz P, et al. Hypoxia Prolongs Monocyte/Macrophage Survival and Enhanced Glycolysis Is Associated with Their Maturation under Aerobic Conditions. The Journal of Immunology 2009; 182(12) 7974-7981.

[88] Quail D, Taylor M, Walsh L, et al. Low Oxygen Levels Induce the Expression of the Embryonic Morphogen Nodal. Mol Biol Cell 2011;22(24):4809-21.

[89] Silván U, Díez-Torre A, Arluzea J, Andrade R, Silió M, Aréchaga J. Hypoxia and Pluripotency in Embryonic and Embryonal Carcinoma Stem Cell Biology. Differentiation 2009;78:159–168.

[90] Amberger-Murphy V. Hypoxia Helps Glioma to Fight Therapy. Curr. Cancer Drug Targets 2009; 9:381–390.

[91] Chan Gao, Weipeng Cao, Lan Bao, et al. Autophagy Negatively Regulates Wnt Signalling by Promoting Dishevelled Degradation. Nature Cell Biology 2010; 12, 781.

[92] Kanamori H, Takemura G, Maruyama R, et al. Functional Significance and Morphological Characterization of Starvation-Induced Autophagy in the Adult Heart. Am J Pathol. 2009; 174(5):1705-14.

[93] Degenhardt K, Mathew R, Beaudoin B, et al. Autophagy Promotes Tumor Cell Survival and Restricts Necrosis, Inflammation, and Tumorigenesis. Cancer Cell 2006; 10(1) 51–64.

[94] White E. Role of Metabolic Stress Responses of Apoptosis and Autophagy in Tumor Suppression. Ernst Schering Found Symp Proc. 2007; (4): 23–34.

[95] Komatsu M, Ichimura Y. Selective Autophagy Regulates Various Cellular Functions. Genes Cells. 2010;15(9):923-33.

[96] Matecic M, Smith DL Jr, Pan X, Maqani N, et al. A Microarray-Based Genetic Screen for Yeast Chronological Aging Factors. PLoS Genet 2010; 6(4): e1000921. doi:10.1371/journal.pgen.1000921.

[97] Boya P, González-Polo R, Casares N, et al. Inhibition of Macroautophagy Triggers Apoptosis. Mol Cell Biol. 2005; 25(3): 1025-1040.

[98] Huang L, Bindra R, Glazer P, Harris A. Hypoxia-Induced Genetic Instability—a Calculated Mechanism Underlying Tumor Progression. Journal of Molecular Medicine 2007; 85(2) 139-148.

[99] Stephens P, Greenman C, Fu B, et al. Massive Genomic Rearrangement Acquired in a Single Catastrophic Event during Cancer Development. Cell, 2011; 144(1) 27-40.

[100] Kloosterman V, Tavakoli-Yaraki M, Roosmalen M. et al. Constitutional Chromothripsis Rearrangements Involve Clustered Double-Stranded DNA Breaks and Nonhomologous Repair Mechanisms. Cell Reports 2012; 1(6) 648-655.

[101] Rich J. Cancer Stem Cells in Radiation Resistance. Cancer Res 2007; 67: 8980-8984

[102] Evans A. Ductal Carcinoma in situ (DCIS): Are We Overdetecting it? Breast Cancer Research 2004; 6: 23.

[103] Stattin P, Holmberg E, Johansson J. et al. Outcomes in Localized Prostate Cancer: National Prostate Cancer Register of Sweden Follow-up Study, JNCI J. Natl. Cancer Inst. 2010; 102(13) 950-958.

Chapter 8

Role of CREB Protein Family Members in Human Haematological Malignancies

Francesca D'Auria and Roberta Di Pietro

Additional information is available at the end of the chapter

1. Introduction

Cyclic AMP Response Element Binding (CREB) protein is a member of the CREB/ATF (Activating Transcription Factor) family of transcription factors playing an important role in the nuclear responses to a variety of external signals that lead to proliferation, differentiation, apoptosis and survival. Other authors' evidences have highlighted a critical role of CREB in the regulation of normal haematopoiesis and leukemogenesis due to the interaction with target genes crucially involved in the cell cycle machinery. Recent findings of our research group have demonstrated that CREB and ATF-1 phosphorylation levels are related to a different sensitivity of T leukaemia cell clones to the cytotoxic action of TNF-related apoptosis inducing ligand (TRAIL) and that low dose radiation treatment of erythroleukaemia cells (K562) can trigger CREB activation and deliver a survival signal. Since one fundamental problem of most malignancies, including those of haematological origin, is the development of multiple mechanisms of resistance, which progressively reduce or suppress the therapeutic efficacy of anticancer treatment, the early identification of biological markers of responsiveness/unresponsiveness and the follow-up of individual response are highly desirable to adjust therapeutic treatments. In light of all these considerations and of the complex molecular interactions involving CREB/ATF family members, the present chapter is aimed at revising literature focusing, in particular, on the involvement of CREB/ATF family members in leukemogenesis and lymphomagenesis, in order to gain more insight into this matter that could result useful to the treatment of leukaemia and lymphoma diseases.

2. CREB family members

The CREB or CREB/ATF multigenic family is composed by several nuclear transcription factors. The prototype of this family is CREB, a 43 kDa – basic-region leucine zipper (bZIP)

transcription factor that elicits responses to a variety of extracellular signals, including stress and growth factors, and that is involved in several cellular processes such as glucose homeostasis, proliferation, ageing and differentiation, survival and apoptosis, memory and learning [1]. The CREB/ATF family of transcription factors includes three homologous genes: cAMP response element binding (*CREB*), cAMP response element modulator (*CREM*), and activating transcription factor-1 (*ATF-1*), whose structure domains are illustrated in a recent review [2]. These genes generate a group of highly homologous proteins that have been named after their prototypes: CREB, CREM, and ATF-1, respectively [3].

CREB/ATF proteins were initially identified for their binding to the cyclic AMP response element (CRE) in various gene promoters that contain the octanucleotide consensus sequence TGACGTCA [4]. Over the years, cDNA clones encoding identical or homologous proteins have been isolated. Up to now, at least 20 different mammalian proteins with the prefix CREB or ATF have been characterized and grouped into subgroups on the basis of their amino acid similarity [5, 6]. CREB/ATF family members include CREB-1 (also known as CREB), CREB-2 (recently named ATF-4), CREB-3, CREB-5, CREM, ATF-1 (also known as TREB36), ATF-2 (also known as CRE-BP1), ATF-3, ATF-4 (previously named CREB-2), ATF-5 (also known as ATFX), ATF-6, ATF-7 and B-ATF subgroups [7, 8]. Proteins belonging to this class represent a large group of bZIP transcription factors containing highly divergent N-terminal domains, but sharing a C-terminal leucine zipper domain. The basic region in the bZIP domain is rich in basic amino acids and is responsible for specific DNA binding, while the leucine zipper region contains leucine residues and is responsible for dimerization of the proteins by resembling a zipper. Based on the sequence of each bZip domain, these proteins form homodimers or heterodimers both with other members of the family and with other bZIP containing proteins like the activator protein-1 (AP-1), C/EBP, Fos, Jun or Maf family proteins [8]. That implies the expansion of the repertoire and different opportunities of target gene regulation that are further increased by the alternative splice products of *CREB* and *CREM* genes that show repressor or activator properties [5, 7]. Whereas CREB, CREM, and ATF-1 are relatively well characterized and known to regulate gene transcription via binding to CRE sites, ATF-2, ATF-3, and ATF-4 are structurally more distant and their functional properties remain poorly understood. Rather than being activated by the cAMP cascade, ATF-2 is activated by c-Jun N-terminal kinase (JNK) and can dimerize with members of the AP-1 family such as c-Jun to bind to CRE or AP-1 sites [9, 10]. Additionally, ATF-2 homodimers and ATF-2/c-Jun heterodimers can bind to certain CRE-like sites that are insensitive to CREB [11]. ATF-3 and ATF-4 also dimerize with various Jun species and can shift c-Jun DNA binding site preferences from AP-1 to CRE, thereby promoting crosstalk among AP-1 and CREB protein families [9]. In addition, ATF-4 is able to dimerize with Nrf1 (NF-E2 related factor 1) and Nrf2 (NF-E2 related factor 2) and then interact with the antioxidant responsive element (ARE) present in the promoters of many antioxidant genes [12]. ATF-2, ATF-3, and ATF-4 have been considered as cellular stress response proteins [5, 13, 14] but recently they have been also involved in non-stress adaptations. In fact, extensive studies have demonstrated that ATF-3 is an adaptive response gene that is activated by a wide variety of signals including those initiated by cytokines, genotoxic agents or physiological stresses [15]. Interestingly, unlike other ATF family members, emerging evidences have implicated ATF-3 in the host defence against invading pathogens and cancer. These processes are controlled by the efficient coordination of cell responses and genetic regulatory networks which allow this key transcription factor to modulate the expression of a diverse set of target genes, depending on the cell type and/or the nature of the stimuli [16, 17].

While both CREBs and ATF-1 are ubiquitously expressed, CREMs are mainly present in spermatids [6] and in the neuroendocrine system [18]. Interestingly, a recently published paper on the effects of traumatic brain injury demonstrated the nuclear co-localization of CREM-1 and active caspase-3 in the ispilateral cortex of adult rats, suggesting a possible role for CREM-1 in neuronal apoptosis [19]. In a recent report of our research group on Jurkat leukaemia cells [20], we observed a different cell compartmentalization of CREB protein in dependence of the TRAIL dose employed and induced cytotoxicity. Indeed, both under normal or low serum culture conditions an evident nuclear translocation of phospho-CREB was detected after 1 h treatment only with the lower dose of TRAIL (100 ng/mL) and prevented in the presence of PI3K/Akt and p38 mitogen-activated protein kinase (MAPK) specific inhibitors [20]. In another model under investigation in our laboratories and represented by K562 erythroleukaemia cells induced to differentiation [21], the nuclear localization of the active form of CREB was clearly evident after only 1 h treatment with haemin. Interestingly, CREB positive nuclei resembled the features of apoptotic nuclei, suggesting that CREB phosphorylation is possibly required to determine the nuclear structural changes occurring during erythroblast maturation [21, 22]. Concerning other family members, it has been recently shown that ATF-2 is a nucleocytoplasmic shuttling protein and that its subcellular localization is regulated by AP-1 dimerization [23]. ATF-3 is ubiquitously expressed and localized in the nucleus but maintained at low levels in the absence of cellular stresses. Instead, it is rapidly transcriptionally induced under different conditions, among which hypoxia, DNA damage (induced by UV radiation, ionizing radiation, etoposide), heat or cold shock, serum starvation or stimulation [13, 15]. ATF-4 is of particular interest since it has been demonstrated to translocate from the cytoplasmic membrane to the nucleus in neuronal cells upon γ aminobutyric acid (GABA) receptor activation, to be likely involved in neuronal plasticity by coupling receptor activity to gene expression [24]. Finally, a number of immunofluorescent and cell fractionation experiments indicate that ATF-6 is linked to the endoplasmic reticulum (ER) chaperone Bip/Crp78 and localizes in the precursor form on the ER membrane [25]. Upon ER stress induced by prolonged nutrient deprivation, it translocates to the Golgi where it is cleaved by resident proteases to liberate its active N-terminal domain. In this active form it translocates to the nucleus where it up-regulates a number of target genes involved in energy homeostasis [25].

3. CREB binding proteins

The human CREB-binding protein (CBP) and its paralogue, p300, are highly related proteins that are well conserved amongst mammals. Due to their high degree of sequence similarity, these two proteins are most often functionally interchangeable although they also possess unique functions [26, 27]. CBP was initially recognized as an interaction partner for CREB nuclear transcription factor [28], whereas p300 cDNA was cloned encoding the 300 kDa protein known to be associated with the adenoviral protein E1A [29]. Though encoded by different genes, CBP/p300 share several conserved regions that constitute most of their known functional domains [for details see 27]. Both CBP and p300 have originally been described as transcriptional co-activators that bridge DNA-binding transcription factors to components of the basal transcriptional machinery, including the TATA-box-binding protein (TBP) [30], TFIIB [31] and, via RNA helicase A, also RNA polymerase II [32]. Due to the huge size of over 2400 amino acids, CBP/p300 can also behave as a scaffold, bridging together a variety of cofactor proteins at the same time and leading to the assembly of multi-competent co-activator complexes [26, 27]. In addition, CBP/p300 interact with protein kinases such as the MAPKs and the cyclin E-Cdk2 complex, thus mediating the phosphorylation of CBP/p300-interacting transcription factors such as ER81 and E2F family members. Both CBP and p300 have been found originally to possess histone acetyltransferase (HAT) activity [33]. This acetyltransferase function has profound consequences for nucleosomal structure and the activity of transcription factors, and thereby affects gene activity in multiple ways. In fact, it is well known that acetylation of multiple sites in the histone tails has been directly associated with transcriptional up-regulation, whereas de-acetylation correlates with transcriptional repression. Mechanistically, histone acetylation promotes the accessibility of DNA to transcription protein complexes, by facilitating the "unwiring" of the chromatin structure. During the last years, both CBP and p300 have been regarded as protein acetyltransferases rather than only HAT since they have shown the capacity to acetylate a number of non-histone nuclear proteins, including the tumour suppressor protein p53, dTCF, EKLF (erythroid Kruppel-like factor), GATA-1, NF-Y and other basal transcription factors [34, 35]. Thus, in light of the number of proteins interacting with CBP/p300, it is not surprising to find that many physiological processes, including cell growth, cell division, cell differentiation, cell transformation, embryogenesis and apoptosis, are dependent on CBP/p300 function [27, 28, 34]. Moreover, the importance of CBP/p300 is underscored by the fact that genetic alterations as well as their functional dysregulation are strongly linked to human diseases [36, 37].

Previous studies have shown that CBP and p300 play distinct roles in haematopoiesis and act non-redundantly in microenvironment-mediated haematopoietic regulation in spite of their high homology [38-40]. It has been widely documented that both proteins interact with crucial transcriptional regulators in virtually all haematopoietic lineages. Intriguingly, CBP/p300 can promote, on one hand, normal differentiation and cell cycle arrest (by cooperating with GATA-1) and, on the other hand, cell cycle progression and transformation by cooperating with c-Myb and PU.1, an Ets family transcription factor. It is conceivable that an overexpressed oncoprotein might compete with differentiation-inducing factors for CBP/p300 function. Furthermore, during normal development, CBP/p300 could differentially partition among transcriptional regulators with opposing functions, thus controlling the balance between proliferation and differentiation. As an example, the down-modulation of the proto-oncoproteins PU.1 and c-Myb during the erythroleukaemia MEL cell line maturation might increase availability of CBP/p300 for differentiation-associated factors such as GATA-1, NF-E2 and EKLF. Moreover, besides the involvement in erythroid cell lineage differentiation, CBP and, very likely, p300 target a broad range of myeloid and lymphoid expressed transcription factors [38-40].

Because of its central role in transcription, it is not surprising that aberrations in CREBBP can affect many tissues [17]. In humans, chromosomal translocations involving the CREBBP gene have been observed in leukaemia and myelodysplastic syndrome [38]. Mutations of CREBBP in the germline have been associated to the Rubinstein-Taybi syndrome (RTS), an autosomal dominant disease characterized by mental retardation, skeletal abnormalities and a high propensity to develop cancer, including leukaemia [36]. Similarly, CREBBP(+/-) mice show abnormalities in bone, haematopoietic tissues and neural tissues and an increased tendency to develop haematological malignancies with age [41]. In earlier studies, in CREBBP(+/-) HSCs (haematopoietic stem cells) a number of cell-intrinsic defects have been described, including diminished HSC self-renewal and excessive myeloid differentiation [42]. The combination of skeletal and haematopoietic defects in CREBBP(+/-) mice suggests the involvement of the bone marrow (BM) microenvironment in the haematopoietic phenotype of these mice. One of the genes whose transcription is directly regulated by CBP is matrix metalloproteinase 9 (MMP9) that was reported to be a microenvironmental regulator of haematopoiesis [43]. Interestingly, CREBBP heterozygosity in the BM microenvironment results in reduced levels of MMP9 and soluble kit ligand (KITL) and increased expression of endothelial cell adhesion molecule 1 (ESAM1) and cadherin 5 (CDH5) on a subset of endothelial cells. In addition, it has been reported that the loss of a single CREBBP allele is deleterious for the BM microenvironment, leading to defective haematopoiesis. In fact, the CREBBP(+/-) microenvironment poorly supports HSCs, promotes excessive myelopoiesis and reduces lymphopoiesis. Furthermore, it has been reported that CREBBP(+/-) mice have reduced bone volume due to increased osteoclastogenesis. A concomitant reduction in CFU-fibroblasts (CFU-Fs) and osteoblasts per tissue area was also identified and likely contributes to fewer HSC niches [41]. Thus, all these findings reveal the importance of CBP in the development and function of the BM microenvironment and underscore the multiple levels at which this protein acts to regulate haematopoiesis. Indeed, half of the normal complement of CREBBP, but not of EP300, in the BM microenvironment has a deleterious effect on haematopoiesis via multiple mechanisms, leading to the development of excessive myelopoiesis, disrupting the proper architecture of the BM and resulting in poor maintenance of HSC number and quality.

4. CREB physiological roles and signalling pathways

CREB is a multi-functional transcriptional activator that is involved in many signalling pathways under normal and pathologic conditions. CREB mediates its transcriptional responses following phosphorylation at Ser133 [7] and the consequent association with the 256 kDa co-activator CBP [28] or related family members like p300 [29]. Both Ser133 phosphorylation and CBP association play an essential role for gene transactivation mediated by an octanucleotide CRE consensus sequence placed in the promoters of many cellular genes [29]. In more detail, CREB transactivation domain, that is the site able to interact with other nuclear factors, contains a constitutive glutamine rich domain termed Q2 and an inducible domain, termed the kinase-inducible domain (KID), regulated by cellular kinases [2]. The Q2 domain interacts with a TATA binding protein-associated factor and is constitutively active; instead, the KID region promotes isomerization by recruiting the co-activator factors CBP and p300 to the gene promoters and is active only when it is phosphorylated at Ser133 by a variety of cellular kinases. Recent studies using a genome-wide analysis showed that the number of putative target genes for CREB is about 5000, among which immediate-early genes, including c-FOS, AP-1/JunB and early growth response protein 1 (EGR-1) [44], as well as genes crucially involved in the cell cycle machinery, namely *Cyclin A1* and *D1* [7]. In this respect, it has been found that Cyclin A is up-regulated in cell lines, transgenic mice and patient bone marrow that show increased CREB levels [44]. It is still to unravel whether this occurs through a direct or indirect mechanism. To address this issue or, in other words, to determine whether CREB overexpression results in target gene activation through increased occupancy of binding sites or by altering levels of Ser133 phosphorylation, several authors proposed to use chromatin immunoprecipitation assays. Moreover, microarray analysis of potential CREB target genes will help in understanding the downstream pathways through which CREB contributes to normal and aberrant haematopoiesis. By interacting with its huge number of target genes CREB plays a critical role in the regulation of various biological processes including haema-topoiesis, liver gluconeogenesis, pituitary gland physiology, circadian rhythm, spermatogen-esis, learning and memory [1, 45, 46]. Concerning haematopoiesis, CREB is a downstream target of haematopoietic growth factor signalling activated by granulocyte-macrophage–colony stimulating factor (GM-CSF) and interleukin-3 (IL-3), thus resulting a crucial factor for normal myelopoiesis [44]. In addition, it appears to play a role in primary erythroblast differentiation [47] as well as in megacaryocyte differentiation where it is activated in a MAPK-dependent manner [48]. More recently, it has also been involved in HSC and uncommitted progenitor proliferation and survival through its effects on cell cycle control [45, 46]. A growing body of evidences is unravelling the role of CREB in the regulation of the immune system [49]. Indeed, several immune-related genes contain a cAMP responsive element, as in the case of IL-2, IL-6, IL-10 and TNF-α. In monocytes and macrophages CREB exerts anti-apoptotic survival effects. Moreover, CREB promotes normal B and T cell survival and proliferation when it is phosphorylated in response to signalling by the B-cell receptor or different kinases [49]. Particularly well characterized is the regulatory role that CREB plays in the nervous system. Actually, numerous papers have demonstrated CREB involvement in promoting neuronal survival, precursor proliferation, neurite outgrowth and neuronal differentiation in certain neuronal populations [50], highlighting the importance of CREB signalling in learning and memory processes in several organisms [2, 51].

In the late 1980s, it was discovered that cAMP mediates the hormonal stimulation of several cellular processes by regulating the phosphorylation of critical proteins among which CREB transcription factor [52]. Although it was initially identified as a target of the cAMP signalling pathway, studies on activation of immediate-early genes revealed that CREB is a substrate for kinases other than cAMP-dependent protein kinase A (PKA) and that various signalling routes converge on CREB and CREM, controlling their function by modulating their phosphorylation states [52, 53]. As above mentioned, almost all the signalling pathways that activate CREB lead to the phosphorylation of Ser133, which is required for CREB-induced gene transcription, but additional sites on CREB or on linked proteins can be phosphorylated exerting a modulation of CREB activity [35]. For example, Ser133 phosphorylation primes CREB for phosphorylation by Glycogen synthase kinase 3 (GSK-3) at Ser129. However, unlike Ser133 phosphorylation, the physiologic consequences of Ser129 phosphorylation are not well defined, although evidence suggests that it is also linked to CREB activation [54]. In different systems a number of different kinases have been shown to stimulate CREB phosphorylation and several CREB kinase candidates have been identified so far. PKA, which is activated by cAMP, is the major kinase that targets Ser133 in many processes [1, 3]. Other signalling molecules responsible for CREB Ser133 phosphorylation include mitogen- and stress-activated kinase 1 (MSK-1), extracellular signal-regulated kinase (ERK), calcium/calmodulin-dependent kinases (CaMKs), p90 ribosomal S6 kinase (RSK), MAPKs and Akt/protein kinase B (PKB) [1, 3, 7, 55, 56]. Both MAPK and Akt have been shown to enhance the survival of cultured cells by stimulating CREB-dependent target gene expression [56]. CREB activity is also regulated by a family of cytoplasmic co-activators known as transducers of regulated CREB activity (TORCs) and including TORC1, TORC2 and TORC3. TORCs are activated by extracellular stimuli represented by nutrients (glucose) and hormones. Once activated, they translocate into the nucleus where they bind to the bZIP domain of CREB exerting its activation through a phospho-Ser133-independent mechanism. All TORCs are regarded as strong activators of CREB-dependent transcription [57].

In Fig. 1 the main factors and signalling molecules leading to CREB activation in haematopoietic cells are schematically represented.

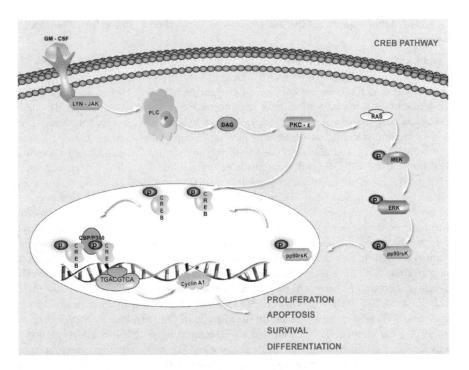

Figure 1. Schematic representation of the main factors and signalling molecules leading to CREB activation in haematopoietic cells. A various array of extracellular stimuli promote CREB activation through phosphorylation or through interaction with CREB co-activators to enhance the expression of CREB responsive genes. CREB target genes, including Cyclin A1, are able to mediate effects on cellular proliferation, apoptosis, survival and differentiation. PLC: phospholipase-C; DAG: 1,2-diacylglycerol; PKC-ε: protein kinase C-ε.

5. CREB family members and leukemogenesis

Recent data suggest that CREB acts as a proto-oncogene in haematopoietic cells and contributes to the leukaemia phenotype [37, 38, 45, 46]. It has been shown anyway that CREB is able to promote tumour formation only when other oncogenes are also activated. In fact, its overexpression is not sufficient to induce acute leukaemia *in vivo*. This is consistent with similar observations obtained with translocations, such as AML1-ETO (Acute Myeloid Leukaemia Eight-Twenty-One), a chimeric protein that requires additional mutations to develop leukaemia in mouse models [58]. In previous works different strategies have been delineated to identify the oncogenes cooperating with CREB to drive leukemogenesis: one way is represented by crossing different transgenic mice of known oncogenes such as *K-RAS*, *MEIS 1*, *PML/ RARα* etc. to *CREB* transgenic mice; another approach consists in infecting *CREB* transgenics with a retrovirus such as the Molony murine leukaemia virus to insertionally activate cooperating oncogenes. The latter approach has also the potential to identify novel collaborators of CREB besides the already known CBP and p300. Identifying novel oncogenic alterations that cause leukaemia and discovering the signalling pathways involved will be of great value to gain a better knowledge of the disease and to lead to novel and more efficient therapeutic measures.

Several CREB family members have been implicated in different malignant conditions. The first malignancy to be discovered was the clear cell sarcoma of the soft tissue (CSST). In this solid tumour, the cells are induced to proliferation by an Ewing's Sarcoma (EWS)-ATF-1 fusion oncoprotein derived by a chromosomal translocation that fuses the DNA-binding and bZip domain of ATF-1 to the EWS gene. In haematological malignancies, CREB has been implicated in the pathogenesis of human T lymphotropic virus I (HTLV-I) related T-cell leukaemia [59] and also associated with the genesis of follicular lymphoma, where CREB binds to the CRE site in the promoter of translocated Bcl-2 [46]. Other leukaemia-associated chromosomal translocations involving the CBP and p300 genes were also linked to haematological malignancies. These translocations generally result in fusion products that preserve most of the CBP and p300 molecules, suggesting that the disease mechanism does not simply involve loss of function of CBP, as is the case in Rubinstein-Taybi syndrome, but often implies an altered cofactor function (dominant positive or dominant negative) through fusion to another molecule. The most frequent chromosomal translocations targeting *CREBBP* and *EP300* have been described in specific subtypes of myeloid leukaemia and are represented by Mixed-Lineage Leukaemia 1 (*MLL*)-*EP300*, *MLL-CREBBP*, *MOZ-CREBBP* and *MOZ-EP300* [37, 60]. Interestingly, most translocations involving CREB-related genes result in leukaemia of the myeloid/monocytic lineage, highlighting the importance of CREB and CREB-interacting proteins in the regulation of haematopoietic cell differentiation and proliferation [45, 46]. Actually, previous work demonstrated that bone marrow cells from patients with acute myeloid or lymphoid leukaemia expressed higher levels of CREB compared to patients not affected by leukaemia or with normal bone marrow [60]. Moreover, it appears that an elevated CREB expression is associated with an increased risk of relapse or persistent disease and decreased event-free survival [45]. This is consistent with the observation that leukaemia cell lines expressing CREB at elevated levels show an increased growth/proliferation rate in normal conditions and an increased survival when exposed to stress like serum starvation [61]. On the contrary, down-regulation of endogenous CREB in leukaemia cell lines by siRNA resulted in reduced cell viability [20, 45], indicating that CREB is a critical regulator of growth and survival in both myeloid and lymphoid leukaemia cells. Unfortunately, chromosomal translocations have also been involved in drug-induced leukaemia. For instance, the involvement of 11q23-balanced translocations in acute leukaemia after treatment with drugs that inhibit the function of DNA topoisomerase II (topo II) is being recognized with increasing frequency. It has been shown that the gene at 11q23, involved in all of these treatment-related leukaemias, is *MLL* (also called ALL1, Htrx, and HRX). In general, the translocations occurring in these leukaemias are the same as those occurring in *de novo* leukaemia [eg. t(9;11), t(11;19), and t(4;11)]. Interestingly, the t(11;16)(q23;p13.3) has been cloned and has been shown to involve both *MLL* and *CREBBP* [62]. Besides chromosomal translocations, another way for CREB to contribute to tumorigenesis is through the suppression of cellular genes either by competing with or binding to sites occupied by other transcription factors or by confiscating the transcriptional machinery [63].

5.1. Acute myeloid leukaemia

Acute leukaemia derives from the clonal expansion of haematopoietic stem/progenitor cells that have lost their ability to undergo terminal differentiation. Since transcription factors control HSC production and differentiation, it is conceivable that disorders of the haematopoietic system often involve alterations of the regulatory network of transcription factors. In haematological malignancies transcription factors can be overexpressed, involved in chromosomal translocations or become targets of somatic mutations that disrupt their normal function [37, 60-63]. Previous studies have demonstrated that *CREB* is a proto-oncogene whose overexpression promotes cellular proliferation in haematopoietic cells [1, 3]. The abnormal proliferation and survival of myeloid cells *in vitro* and *in vivo* appears to be due to the upregulation of CREB target genes such as *Cyclin A1* [60, 63]. Transgenic mice that overexpress CREB in myeloid cells develop a myeloproliferative disease with splenomegaly and aberrant myelopoiesis. However, CREB overexpressing mice do not spontaneously develop acute myeloid leukaemia (AML) [61]. To identify genes that accelerate leukaemia in CREB transgenic mice retroviral insertional mutagenesis has been used. The mutagenesis screen identified several integration sites, including oncogenes *Gfi1*, *Myb*, and *Ras*. Among transcription factors, *Sox4* was identified with the screen as a gene that cooperates with *CREB* in myeloid leukemogenesis by contributing to increased proliferation of haematopoietic progenitor cells [64]. Moreover, chromatin immunoprecipitation assays have demonstrated that *CREB* is a direct target of *Sox4*. In fact, it has been shown that the transduction of *CREB* transgenic mouse bone marrow cells with a Sox4 retrovirus increases survival and self-renewal of cells *in vitro* and results in increased expression of CREB target genes. Consistently, leukaemia blasts from the majority of AML patients have higher levels of CREB, phospho-CREB, and Sox4 protein expression in the bone marrow [64]. The increase in both CREB protein and mRNA levels in primary AML cells is possibly due to *CREB* gene amplification in the blast cells. Furthermore, a higher level of CREB has been found to correlate with a less favourable prognosis and an increased risk of relapse and decreased event-free survival in a small cohort of AML patients [45, 61]. Generally, AML in adults has a 20% five-year disease free survival despite treatment with aggressive cytotoxic chemotherapy and two thirds of AML patients do not experience significant periods of remission. Therefore, in light of its important role in the pathogenesis of leukaemia, CREB has been indicated as a potential prognostic marker of disease progression in AML and a molecular target for future treatment of leukaemia.

Clinical and experimental findings underline that AML is induced by numerous functionally cooperating genetic alterations, including chromosomal translocations that lead to the expression of fusion proteins often behaving as aberrant transcription factors. Several AML-associated lesions target chromatin regulators like histone methyltransferases or histone acetyltransferases, including MLL1 or CBP/p300 [65]. As already mentioned, CBP is an adapter protein that is involved in regulating transcription and histone acetylation, through which it is thought to contribute to an increased level of gene expression. The *CBP* gene was recently identified as a partner gene in the t(8;16) that occurs in *de novo* acute myelomonocytic leukae-mia (AML-M4) and rarely in treatment-related AML [66]. The fusion gene could alter the CBP protein so that it becomes constitutively active or, alternatively, it could modify the chromatin-association functions of *MLL* gene [38, 40]. *MLL* and *HOXB4*, a member of the homeobox domain transcription factors, have been identified as regulators of HSC maturation during early haematopoiesis [67]. *HOXB4* belongs to the *HOX* genes, a family of oncogenes implicated in the pathogenesis of various human cancers and highly expressed in the majority of AML. In a recent report Wang et al. [54] demonstrated the association of CREB and its co-activators TORC and CBP with homeodomain protein MEIS1, a HOX DNA-binding cofactor and critical downstream mediator of the *MLL* oncogenic program. This MEIS-CREB nexus is regulated by GSK-3, a multi-functional serine/threonine kinase that impairs the proliferation and induces the differentiation of a variety of cancers, including leukaemias, induced by *MLL* oncogenes. This kinase mediates CREB activation through phosphorylation at Ser129. In fact, CREB Ser129 mutation antagonizes *HOX/MEIS* activity and decreases colony-forming abilities of *HOX/ MEIS* or *MLL* transformed cells. These and other similar observations provide a molecular rationale for targeting *HOX*-associated transcription through GSK-3 inhibition in a subset of leukaemias.

Myelodysplastic syndromes (MDS) include a heterogeneous group of clonal haematopoietic stem cell malignancies with significant morbidity and high mortality. The incidence of MDS increases markedly with age and the disease is most prevalent in individuals who are white and male. Because of an ageing population and an improving awareness of the disease, the documented disease burden is expected to worsen in the near future. Due to the poor survival of individuals with MDS, it is important to identify prognostic factors to better risk-stratify patients for more effective treatments [68]. Genomic instability is associated with progression of the disease so that a part of patients develops AML. It has been reported that an increased incidence of haematological malignancies occurs in *CREBBP* heterozygous mice and other authors have shown that *CREBBP* is one of the genes altered by chromosomal translocations in patients suffering from therapy-related myelodysplastic syndrome [69]. Moreover, it has been demonstrated that *CREBBP*(+/-) mice invariably develop myelodysplastic/myeloproliferative neoplasm within 9-12 months of age. They are also hypersensitive to ionizing radiation and show a marked decrease in poly(ADP-ribose) polymerase-1 activity after irradiation. In addition, protein levels of XRCC1 (X-ray repair complementing defective repair in Chinese hamster cells 1) and APEX1 (APEX nuclease), key components of base excision repair machinery, are reduced in un-irradiated CREBBP(+/-) cells or upon targeted knockdown of CREBBP levels. These results provide validation of a new myelodysplastic/myeloproliferative neoplasm mouse model and, more importantly, point at a defective repair of DNA damage as a contributing factor to the pathogenesis of this currently incurable disease [46].

5.2. Acute lymphoblastic leukaemia

Acute lymphoblastic leukaemia (ALL) is a heterogeneous disease characterized by the predominance of immature haematopoietic cells, in which malignant cells express phenotypes of either T-cell or B-cell lineages [61]. ALLs account for the 25-30% of all cancer diagnoses in children. CREB involvement in the molecular events related to *in vitro* and *in vivo* lymphoblastic proliferation is still little known, whereas a lot of evidences disclose a role of CREB as a proto-oncogene in haematopoiesis and in AML. CREB can be overexpressed in the 84% of ALL patients (73/86) at diagnosis but neither in remission nor in non-leukaemia samples [70]. By contrast, the parallel expression of the cAMP early inducible repressor (ICER), which represses CREB activity by competing for the CRE consensus site, appears down-regulated at diagnosis but neither in remission nor in control samples [70]. Thus, it is presumable that CREB overexpression leads to target gene up-regulation and increase in cell proliferation and survival that are not counteracted by the insufficient level of ICER expression. Besides this hypothesis, Pigazzi et al. [71] have also demonstrated the co-expression of miR34b in CREB overexpressing myeloid leukaemia cells providing new information about myeloid transformation and therapeutic strategies. Despite the apparently good prognosis, the 15% of high hyper-diploid (HD) childhood ALL cases relapse [72, 73]. Relapsed ALL is a leading cause of death due to disease in young people, but the molecular mechanisms of treatment failure are still to be elucidated. Genome-wide profiling of structural DNA alterations in ALL identified multiple sub-microscopic somatic mutations targeting key cellular pathways and demonstrated evolution in genetic alterations from diagnosis to relapse [74]. Many of the mutations that have been identified concern the transcriptional co-activators CREBBP and NCOR1, the transcription factors ERG, SPI1, TCF4 and TCF7L2, components of the Ras signalling pathway, histone genes, genes involved in histone modification (CREBBP and CTCF) and genes target of DNA copy number alterations [74]. The parallel analysis of an extended cohort of diagnosis-relapsed cases and acute leukaemia cases that did not relapse showed that the 18.3% of relapsed cases had sequence or deletion mutations of CREBBP [72, 74]. CREBBP is expressed in leukaemia cells and normal B-cell progenitors, and the mutant CREBBP alleles are expressed in ALL cell lines harbouring mutations. Mutations at diagnosis or acquired at relapse consist in truncated alleles or deleterious substitutions in conserved residues of the histone acetyltransferase domain, impairing histone acetylation and transcriptional regulation of CREBBP targets, including glucocorticoid responsive genes. In mice the homozygous deletion of CREBBP or EP300 is lethal due to developmental abnormalities whereas CREBBP(+/−) mice show defects in B lymphoid development and an increased incidence of haematopoietic tumours [75]. Both *CREBBP* and *EP300* sequence mutations have been reported in solid tumours and, more recently, also in haematological malignancies, whereas rare *EP300* mutations have been detected in an ALL cell lines and myelodysplasia [74, 76]. A lot of detected mutations at relapse, the same identified at diagnosis in other clones, prove that mutations confer resistance to therapy. Many identified mutations are target in transcriptional and epigenetic regulation as a mechanism of resistance in ALL. It is worth outlining that the high incidence of *CREBBP* mutations found in relapse-prone HD ALL cases discloses the possibility of a targeted customized treatment in this genetic subgroup [73].

In our laboratory we have investigated the role of PI3K/Akt pathway and CREB family members in a number of lymphoid and erythroleukaemia cell lines treated with chemical and physical agents inducing cell death by apoptosis or necrosis [20, 21, 47, 77-80]. We first detected with Western Blotting a high constitutive level of CREB phosphorylation at Ser133 in Jurkat T cells under normal serum culture conditions [20]. Under low serum culture conditions, an early (within 1 h) and transient increase in CREB phosphorylation was observed in response to TRAIL treatment and reduced upon pre-treatment with LY294002 or SB253580, demonstrating the PI3K/Akt- and p38 MAPK-dependency of this effect. Interestingly, both phospho-CREB and phospho-ATF-1 were down-regulated in response to TRAIL treatment of normal primary cells derived from haematopoietic precursors (HUVEC, HEMA), whereas both of them were up-regulated in the neoplastic counterparts (K562 cell line) [20, 21]. The PI3K/Akt pathway dependency of CREB/ATF-1 phosphorylation induced by TRAIL treatment was demonstrated both in primary cells and in leukaemia cell lines of different origin and TRAIL sensitivity, showing that the observed phenomenon is a general feature of TRAIL action in leukaemia [77, 80]. In addition, the observation of CREB cleavage products upon TRAIL/LY294002 combined treatment of sensitive leukaemia cells was consistent with previous reports on other neoplastic cell lines [81] and compatible with the TRAIL-mediated activation of the caspase cascade and cleavage of anti-apoptotic molecules. The parallel analysis with immune fluorescence demonstrated the nuclear translocation of the phosphorylated form of CREB upon treatment with 100 ng/mL TRAIL, whereas the immune labelling was mainly detectable in the cytoplasm compartment upon the higher more cytotoxic dose (1000 ng/mL) as shown in Fig. 2. A further enhancement of apoptotic cell death was obtained with the use of CREB1 siRNA technology leading us to hypothesize that CREB activation can have an important role in the complex crosstalk among pro- and anti-apoptotic pathways in Jurkat T cells [20, 80].

5.3. Chronic myelogenous leukaemia

Chronic myelogenous leukaemia (CML) is characterized in the 85-90% of the cases by the presence of the Philadelphia (Ph) chromosome and the *BCR-ABL* fusion gene. A further 5-10% of the cases display other translocations, most commonly complex variants, that involve one or more chromosomal regions in addition to bands 9q34 and 22q11, but also simple variants that typically involve 22q11 and a chromosome other than 9q34. However, genes that cooperate with *BCR-ABL* leading to acute leukaemia are not well understood neither the role played by CREB in CML has been clarified. Preliminary observations of the group of Kathleen Sakamoto indicate that CREB is highly expressed in blood and bone marrow cells from patients with CML in chronic phase, but not in normal bone marrow cells

[82]. The same authors previously showed that inhibition of CREB by using RNA interference (RNAi) technology resulted in decreased proliferation and survival of bcr-abl-expressing K562 cells [45, 83], whereas other authors reported that CREB antisense oligonucleotides were able to induce death of human leukaemia cells and bone marrow cells from patients affected with both AML and CML [84]. A critical factor for the genesis of acute leukaemia or acute transformation of CML appears to be the formation of fusion genes between *NUP98* and members of the *HOX* gene family [85]. Interestingly, all the NUP98-HOX-involved fusion products exhibit dual binding ability to both CREB binding protein, a co-activator, and histone deacetylase 1, a co-repressor, acting as both trans-activators and trans-repressors and contributing to the genesis of acute leukaemia or acute transformation of CML [86].

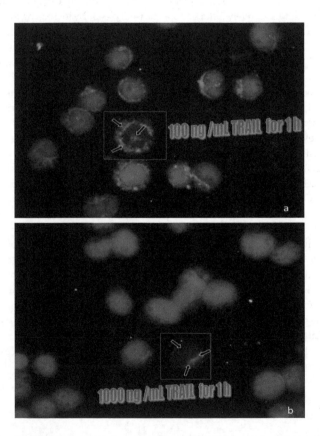

Figure 2. a, b: Phospho-CREB localization in Jurkat T cells upon TRAIL treatment. An evident nuclear translocation of phospho-CREB (green fluorescence) was detected upon 1 h treatment only with the lower dose of TRAIL (panel a), whereas the labelling was located at cytoplasm level upon the higher more cytotoxic dose (panel b). Nuclei were counterstained with 6-diamino-2-phenylindole (DAPI) (blue fluorescence). Green and blue fluorescence single emissions are overlapped in the merge panels. The insets show green fluorescence single emission. Original magnification: 40X. The figure has been adapted from [20].

5.4. Chronic lymphocytic leukaemia

Chronic lymphocytic leukaemia (CLL) originates from the abnormal accumulation of antigen-stimulated B cells that escape normal cell death mechanisms and/or undergo increased proliferation [87]. CLL is the most prevalent adult leukaemia in the Western world, yet no curative treatment exists. Many studies have explored the use of family-specific cyclic nucleotide phosphodiesterase (PDE) inhibitors in light of the potent effects of cAMP signalling on immune system function [88, 89]. Among the 11 currently known families of cyclic nucleotide PDEs, all but three are capable of catabolizing cAMP and at least 5 PDE families (PDE1-4, PDE7 and PDE8) are expressed in lymphoid cells and regulated by either mitogens or agents that induce cAMP-mediated signalling. Previous work has established that inhibition of PDE4 is sufficient to selectively induce apoptosis in CLL cells by increasing the concentration of cAMP [88]. In a recent paper Meyers et al. [89] examined how CLL cells differ from normal haematopoietic cells with regard to their sensitivity to PDE4 inhibitor-mediated cAMP accumulation, CREB phosphorylation and gene expression. Interestingly, it was discovered that upon exposure to rolipram, a prototypical PDE4 inhibitor, cAMP intracellular levels rapidly rose in both CLL and normal B cells, whereas no such increase was detected in T cells. Likewise, ATF-1/CREB Ser63/133 phosphorylation was induced by rolipram in nearly all CLL and B cells, whereas normal T cells displayed a lower response. Based on these findings and on previous observations of a reduced basal cAMP signalling in CLL cells, the authors suggested the involvement of specific PDE or splice isoforms in the reduced basal apoptotic index of CLL cells [89]. Looking for etiological agents, other authors have identified a stromal cell–derived factor-1 (SDF-1)-dependent mechanism as a microenvironmental regulatory mechanism of CLL cell survival [90]. It is known that SDF-1 is a chemokine that plays an important role in B-cell development. In fact, high levels of SDF-1 are produced by stromal cells within the marrow to retain B-cell precursors in close contact with them, within the supportive haematopoietic microenvironment [91], and to prevent their premature release into the circulation. Upon *in vitro* treatment of CLL cells with synthetic SDF-1α, a rapid and transient activation of p44/42 MAPK (ERK1/2) signalling pathway was observed and related to CLL cell survival. Downward MAPK activation transcription-dependent and -independent mechanisms were involved. In fact, MAPK was able to promote cell survival directly by inactivating the pro-apoptotic BAD protein and indirectly by activating CREB, which, in turn, is important for the transcriptional up-regulation of the anti-apoptotic BCL-2 gene [92]. Thus, SDF-1 engages B lineage CLL cells through the stromal cell receptor CXCR4 and affects components of the cell death machinery, leading to the noted resistance of CLL cells to apoptosis.

5.5. Human T Lymphotropic Virus 1 (HTLV-1) related T cell leukaemia

Human T-cell leukaemia virus type-I (HTLV-1) is the first discovered human retrovirus [93]. It has been recognized as the etiological agent of an aggressive malignancy known as adult T-cell leukaemia (ATL) as well as of the neurological syndrome TSP/HAM and of other clinical disorders. *In vitro* HTLV-1 is able to infect a number of different cell types, whereas in natural human infections it generally targets mature CD4+ helper T cells or, less frequently, CD8+ T cells. Although the mechanism of HTLV-1 pathogenicity is not fully understood yet, it is widely believed that a virally encoded trans-activator protein, called Tax, is centrally involved in this mechanism. In a recent review Azran et al. [94] provide valuable insights into the molecular mechanisms of HTLV-1 leukemogenesis. In particular, the authors detail the signalling pathways recruited by Tax to set infected T cells into continuous uncontrolled replication and to destabilize their genome, enabling, thereby, accumulation of mutations that can contribute to the leukemogenic process. Tax is able to modulate the expression of many viral genes via the viral long terminal repeat (LTR) and cellular genes through the CREB/ATF-, AP-1-, serum responsive factor (SRF)- and NF-κB-associated pathways, employing the CBP/p300 and p/CAF (p300/CBP-associated factor) co-activators for achieving the full transcriptional activation competence of each of these pathways. It is worth noting that Tax responsive elements (TxRE) contain a centered sequence TGACG(T/A)(C/G)(T/A) that is imperfectly homologous to the consensus cAMP responsive element (CRE; TGACGTCA). Thus, the presence of Tax is necessary for CREB to form a stable complex with the viral CRE. In fact, by interacting with the bZIP region of CREB, Tax enhances CREB dimerization and increases, thereby, its affinity to CRE. In particular, it has been recently shown that CREB is the most prominent factor that cooperates with Tax in activating HTLV-1 LTR region expression [95]. Moreover, it has been demonstrated that while, in the absence of Tax, CREB can activate HTLV-1 LTR expression only if phosphorylated by PKA, another member of the family, namely CREB2, can markedly activate the viral LTR without phosphorylation and can mediate a much stronger activation of the viral LTR by Tax than CREB does [94, 96]. Interestingly, mutant models disrupting Tax activation of the CREB protein resulted in the preferential immortalization of CD8+ lympho-cytes, rather than CD4+ lymphocytes, whereas the disruption of Tax interaction with CBP did not affect lymphocyte immortalization [97].

5.6. Lymphoma

Lymphomas are haematological malignancies of the lymphoid system. Deregulated gene expression is a hallmark of cancer and is well documented in B-cell lymphomas [98]. B cells are particularly susceptible to malignant transformation since the mechanisms involved in antibody diversification can cause chromosomal translocations and oncogenic mutations. B-cell lymphomas include Hodgkin lymphoma (HL) and non-Hodgkin lymphoma (B-NHL). B-NHL consists of a heterogeneous group of diseases whose pathogenesis is associated with multiple genetic lesions affecting oncogenes and tumour-suppressor genes and whose treatment is related to the different grade of malignancy. The most common type of B-NHL is represented by the diffuse large B-cell lymphoma (DLBCL), which generally arises as a clinical evolution of the follicular lymphoma (FL). A number of papers have demonstrated the involvement of CREB family members in the pathogenesis of lymphoma. It has been previ-ously found that CREB acts as a positive regulator of the translocated BCL-2 allele in FLs with the t(14;18) translocation [60] and that the high constitutive expression of ATF-3 is linked to the viability of Hodgkin/Reed-Sternberg cells and, thus, considered as a molecular hallmark of classical HL [99]. More recently, a number of studies have disclosed the implication of the HAT proteins CBP and p300 as tumour suppressors in B-cell neoplasms [100-102]. Neverthe-less, the various mechanisms through which each of these cofactors specifically contributes to lymphomagenesis are still to be elucidated. As before mentioned, CBP and p300 function as co-activators of transcription factors and acetylate proteins relevant to lymphomagenesis such as p53, NF-κB, Bcl-6 and Hsp90 [100, 103, 104]. In particular, p300 acts as a co-activator of NF-κB, activates p53 but attenuates Hsp90 chaperone functions and, moreover, transcriptional repressor *BCL-6* is frequently translocated and hyper-mutated in DLBCL where it results inversely correlated with p300 [100]. Importantly, de-acetylated Hsp90 represses p53 but maintains *BCL-6* expression, which suppresses p300 and its essential cofactor BAT3, which is necessary for p53 acetylation and activation. Somatic heterozygous mutations or deletions of the *CREBBP* locus occur in more than the 50% of DLBCL and the 32% of FL cases, whereas *EP300* mutations occur in the 10% of DLBCLs. All cases seem to have in common the disruption of the HAT catalytic domain, and the resulting truncated or mutant proteins may have dominant negative or gain of function properties, or may simply result in a reduced dosage of histone acetyltransferases. Structural alterations inactivating *CREBBP* and, less often, *EP300* have been recently documented and linked to the pathogenesis of both most common types of B-NHL [102]. According to Pasqualucci et al. [102] point mutations at the HAT coding domain of *CREBBP* and *EP300* result in specific defects in acetylation-mediated inactivation of the Bcl-6 oncoprotein and activation of the p53 tumour-suppressor, representing major pathogenetic mechanisms shared by the most common forms of B-NHL. Suppression of p300 either through Bcl-6 or inactivating mutations plays a key role in DLBCL. In fact, treatment of DLBCL cells with Bcl-6 inhibitors leads to p300 protein expression and acetyltransferase activity with subsequent acetylation of p53 (which induces p53 transcriptional functions) and Hsp90 (which suppresses Hsp90 chaperone activity) [100]. Moreover, the combination of Bcl-6 and histone deacetylase inhibitors (HDACI) leads to even higher p300 activity and synergistic killing of lymphoma cells *in vitro* and *in vivo* [100]. Interestingly, the direct effect of HDACI on non-histone proteins as DNA binding transcriptional factors (NF-κB, p53, CREB, GATA, c-myc, Bcl-6, E2F, IRF) can also affect cell growth and differentiation [101]. Furthermore, in light of HDACI effects on cell cycle regulatory molecules (Cyclin D1, p21 and p27) there is enough evidence that indicates these novel pleiotropic drugs as promising compounds for the treatment of B- and even T-cell malignancies in addition to conventional chemotherapy [105].

5.7. Multiple myeloma

Multiple myeloma (MM), also known as plasma cell myeloma or Kahler's disease, is a B-cell malignancy characterized by the accumulation in the bone marrow of plasma cells with a low proliferation index and an extended life span. Most cases of myeloma also feature the pro-duction of a paraprotein, an abnormal antibody that can cause kidney problems. MM cell lines as well as *de novo* MM cells express multiple anti-apoptotic proteins, often do not encode functional p53 and frequently contain a dysregulated Akt pathway [104-107]. A number of factors related to MM cell growth and survival and linked to CREB family members have been identified [108]. Among these factors, the myeloid cell leukaemia-1 (Mcl-1) protein, an anti-apoptotic member of the Bcl-2 family, has been considered as a critical regulator of MM cell survival and proposed as an attractive therapeutic target [108]. *Mcl-1* is an immediate early gene activated in response to GM-CSF and IL-3. It has been previously reported that *Mcl-1* activation can occur in dependence of the PI3K/Akt pathway through a transcription factor complex containing CREB [109]. Recent reports have demonstrated that Mcl-1 specific down-regulation or repression is able to initiate apoptosis in MM [110]. To this end, proteasome inhibitors like bortezomib have been used though with contrasting results. In fact, it has been shown that accumulated and cleaved Mcl-1 products by proteasome inhibition have either a pro- or an anti-apoptotic function. In particular, Hu et al. [111] have investigated the role of endoplasmic reticulum unfolded protein response (UPR) in order to unravel the mechanisms underlying Mcl-1 accumulation following treatment with proteasome inhibitors, discovering the enhanced translation of ATF-4, an important effector of UPR, upon proteasome inhibition, and indicating ATF-4 as responsible for bortezomib resistance of MM [111]. Besides Mcl-1, novel factors are being identified as important players in the pathogenesis of MM. Recent studies have suggested that X-box–binding protein 1 (XBP1), a bZIP transcription factor of the CREB/ATF family, has an important role in the survival of MM cells [112]. XBP1 is required for B lymphocyte terminal differentiation to plasma cells and is essential for immunoglobulin secretion. Abundant or deregulated expression of *XBP1* has been detected in MM cells [113, 114] and in hepatocellular carcinomas [115]. Due to the production of abundant immunoglobulins and cytokines, MM cells must be able to survive under conditions of chronic ER stress involving UPR and including constitutive activation of the ER-located transmembrane kinase/endoribonuclease (RNase) protein IRE1α-XBP1 pathway. This pathway, implicated in the proliferation and survival of MM cells, has been considered as a prognostic factor [116] and, moreover, as a possible target of chemo/immunotherapy [114, 117]. A growing body of evidence attributes a pathogenetic role to several microRNAs (miRNA) resulting up-regulated in MM and targeting p/CAF, a positive regulator of p53 [118]. Other authors have indicated a possible role of CREB family members in IL-6-mediated effects on myeloma cell growth and survival [119].

6. Concluding remarks

CREB/ATF family is a growing family of transcription factors involved in a number of physiological and pathological processes. Day by day, new family members are being identified for their primary role in normal or aberrant haematopoiesis and proposed as therapeutic targets of anticancer drugs [112]. In fact, by regulating gene expression, transcription factors are often the final mediators of such central processes as proliferation, survival, self-renewal and invasion. Based on these effects, it is conceivable that inhibition of transcription factors can revert the malignant behaviour of many tumour types and can potentially achieve a very high therapeutic index [86]. Actually, in light of its important role in the pathogenesis of leukaemia, CREB has been indicated as a potential prognostic marker of disease progression in AML and a molecular target for future treatment of leukaemia. In addition, CREB has also been implicated in many solid tumours including hepatocellular carcinoma, osteosarcoma, lung adenocarcinoma, melanoma and lymphoma [46]. Indeed, since *CREB* overexpression results in a poor prognosis for the patient, the regulation of CREB activity might represent a useful strategy to treat solid tumours like prostate, breast and lung cancer, as well as haematological malignancies like AML and lymphoma. However, a key question concerns whether the activation of CREB (or other transcription factors) seen in cancer cells is directly driving the cell malignant phenotype, or whether it is merely a by-product of activation of one of the upstream pathways or only a partner in a more complex scenario. This is a crucial point, since CREB would represent a good molecular target only if it were a main player in the specific tumour biology. Unfortunately, clinical and experimental evidences suggest that several functionally cooperating genetic alterations, including chromosomal translocations, lead to the expression of fusion proteins that play a key role in the pathogenesis of the leukaemia phenotype. CREB itself can promote cellular transformation as a fusion protein or by cooperating with other oncogenes or transcription factors. Furthermore, due to the recruitment of chromatin modulating mechanisms in the transforming activity of leukemogenic factors, transcriptional therapies aimed at inhibiting DNA methyltransferases, histone deacetylases or acetyltransferases, like CBP and p300, are emerging as new frontiers for cancer treatment. Unlike HDACI, which have been used in several phase I/II clinical trials, HAT inhibitors have been less extensively investigated for their potential use in cancer therapy. Indeed, interesting results obtained with clinical treatment of solid tumours [120] suggest that p300 inhibition may be a promising anticancer approach. To overcome the numerous side effects and the mostly transient clinical responses exerted by epigenetic compounds used as a single treatment [121], combinatorial therapy involving epigenetic agents together with conventional or targeted agents is increasingly seen as a more attractive opportunity. Therefore, further preclinical investigations aimed at better dissecting epigenetic mechanisms driving induction, maintenance and potential reversibility of the leukaemia state are welcome and functional to select the most potent drugs and combinations and to develop more efficient and long-lasting targeted therapeutic strategies. We hope to have contributed with this chapter to make the state of the art on the role of CREB in leukaemia and lymphoma neoplasms in order to allow further steps moving ahead from bench to bedside.

Acknowledgements

This book chapter was supported by funds of the Italian Ministry of University and Research (MIUR) granted in 2011 to Prof. Roberta Di Pietro.

Author details

Francesca D'Auria[1] and Roberta Di Pietro[2*]

*Address all correspondence to: r.dipietro@unich.it

1 Department of Cardiac and Vascular Surgery, Campus Bio-Medico University of Rome, Italy

2 Department of Medicine and Ageing Sciences, G. d'Annunzio University of Chieti-Pescara, Italy

References

[1] Sassone-Corsi P. Transcription factors responsive to cAMP. Annu Rev Cell Dev Biol. 1995;11: 355-77.

[2] Alberini CM. Transcription factors in long-term memory and synaptic plasticity. Physiol Rev. 2009;89(1): 121-45.

[3] Montminy M. Transcriptional regulation by cyclic AMP. Annu Rev Biochem.1997;66: 807–22.

[4] Persengiev SP, Green MR. The role of CREB/ATF family members in cell growth, survival and apoptosis. Apoptosis. 2003;8(3): 225-28.

[5] Lu D, Wolfgang CD, Hai T. Activating transcription factor 3, a stress-inducible gene, suppresses Ras-stimulated tumorigenesis. J Biol Chem. 2006;281(15): 10473-81.

[6] Don J, Stelzer G. The expanding family of CREB/CREM transcription factors that are involved with spermatogenesis. Mol Cell Endocrinol. 2002;187(1-2): 115-24.

[7] Mayr B, Montminy M. Transcriptional regulation by the phosphorylation-dependent factor CREB. Nat Rev Mol Cell Biol. 2001;2: 599-609.

[8] Salameh A, Galvagni F, Anselmi F, De Clemente C, Orlandini M, Oliviero S. Growth factor stimulation induces cell survival by c-Jun. ATF2-dependent activation of Bcl-XL. J Biol Chem. 2010;285(30): 23096-104.

[9] Hai T, Curran T. Cross-family dimerization of transcription factors Fos/Jun and ATF/CREB alters DNA binding specificity. Proc Natl Acad Sci U S A. 1991;88(9): 3720-24.

[10] De Cesare D, Vallone D, Caracciolo A, Sassone-Corsi P, Nerlov C, Verde P. Heterodimerization of c-Jun with ATF-2 and c-Fos is required for positive and negative regulation of the human urokinase enhancer. Oncogene. 1995;11(2): 365-76.

[11] Benbrook DM, Jones NC. Different binding specificities and transactivation of variant CRE's by CREB complexes. Nucleic Acids Res. 1994;22(8): 1463-69.

[12] Hayes, JD, McMahon M. Molecular basis for the contribution of the antioxidant response element to cancer chemoprevention. Cancer Letters. 2001;174(2): 103-13.

[13] Hai T, Wolfgang CD, Marsee DK, Allen AE, Sivaprasad U. ATF3 and stress responses. Gene Expr. 1999;7(4-6): 321-35.

[14] Wek RC, Anthony TG. EXtENDINg beta cell survival by UPRegulating ATF4 translation. Cell Metab. 2006;4(5): 333-34.

[15] Hai T, Wolford CC, Chang YS. ATF3, a hub of the cellular adaptive-response network, in the pathogenesis of diseases: is modulation of inflammation a unifying component? Gene Expr. 2010;15(1): 1-11.

[16] Han SI, Yasuda K, Kataoka K. ATF2 interacts with beta-cell-enriched transcription factors, MafA, Pdx1, and beta2, and activates insulin gene transcription. J Biol Chem. 2011;286(12): 10449-56.

[17] Conkright MD, Canettieri G, Screaton R, Guzman E, Miraglia L, et al. TORCs: transducers of regulated CREB activity. Mol Cell. 2003;12: 413-23.

[18] Drozdov I, Svejda B, Gustafsson BI, Mane S, Pfragner R, Kidd M, Modlin IM. Gene network inference and biochemical assessment delineates GPCR pathways and CREB targets in small intestinal neuroendocrine neoplasia. PLoS One. 2011;6(8): e22457.

[19] Wu X, Jin W, Liu X, Fu H, Gong P, et al. Cyclic AMP response element modulator-1 (CREM-1) involves in neuronal apoptosis after traumatic brain injury. J Mol Neurosci. 2012;47(2): 357-67.

[20] Caravatta L, Sancilio S, di Giacomo V, Rana R, Cataldi A, Di Pietro R. PI3-K/Akt-dependent activation of cAMP-response element-binding (CREB) protein in Jurkat T leukemia cells treated with TRAIL. J Cell Physiol. 2008;214(1): 192-200.

[21] Di Pietro R, di Giacomo V, Caravatta L, Sancilio S, Rana RA, Cataldi A. Cyclic nucleotide response element binding (CREB) protein activation is involved in K562 erythroleukemia cells differentiation. J Cell Biochem. 2007;100(4): 1070-79.

[22] Migliaccio G, Di Pietro R, di Giacomo V, Di Baldassarre A, Migliaccio AR, et al. In vitro mass production of human erythroid cells from the blood of normal donors and of thalassemic patients. Blood Cells Mol Dis. 2002;28(2): 169-80.

[23] Lau E, Ronai ZA. ATF2 - at the crossroad of nuclear and cytosolic functions. J Cell Sci. 2012;125(Pt 12): 2815-24.

[24] Hai T, Hartman MG. The molecular biology and nomenclature of the activating transcription factor/cAMP responsive element binding family of transcription factors: activating transcription factor proteins and homeostasis. Gene. 2001;273: 1–11.

[25] Llarena M, Bailey D, Curtis H, O'Hare P. Different mechanisms of recognition and ER retention by transmembrane transcription factors CREB-H and ATF6. Traffic. 2010;11(1): 48-69.

[26] Chan HM, La Thangue NB. p300/CBP proteins: HATs for transcriptional bridges and scaffolds. J Cell Sci. 2001;114(Pt 13): 2363-73.

[27] Janknecht R. The versatile functions of the transcriptional coactivators p300 and CBP and their roles in disease. Histol Histopathol. 2002;17(2): 657-68.

[28] Chrivia JC, Kwok RP, Lamb N, Hagiwara M, Montminy MR, Goodman RH. Phosphorylated CREB binds specifically to the nuclear protein CBP. Nature. 1993;365(6449): 855-59.

[29] Arany Z, Sellers WR, Livingston DM, Eckner R. E1A-associated p300 and CREB-associated CBP belong to a conserved family of coactivators. Cell. 1994;77(6): 799-800.

[30] Yuan W, Condorelli G, Caruso M, Felsani A, Giordano A. Human p300 protein is a coactivator for the transcription factor MyoD. J Biol Chem. 1996;271: 9009-13.

[31] Kwok RP, Lundblad JR, Chrivia JC, Richards JP, Bächinger HP, et al. Nuclear protein CBP is a coactivator for the transcription factor CREB. Nature. 1994;370(6486): 223-26.

[32] Nakajima T, Uchida C, Anderson SF, Parvin JD, Montminy M. Analysis of a cAMP-responsive activator reveals a two-component mechanism for transcriptional induction via signal-dependent factors. Genes Dev. 1997;11(6): 738-47.

[33] Ogryzko VV, Schiltz RL, Russanova V, Howard BH, Nakatani Y. The transcriptional coactivators p300 and CBP are histone acetyltransferases. Cell. 1996;87(5): 953-59.

[34] Kalkhoven E. CBP and p300: HATs for different occasions. Biochem Pharmacol. 2004;68: 1145-55.

[35] Fu M, Wang C, Zhang X, Pestell RG. Acetylation of nuclear receptors in cellular growth and apoptosis. Biochem Pharmacol. 2004;68: 1199-208.

[36] Petrij F, Dorsman JC, Dauwerse HG, Giles RH, Peeters T, et al. Rubinstein-Taybi syndrome caused by a de novo reciprocal translocation t(2;16)(q36.3; p13.3). Am J Med Genet. 2000;92: 47-52.

[37] Shima Y, Kitabayashi I. Deregulated transcription factors in leukemia. Int J Hematol. 2011; 94(2): 134-41.

[38] Blobel GA. CREB-binding protein and p300: molecular integrators of hematopoietic transcription. Blood. 2000; 95(3): 745-55.

[39] Kasper LH, Boussouar F, Ney PA, Jackson CW, Rehg J, et al. A transcription-factor-binding surface of coactivator p300 is required for haematopoiesis. Nature. 2002; 419(6908): 738-43.

[40] Blobel GA. CBP and p300: versatile coregulators with important roles in hematopoietic gene expression. J Leukoc Biol. 2002; 71(4): 545-56.

[41] Zimmer SN, Zhou Q, Zhou T, Cheng Z, Abboud-Werner SL, et al. Crebbp haploinsufficiency in mice alters the bone marrow microenvironment, leading to loss of stem cells and excessive myelopoiesis. Blood. 2011;118(1): 69-79.

[42] Rebel VI, Kung AL, Tanner EA, Yang H, Bronson RT, Livingston DM. Distinct roles for CREB-binding protein and p300 in hematopoietic stem cell self-renewal. Proc Natl Acad Sci U S A. 2002;99(23): 14789-94.

[43] Heissig B, Hattori K, Dias S, Friedrich M, Ferris B, et al. Recruitment of stem and progenitor cells from the bone marrow niche requires MMP-9 mediated release of kit ligand. Cell. 2002;109(5): 625-37.

[44] Kwon EM, Raines MA, Blenis J, Sakamoto KM. Granulocyte-macrophage colony-stimulating factor stimulation results in phosphorylation of cAMP response element-binding protein through activation of pp90RSK. Blood. 2000;95: 2552-58.

[45] Cheng JC, Kinjo K, Judelson DR, Chang J, Wu WS, et al. CREB is a critical regulator of normal hematopoiesis and leukemogenesis. Blood. 2008;111(3): 1182–92.

[46] Sandoval S, Pigazzi M, Sakamoto KM. CREB: A Key Regulator of Normal and Neoplastic Hematopoiesis. Adv Hematol. 2009; 2009: 634292-300.

[47] di Giacomo V, Sancilio S, Caravatta L, Rana RA, Di Pietro R, Cataldi A. Regulation of CREB activation by p38 MAPKinase during human primary erythroblasts differentiation. Int J Immunopathol Pharmacol, 2009;22(3): 679-88.

[48] Zauli G, Gibellini D, Vitale M, Secchiero P, Celeghini C, et al. The induction of megakaryocyte differentiation is accompanied by selective Ser133 phosphorylation of the transcription factor CREB in both HEL cell line and primary CD34 cells. Blood. 1998;92: 472–80.

[49] Wen AY, Sakamoto KM, Miller LS. The role of the transcription factor CREB in immune function. J Immunol. 2010;185(11): 6413-19.

[50] Mantamadiotis T, Papalexis N, Dworkin S. CREB signalling in neural stem/progenitor cells: recent developments and the implications for brain tumour biology. Bioessays. 2012;34(4): 293-300.

[51] Hawk JD, Abel T. The role of NR4A transcription factors in memory formation. Brain Res Bull. 2011;85(1-2): 21-29.

[52] Montminy MR, Gonzalez GA, Yamamoto KK. Characteristics of the cAMP response unit. Metabolism. 1990;39(9 Suppl 2): 6-12.

[53] Shaywitz AJ, Greenberg ME. CREB: A Stimulus-Induced Transcription Factor Activated by A Diverse Array of Extracellular Signals. Annual Rev Biochem. 1999;68: 821-61.

[54] Wang Z, Iwasaki M, Ficara F, Lin C, Matheny C et al. GSK-3 promotes conditional association of CREB and its co-activators with MEIS1 to facilitate HOX-mediated transcription and oncogenesis. Cancer Cell. 2010;17(6): 597–608.

[55] Xing J, Kornhauser JM, Xia Z, Thiele EA, Greenberg ME. Nerve growth factor activates extracellular signal-regulated kinase and p38 mitogen-activated protein kinase pathways to stimulate CREB serine 133 phosphorylation. Mol Cell Biol. 1998;18(4): 1946-55.

[56] Brunet A, Bonni A, Zigmond MJ, Lin MZ, Juo P, et al. Akt promotes cell survival by phosphorylating and inhibiting a Forkhead transcription factor. Cell. 1999;19;96(6): 857-68.

[57] Screaton RA, Conkright MD, Katoh Y, Best JL, Canettieri G, et al. The CREB coactivator TORC2 functions as a calcium- and cAMP-sensitive coincidence detector. Cell. 2004;119(1): 61-74.

[58] Wang L, Gural A, Sun XJ, Zhao X, Perna F, et al. The Leukemogenicity of AML1-ETO Is Dependent on Site-Specific Lysine Acetylation. Science. 2011;333(6043): 765–69.

[59] Chevalier SA, Durand S, Dasqupta A, Radonovic M, Cimarelli A, et al. The Transcription Profile of Tax-3 Is More Similar to Tax-1 than Tax-2: Insights into HTLV-3 Potential Leukemogenic Properties. PLoS One. 2012;7(7): e41003.

[60] Shankar DB, Cheng JC, Kinjo K, Federman N, Moore TB, et al. The role of CREB as a proto-oncogene in hematopoiesis and in acute myeloid leukemia. Cancer Cell. 2005;7(4): 351-62.

[61] Cho EC, Mitton B, Sakamoto KM. CREB and Leukemogenesis. Crit Rev Oncog. 2011;16(1-2): 37–46.

[62] Sobulo OM, Borrow J, Tomek R, Reshmi S, Harden A, et al. MLL is fused to CBP, a histone acetyltransferase, in therapy-related acute myeloid leukemia with at(11;16) (q23;p13.3). Proc Natl Acad Sci U S A. 1997;94(16): 8732–37.

[63] Kinjo K, Sandoval S, Sakamoto KM, Shankar DB. The role of CREB as a proto-oncogene in hematopoiesis. Cell Cycle. 2005;4(9): 1134-35.

[64] Sandoval S, Kraus C, Cho EC, Cho M, Bies J, et al. Sox4 cooperates with CREB in myeloid transformation. Blood. 2012;120(1): 155-65.

[65] Peters AH, Schwaller J. Epigenetic mechanisms in acute myeloid leukemia. Prog Drug Res. 2011;67: 197-219.

[66] Rowley JD, Reshmi S, Sobulo O, Musvee T, Anastasi J, et al. All patients with the T(11;16)(q23;p13.3) that involves MLL and CBP have treatment-related hematologic disorders. Blood. 1997;90(2): 535-41.

[67] Ernst P, Mabon M, Davidson AJ, Zon LI, Korsmeyer SJ. An Mll-dependent Hox program drives hematopoietic progenitor expansion. Current Biology. 2004;14(22): 2063-69.

[68] Ma X. Epidemiology of myelodysplastic syndromes. Am J Med. 2012;125(7 Suppl): S2-5.

[69] Zimmer SN, Lemieux ME, Karia BP, Day C, Zhou T, et al. Mice heterozygous for CREB binding protein are hypersensitive to γ-radiation and invariably develop myelodysplastic/myeloproliferative neoplasm. Exp Hematol. 2012;40(4): 295-306.

[70] Pigazzi M, Manara E, Baron E, Basso G. ICER expression inhibits leukemia phenotype and controls tumor progression. Leukemia. 2008;22(12): 2217–25.

[71] Pigazzi M, Manara E, Baron E, Basso G. miR-34b targets cyclic AMP-responsive element binding protein in acute myeloid leukemia. Cancer Res. 2009;69(6): 2471-78.

[72] Pui CH, Mullighan CG, Evans WE, Relling MV. Pediatric acute lymphoblastic leukemia: where are we going and how do we get there? Blood. 2012;120(6): 1165-74.

[73] Inthal A, Zeitlhofer P, Zeginigg M, Morak M, Grausenburger R, et al. CREBBP HAT domain mutations prevail in relapse cases of high hyperdiploid childhood acute lymphoblastic leukemia. Leukemia. 2012;26(8): 1797-803.

[74] Mullighan CG, Zhang J, Kasper LH, Lerach S, Payne-Turner D, et al. CREBBP mutations in relapsed acute lymphoblastic leukaemia. Nature. 2011;471(7337): 235-39.

[75] Kung AL, Rebel VI, Bronson RT, Ch'ng LE, Sieff CA, et al. Gene dose-dependent control of hematopoiesis and hematologic tumor suppression by CBP. Genes Dev. 2000;14(3): 272-77.

[76] Shigeno K, Yoshida H, Pan L, Luo J.M, Fujisawa S, et al. Disease-related potential of mutations in transcriptional cofactors CREB-binding protein and p300 in leukemias. Cancer Lett. 2004;213(1): 11-20.

[77] Di Pietro R, Zauli G. Emerging non-apoptotic functions of Tumor necrosis factor-Related Apoptosis Inducing Ligand (TRAIL)/Apo2L. J Cell Physiol. 2004;201(3): 331-40.

[78] Sabatini N, Di Pietro R, Rapino M, Sancilio S, Comani S, Cataldi A. PI-3-kinase/NF-κB mediated response of Jurkat T leukemic cells to two different chemotherapeutic drugs, Etoposide and TRAIL. J Cell Biochem. 2004;93(2): 301-11.

[79] Zauli G, Sancilio S, Cataldi A, Sabatini N, Bosco D, Di Pietro R. PI-3K/Akt and NF-κB/IκBα pathways are activated in Jurkat T cells in response to TRAIL treatment. J Cell Physiol. 2005;202(3): 900-11.

[80] R. Di Pietro. Signalling pathways leading to TRAIL resistance. In Advances in Cancer Therapy, Book 3, ISBN 979-953-307-209-7, Eds. Hala Gali-Muhtasib, 2011; 201-26.

[81] Milani D, Zauli G, Rimondi E, Celeghini C, Marmiroli S, et al. Tumour necrosis factor–related apoptosis-inducing ligand (TRAIL) sequentially activates pro-survival and pro-apoptotic pathways in SK-N-MC neuronal cells. J Neurochem. 2003;86: 126-35.

[82] Cheng HC, Sakamoto KM. Report on the workshop "New Technologies in Stem Cell Research" Society for Pediatric Research, San Francisco, California. Stem Cells. 2007;25: 1070-88.

[83] Pellegrini M, Cheng JC, Voutila J, Judelson D, Taylor J, et al. Expression profile of CREB knockdown in myeloid leukemia cells. BMC Cancer. 2008;8: 264-76.

[84] Saeki K, Yuo A, Koizumi M, Fujiwara K, Kaneko M, et al. CREB antisense oligonucleotides induce non-apoptotic cell death in proliferating leukemia cells, but not nor-

mal hematopoietic cells, by a bizarre non-antisense mechanism. Leukemia. 2001;15: 238-45.

[85] Bai XT, Gu BW, Yin T, Niu C, Xi XD, et al. Trans-repressive effect of NUP98-PMX1 on PMX1-regulated c-FOS gene through recruitment of histone deacetylase 1 by FG repeats. Cancer Res. 2006;66(9): 4584-90.

[86] Sakamoto KM, Frank DA. CREB in the Pathophysiology of Cancer: Implications for Targeting Transcription Factors for Cancer Therapy. Clin Cancer Res. 2009;15: 2583-87.

[87] Chiorazzi N, Hatzi K, Albesiano E. B-cell chronic lymphocytic leukemia, a clonal disease of B lymphocytes with receptors that vary in specificity for (auto)antigens. Ann N Y Acad Sci. 2005;1062: 1-12.

[88] Lerner A, Epstein PM. Cyclic nucleotide phosphodiesterases as targets for treatment of haematological malignancies. Biochem J. 2006;393(Pt 1): 21-41.

[89] Meyers JA, Su DW, Lerner A. Chronic lymphocytic leukemia and B and T cells differ in their response to cyclic nucleotide phosphodiesterase inhibitors. J Immunol. 2009;182(9): 5400-11.

[90] Burger JA, Tsukada N, Burger M, Zvaifler NJ, Dell'Aquila M, Kipps TJ. Blood-derived nurse-like cells protect chronic lymphocytic leukemia B cells from spontaneous apoptosis through stromal cell-derived factor-1. Blood. 2000;96(8): 2655-63.

[91] Ma Q, Jones D, Springer TA. The chemokine receptor CXCR4 is required for the retention of B lineage and granulocytic precursors within the bone marrow microenvironment. Immunity. 1999;10: 463-71.

[92] Bonni A, Brunet A, West AE, Datta SR, Takasu MA, Greenberg ME. Cell survival promoted by the Ras-MAPK signaling pathway by transcription-dependent and -independent mechanisms. Science. 1999;286(5443): 1358-62.

[93] Poiesz BJ, Ruscetti FW, Gazdar AF, Bunn PA, Minna JD, Gallo RC. Detection and isolation of type C retrovirus particles from fresh and cultured lymphocytes of a patient with cutaneous T-cell lymphoma. Proc Natl Acad Sci USA. 1980;77: 7415–19.

[94] Azran I, Schavinsky-Khrapunsky Y, Aboud M. Role of Tax protein in human T-cell leukemia virus type-I leukemogenicity. Retrovirology. 2004;1: 20-44.

[95] Ching YP, Chun ACS, Chin KT, Jeang KT, Jin DY. Specific TATAA and bZIP requirements reveal that HTLV-I Tax has transcriptional activity subsequent to the assembly of an initiation complex. Retrovirology. 2004;1: 18-30.

[96] Gachon F, Thebault S, Peleraux A, Devaux C, Mesnard JM. Molecular interactions involved in the transactivation of the human T-cell leukemia virus type 1 promoter mediated by Tax and CREB-2 (ATF-4). Mol Cell Biol. 2000;20: 3470-81.

[97] Robek MD, Ratner L. Immortalization of T Lymphocytes by Human T-Cell Leukemia Virus Type 1 Is Independent of the Tax-CBP/p300 Interaction. J Virol. 2000;74(24): 11988-92.

[98] Shaknovich R, Melnick A. Epigenetics and B-cell lymphoma. Curr Opin Hematol. 2011;18(4): 293-99.

[99] Janz M, Hummel M, Truss M, Wollert-Wulf B, Mathas S, et al. Classical Hodgkin lymphoma is characterized by high constitutive expression of activating transcription factor 3 (ATF3), which promotes viability of Hodgkin/Reed-Sternberg cells. Blood. 2006;107(6): 2536-39.

[100] [100] Cerchietti LC, Hatzi K, Caldas-Lopes E, Yang SN, Figueroa ME, et al. BCL6 repression of EP300 in human diffuse large B cell lymphoma cells provides a basis for rational combinatorial therapy. J Clin Invest. 2010;120(12): 4569–82.

[101] Zain J, O'Connor OA. Targeting histone deacetyalses in the treatment of B- and T-cell malignancies. Invest New Drugs. 2010;Suppl 1: S58-78.

[102] Pasqualucci L, Trifonov V, Fabbri G, Ma J, Rossi D, et al. Analysis of the coding genome of diffuse large B-cell lymphoma. Nat Genet. 2011;43(9): 830-37.

[103] Gu W, Roeder RG. Activation of p53 sequence-specific DNA binding by acetylation of the p53 c-terminal domain. Cell. 1997;90(4): 595–606.

[104] Rothgiesser KM, Fey M, Hottiger MO. Acetylation of p65 at lysine 314 is important for late NF-κB-dependent gene expression. BMC Genomics. 2010;11: 22-33.

[105] Zain J. Role of histone deacetylase inhibitors in the treatment of lymphomas and multiple myeloma. Hematol Oncol Clin North Am. 2012;26(3): 671-704, ix.

[106] Portier M, Moles JP, Mazars GR, Jeanteur P, Bataille R, et al. p53 and RAS gene mutations in multiple myeloma. Oncogene. 1992;7: 2539-43.

[107] Hyun T, Yam A, Pece S, Xie X, Zhang J, et al. Loss of PTEN expression leading to high Akt activation in human multiple myelomas. Blood. 2000;96: 3560-68.

[108] Zhang B, Fenton RG. Proliferation of IL-6-independent multiple myeloma does not require the activity of extracellular signal-regulated kinases (ERK1/2). J Cell Physiol. 2002;193(1): 42-54.

[109] Wang JM, Chao JR, Chen W, Kuo ML, Yen JJ, Yang-Yen HF. The antiapoptotic gene mcl-1 is up-regulated by the phosphatidylinositol 3-kinase/Akt signaling pathway through a transcription factor complex containing CREB. Mol Cell Biol. 1999;19: 6195-206.

[110] Gomez-Bougie P, Wuillème-Toumi S, Ménoret E, Trichet V, Robillard N, et al. Noxa up-regulation and Mcl-1 cleavage are associated to apoptosis induction by bortezomib in multiple myeloma. Cancer Res. 2007;67(11): 5418-24.

[111] Hu J, Dang N, Menu E, De Bryune E, Xu D, et al. Activation of ATF4 mediates un-
wanted Mcl-1 accumulation by proteasome inhibition. Blood. 2012;119(3): 826-37.

[112] Ri M, Tashiro E, Oikawa D, Shinjo S, Tokuda M, Yokouchi Y, et al. Identification of
Toyocamycin, an agent cytotoxic for multiple myeloma cells, as a potent inhibitor of
ER stress-induced XBP1 mRNA splicing. Blood Cancer J. 2012;2(7): e79.

[113] Carrasco DR, Sukhdeo K, Protopopova M, Sinha R, Enos M, et al. The differentiation
and stress response factor XBP-1 drives multiple myeloma pathogenesis. Cancer Cell.
2007;11(4): 349-60.

[114] Bae J, Carrasco R, Lee AH, Prabhala R, Tai YT, et al. Identification of novel myeloma-
specific XBP1 peptides able to generate cytotoxic T lymphocytes: a potential therapeutic application in multiple myeloma. Leukemia. 2011;25: 1610-19.

[115] Shuda M, Kondoh N, Imazeki N, Tanaka K, Okada T, et al. Activation of the ATF6,
XBP1 and grp78 genes in human hepatocellular carcinoma: a possible involvement of
the ER stress pathway in hepatocarcinogenesis. J Hepatol. 2003;38(5): 605-14.

[116] Bagratuni T, Wu P, Gonzalez de Castro D, Davenport EL, Dickens NJ, et al. XBP1s
levels are implicated in the biology and outcome of myeloma mediating different
clinical outcomes to thalidomide-based treatments. Blood. 2010;116: 250–53.

[117] Papandreou I, Denko NC, Olson M, Van Melckebeke H, Lust S, et al. Identification of
an Ire1alpha endonuclease specific inhibitor with cytotoxic activity against human
multiple myeloma. Blood 2011;117: 1311–14.

[118] Pichiorri F, Suh SS, Ladetto M, Kuehl M, Palumbo T, et al. MicroRNAs regulate critical genes associated with multiple myeloma pathogenesis. Proc Natl Acad Sci U S A.
2008;105(35): 12885-90.

[119] Xiao W, Hodge DR, Wang L, Yang X, Zhang X, Farrar WL. NF-kappaB activates IL-6
expression through cooperation with c-Jun and IL6-AP1 site, but is independent of
its IL6-NFkappaB regulatory site in autocrine human multiple myeloma cells. Cancer
Biol Ther. 2004;3(10): 1007-17.

[120] Santer FR, Höschele PP, Oh SJ, Erb HH, Bouchal J, et al. Inhibition of the acetyltransferases p300 and CBP reveals a targetable function for p300 in the survival and invasion pathways of prostate cancer cell lines. Mol Cancer Ther. 2011;10(9): 1644-55.

[121] Boumber Y, Issa JP. Epigenetics in cancer: what's the future? Oncology (Williston
Park). 2011;25(3): 220-6, 228.

Permissions

The contributors of this book come from diverse backgrounds, making this book a truly international effort. This book will bring forth new frontiers with its revolutionizing research information and detailed analysis of the nascent developments around the world.

We would like to thank Prof. Letícia Rangel, for lending her expertise to make the book truly unique. She has played a crucial role in the development of this book. Without her invaluable contribution this book wouldn't have been possible. She has made vital efforts to compile up to date information on the varied aspects of this subject to make this book a valuable addition to the collection of many professionals and students.

This book was conceptualized with the vision of imparting up-to-date information and advanced data in this field. To ensure the same, a matchless editorial board was set up. Every individual on the board went through rigorous rounds of assessment to prove their worth. After which they invested a large part of their time researching and compiling the most relevant data for our readers. Conferences and sessions were held from time to time between the editorial board and the contributing authors to present the data in the most comprehensible form. The editorial team has worked tirelessly to provide valuable and valid information to help people across the globe.

Every chapter published in this book has been scrutinized by our experts. Their significance has been extensively debated. The topics covered herein carry significant findings which will fuel the growth of the discipline. They may even be implemented as practical applications or may be referred to as a beginning point for another development. Chapters in this book were first published by InTech; hereby published with permission under the Creative Commons Attribution License or equivalent.

The editorial board has been involved in producing this book since its inception. They have spent rigorous hours researching and exploring the diverse topics which have resulted in the successful publishing of this book. They have passed on their knowledge of decades through this book. To expedite this challenging task, the publisher supported the team at every step. A small team of assistant editors was also appointed to further simplify the editing procedure and attain best results for the readers.

Our editorial team has been hand-picked from every corner of the world. Their multi-ethnicity adds dynamic inputs to the discussions which result in innovative outcomes. These outcomes are then further discussed with the researchers and contributors who give their valuable feedback and opinion regarding the same. The feedback is then collaborated with the researches and they are edited in a comprehensive manner to aid the understanding of the subject.

Apart from the editorial board, the designing team has also invested a significant amount of their time in understanding the subject and creating the most relevant covers. They scrutinized every image to scout for the most suitable representation of the subject and create an appropriate cover for the book.

The publishing team has been involved in this book since its early stages. They were actively engaged in every process, be it collecting the data, connecting with the contributors or procuring relevant information. The team has been an ardent support to the editorial, designing and production team. Their endless efforts to recruit the best for this project, has resulted in the accomplishment of this book. They are a veteran in the field of academics and their pool of knowledge is as vast as their experience in printing. Their expertise and guidance has proved useful at every step. Their uncompromising quality standards have made this book an exceptional effort. Their encouragement from time to time has been an inspiration for everyone.

The publisher and the editorial board hope that this book will prove to be a valuable piece of knowledge for researchers, students, practitioners and scholars across the globe.

List of Contributors

Khanh vinh quoc Luong and Lan Thi Hoang Nguyen
Vietnamese American Medical Research Foundation, Westminster, California, USA

Júlio César Nepomuceno
Universidade Federal de Uberlândia/ Instituto de Genética e Bioquímica, Centro Universitário de Patos de Minas /Laboratório de Citogenética e Mutagênese, Brazil

R. Saggini and M. Calvani
Dept. of Neuroscience and Imaging, "G. d'Annunzio" University, Chieti, Italy
Specialitation school of Physical Medicine and Rehabilitation, "G. d'Annunzio" University, Chieti, Italy

Kenny A. Rodriguez-Wallberg
Clinical Responsible of Fertility Preservation Programme, Karolinska University Hospital, Stockholm, Sweden
Karolinska Institutet, Department of Clinical Science, Intervention and Technology, Division of Obstetrics and Gynecology, Sweden
Karolinska University Hospital Huddinge, Fertility Unit, Stockholm, Sweden

Bassam Abdul Rasool Hassan, Zuraidah Binti Mohd Yusoff and Saad Bin Othman
Clinical Pharmacy Discipline, School of Pharmaceutical Sciences, Universiti Sains Malaysia, Minden, Penang, Malaysia

Mohamed Azmi Hassali
Discipline of Social and Administrative Pharmacy, School of Pharmaceutical Sciences, Universiti Sains Malaysia, Minden Penang, Malaysia

Takanori Moriyama
Medical Laboratory Science, Faculty of Health Sciences, Hokkaido University, Kitaku, Sapporo, Japan

Marina Shaduri and Marc Bouchoucha
Center of Bioholography, Tbilisi, Georgia

Marina Shaduri
Advanced BioResearch & Technology, Luxemburg

Francesca D'Auria
Department of Cardiac and Vascular Surgery, Campus Bio-Medico University of Rome, Italy

Roberta Di Pietro
Department of Medicine and Ageing Sciences, G. d'Annunzio University of Chieti-Pescara, Italy

Printed in the USA
CPSIA information can be obtained
at www.ICGtesting.com
JSHW011421221024
72173JS00004B/621

9 781632 411273